Recent Results in Cancer Research

Fortschritte der Krebsforschung

Progrès dans les recherches sur le cancer

8

Springer-Verlag New York Inc. 1967

Recent Results in Cancer Research

Fortschritte der Krebsforschung

Progrès dans les recherches sur le cancer

8

Edited by

V. G. Allfrey, New York · M. Allgöwer, Chur · C. P. Dagg, Freiburg · K. H. Bauer,
Heidelberg · I. Berenblum, Rehovoth · F. Bergel, London · J. Bernard, Paris · W. Bernhard,
Villejuif · N. N. Blokhin, Moskva · H. E. Bock, Tübingen · P. Bucalossi, Milano · A. V. Chaklin,
Moskva · M. Chorazy, Gliwice · G. J. Cunningham, London · W. Dameshek, Boston ·
M. Dargent, Lyon · G. Della Porta, Milano · P. Denoix, Villejuif · R. Dulbecco, La
Jolla · H. Eagle, New York · R. Eker, Oslo · P. Grabar, Paris · H. Hamperl, Bonn ·
R. J. C. Harris, London · E. Hecker, Heidelberg · R. Herbeuval, Nancy · J. Higginson,
Lyon · W. C. Hueper, Bethesda · H. Isliker, Lausanne · T. H. Kawachi,
Tokyo · J. Kieler, København · G. Klein, Stockholm · H. Koprowski, Philadelphia ·
L. G. Koss, New York · G. Martz, Zürich · G. Mathé, Villejuif · O. Mühlbock,
Amsterdam · J. Roth, New York · W. R. Pollard, Madison · A. A. Sandberg,
Buffalo · L. Sachs, Rehovoth · E. A. Saxén, Helsinki · W. Szybalski, Madison ·
H. Tagnon, Bruxelles · R. M. Taylor, Toronto · A. Tissières, Genève · P. Theologides,
Minneapolis · R. H. Wissler, Chicago · T. Yoshida, Tokyo · A. Zuppinger, Bern

Editor in chief

P. Rentchnick, Genève

Springer-Verlag New York Inc. 1966

New Trends
in the Treatment of Cancer

Edited by

L. Manuila   S. Moles   P. Rentchnick

With 37 Figures

Springer-Verlag New York Inc. 1967

L. Manuila, M.D., F.M.H. Derm.; S. Moles, M.B., B.Ch., B.A.O., D.R.C.O.G.;
P. Rentchnick, M.D.P.D., F.M.H. Med. int., 13, Cours des Bastion, CH 1200 Genève

Sponsored by the Swiss League against Cancer

ISBN 978-3-642-87622-6   ISBN 978-3-642-87620-2 (eBook)
DOI 10.1007/978-3-642-87620-2

Preface

> While it is true that certain types of neoplasms, such as those of the pancreas and brain, are still lesions with a grave prognosis, there are many other common cancers for which appropriate treatment can be curative in substantial numbers of patients... This hopeful aspect of cancer is insufficiently appreciated, even by the medical profession itself; too many pessimistic patients find themselves consulting equally pessimistic physicians.
>
> WHO Expert Committee on Cancer Treatment *.

The aim of this monograph is to present the latest information on the treatment of cancer, and the words quoted above from the report of a WHO Expert Committee on Cancer Treatment form an appropriate introduction to the subject. The pessimism to which they refer is still all too often characteristic of the attitude towards cancer and its treatment.

The various chapters have been specially written for this monograph by specialists of international repute, and it will be noted that some of them were participants in the meeting of the WHO Expert Committee on Cancer Treatment mentioned above. A special effort has been made to choose experts over a wide geographical area, so as to make the monograph as internationally representative as possible. This has the advantage of bringing out differences of emphasis in the approach to the treatment of cancer that are found in different countries. Areas of disagreement among the various contributions will readily be discovered by the reader, but no attempt has been made to eliminate them, for the treatment of cancer is a field in which opinions and methods are not yet fixed; a brief perusal of this monograph will indicate, indeed, that quite the contrary is the case. These differences in emphasis and in viewpoint will, we hope, be thought-provoking, and demonstrate that the field is far from being static. Nevertheless, the reader will also observe what a remarkable amount of common ground exists in the treatment of cancer among experts from very different parts of the world.

This monograph is not addressed to experts on cancer, though it may well be that some of them could learn something from it, at least in fields other than their own. It is intended rather for the general physician, who is usually the first to diagnose or suspect cancer in a patient and who often has the task of caring for him after he has been under the specialists. It is hoped that this monograph will provide a conspectus of the possibilities of treatment now available and place the physician in a better position to weigh them critically. The advances in this field are such that

---

* Wld Hlth Org. techn. Rep. Ser. 1966, 322.

nowadays the prospects of cure or prolongation of life are far brighter than they
have ever been before. Knowing more and playing a more active part in the care
of the patient, the physician is likely to be less pessimistic in his attitude towards
cancer, and his greater optimism should in turn be communicated to the patient.

L. Manuila
S. Moles
P. Rentchnick

Table of Contents

Introduction

David A. Karnofsky

The literature on cancer is so vast that it has become difficult for a clinician to maintain a proper understanding of the diagnosis, course, and treatment of the many forms of the disease in man. Cancer research ranges from virology to geographic pathology, from the functions of nucleic acids to the development of prostheses for jaw resections, from the genetics of tumor transplantation to the surgical approach to total pancreatectomy, from electron microscopy to the metabolism of steroid hormones in breast cancer. Confronted with these extraordinarily diversified aspects, all of which he cannot hope to master, the serious oncologist concentrates his attention on a particular segment of the field; but in doing so he loses much that may be of relevance to his work. Intensive research is the major source of clinical progress, but the connections between the different facets of cancer research are not always apparent, and the transfer of laboratory observations to the clinic has not been notably successful thus far. The reality of the cancer problem in man must continue to be presented by clinicians who are either experienced in some phase of cancer research or are making strenuous efforts to keep closely associated with the sources of new information and ideas.

This book is written by international authorities, and it is a tribute to the wide and vigorous exchange of ideas and data in the cancer field that, despite the fact that the authors work in France, Russia, the United States, Italy, and Belgium, each has an orderly, consistent, and eclectic approach to his subject. This international compilation is not a review of what is being done throughout the world for cancer patients, but of what can be done. The elevation of standards of cancer prevention, diagnosis, and therapy for all patients by utilizing presently available techniques would, to a substantial degree, prevent the disease in some, cure others, and alleviate suffering and prolong life in those who cannot be cured. The advances in cancer diagnosis and management make it mandatory to train more physicians, improve medical facilities, provide funds, and educate people on an international basis to appreciate the principles of cancer prevention and early diagnosis and demand medical help when it will do the most good. It is a challenge to the medical profession and public health authorities to bring the therapeutic advances described in this work to those of the three thousand million people on this planet threatened by cancer or living with the disease, who will require treatment and support during their lifetime.

Denoix, in the first chapter, stresses a fundamental point in the organization of a cancer center: the plan of treatment of an individual patient must be a team effort and the decision represent the considered opinion of competent specialists in different fields of cancer diagnosis and therapy. Each treatment plan, however, should be based on guiding principles that have been established for each type of tumor. DENOIX goes on to examine the practical aspects of cancer management in both specialized cancer institutes and general hospitals.

VERONESI describes the biological factors involved in the clinical course of cancer. A cancer or a precancerous lesion has its own characteristics: growth rate, induction of local tissue reaction, extent of local infiltration, metastatic extension, and preferential growth of metastases in various organs. Cancer, despite its inherent autonomous properties, must interact with the host, who provides it with blood, nourishment, a supporting structure, and an environment which meets its growth requirements to a varying degree. Hormonal and other factors, as yet poorly understood, may be involved in regulating the growth of a cancer, and VERONESI does not underestimate their complexity.

BOCK and DOLD review the importance of the early diagnosis of cancer and describe the most effective methods available to accomplish its control. They make a distinction between early and localized cancer, important since the two terms are not synonymous. In one patient a localized cancer can grow slowly and remain localized for many years, whereas in another metastases may appear even before the primary lesion is detectable by present methods of diagnosis. It is generally true, however, that the earlier the diagnosis of localized cancer, the higher the cure rate.

An early presumptive diagnosis of a localized precancerous lesion leads to the question of how best to treat it. DARGENT discusses the types of treatment recommended and under what circumstances they should be modified. As patients come under observation earlier in the disease, the clinical dilemmas presented become increasingly more complicated. One cannot overemphasize the need for a competent team in order to make the most correct decisions.

DENOIX further comments on the need to appreciate the natural history of a cancer (that is, its inherent rate of growth and interaction with the host) in estimating the prognosis and thus in planning treatment.

If the cancer evolves rapidly and the prognosis appears to be poor, less drastic treatment may be recommended than for the patient for whom the outlook is more favorable. While DENOIX notes in his earlier chapter that a "protocol treatment is desirable for each type of cancer and each clinical situation", he modifies this position by the statement "an over-systematic approach to the treatment of cancer is a lazy attitude that abolishes every stimulus toward the search for something simpler and better". This is another dilemma that arises in many situations; for while set procedures can be drawn up for the management of certain problems, external factors may modify them, such as the training of the responsible physician, the therapeutic facilities available, and the patient's own attitude to the treatment proposed. Many of the arguments about the management of a particular clinical situation become matters of opinion, not of science, and it may be necessary to review a whole gamut of approaches for each patient, from local excision of the lesion to radiotherapy or radical surgery with or without pre- or post-operative radiotherapy. Furthermore, the physician's judgment is not necessarily consistent, logical, or correct, and deferring to an authority does not necessarily lead to the most enlightened recommendation. Protocols and principles of management must be established for each situation, but they should be sufficiently flexible so that they can be changed for objective reasons; as and when a new idea or technical development makes it advisable to alter the approach to a therapeutic problem, the protocol can be changed, the new one then being in force. In this way, it will be possible constantly to evaluate the results of defined methods of treatment and the benefits gained by the introduction of new procedures.

The three major types of cancer treatment are skilfully reviewed by leading practitioners of their art. PACK systematically describes the indications for surgery as the major method of curing resectable cancer, and this includes the use of radical procedures for extensive regional cancers. PACK is a confident surgeon, convinced that extensive cancer operations are justified despite the fact that serious disability may result and the cure rate is uncertain. While there are differences of opinion as to how far the surgeon can and should go, there is no doubt that any surgeon would gladly abandon his therapeutic approach if a more certain or less mutilating or disabling method of treatment for cancer were found. At present the only hope of cure for the vast majority of patients lies in the judgment, ability, and courage of their surgeons.

TUBIANA and CHASSAGNE review the role of modern radiotherapy in the cure and palliation of cancer. This detailed analysis of radiotherapy provides an excellent counterpoint to the surgical approach, particularly in the management of cancers of the cervix and breast. The authors also consider the use of radiotherapy in combination with surgery and chemotherapy, the aim being to utilize these techniques as effectively as possible in each clinical situation.

The youngest members of the cancer therapy family are the anticancer drugs. LARIONOV, in my opinion, overestimates the value of the drugs presently available. The principles to be considered in the use of anticancer drugs are clearly enunciated, however, in his chapter and the roles of various agents in specific clinical situations are described. As a cure for cancer, drugs are not in the same class as surgery or local radiotherapy; as palliative agents their use is in some instances marginal and subject to considerable differences of opinion. Nevertheless, the search for new effective agents is the most active area in clinical cancer research. As LARIONOV points out, there are no limits to the developments that can be expected in chemotherapy.

The remainder of the book reviews the specific methods that are available for the management of certain of the major types of cancer. BERNARD discusses Hodgkin's disease and acute leukemia and the most recent approaches to these diseases in a concise summary. The temporary complete remissions produced in acute leukemia by the use of several types of drugs have led to considerable optimism that means will soon be available to control the disease permanently, either by using the present drugs in a more effective manner, or by the discovery of more active antileukemic drugs, or by the use of drugs in addition to immunological procedures to eliminate the residual leukemic cells.

TAGNON et al. outline the modern management of disseminated breast cancer. Breast cancer is an extraordinarily complicated illness, and the sequence proposed here should simplify the treatment of the patient with progressive disease.

HODGES and KIRCHHEIM discuss the value of various therapeutic methods in metastatic prostatic cancer. When the disease again becomes active after an initial response to hormonal control measures, clinical studies have not demonstrated appreciable benefit from large doses of estrogens, androgens, prednisone, or medroxyprogesterone acetate. The unhappy conclusion is reached that generalizations based on brilliant responses in isolated patients may lose their significance when subjected to a critical and uncommitted evaluation.

CREECH and KREMENTZ developed the drug perfusion technique for tumors of the extremities, and they summarize their experience with melanomas and sarcomas. The administration of drugs by perfusion has not been generally beneficial in recurrent or local metastatic carcinoma or sarcoma from the point of view of prolonged survival without evidence of disease. The best results appear to have occurred in primary melanomas and sarcomas, where perfusion was used as an adjuvant to wide excision of the tumor. While perfusion has apparently improved the cure rate in these situations, the confirmatory data are still insufficient and the procedure is still an experimental one. The perfusion technique is carefully described, but the recommended anticancer drugs are not included; in most instances an alkylating agent, such as melphalan, has been used.

Cancer consists of many separate diseases, each type with its own clinical manifestations, variations in clinical course, and response to treatment. It is a privilege for me to introduce this broad survey of current thinking on the problems of cancer in man and on recent advances in therapy and to recommend it to all clinical and laboratory workers concerned with cancer.

Early Diagnosis and its Importance for Prognosis and Therapy

H. E. Bock and U. Dold

With 5 Figures

As with few other diseases, the early diagnosis of cancer determines the course of the disease and the prospect of cure. Only with detection and treatment at a time when the cell degeneration is localized is the prospect for complete cure good by radical operation or radiotherapy. If the disease process becomes generalized or begins as a generalized or systemic process, cure can hardly ever be achieved and treatment can only retard the course of the disease and make the rest of the patient's life more bearable. Therefore the physician must make every effort to diagnose a malignant disease at the earliest possible moment.

The prospect of cure by radical surgery is excellent when the cancer has not yet emerged from the so-called precancerous state. In carcinoma of the female genital tract the detection and treatment of such precancerous conditions have happily been very effective. However, a prerequisite for the detection of such early stages is easy access to the affected organ for observation and removal of a biopsy specimen. Thus detection of the precancerous or earliest stages of cancer is possible only with a few types of tumor — as well as cancer of the vagina and uterus, there are bladder papillomatosis, intestinal polyposis, Paget's disease of the breast, Bowen's disease, Queyrat's erythroplasia, xeroderma pigmentosum, etc. In addition, medical checks of people even without pain or symptoms are necessary through regular prophylactic examinations.

The method of examination using exfoliative cytology (Papanicolau) has proved to be reliable and easily practicable for the early detection of cancer. In the localization of cancer other than of the female genital tract, the possibilities of routine prophylactic examination are, of course, made difficult because of the great expenditure of effort with little prospect of success involved in taking samples as, for example, of the sputum, gastric secretion, and urine. On the other hand, treatment may be a problem if the findings are positive and further diagnostic search fails to localize a cancer precisely.

Other diagnostic methods all detect tumors that have already developed. X-ray examination of the chest is compulsory for the whole population of Germany because of the campaign against tuberculosis, and a large number of bronchial carcinomas are discovered, although they cause no symptoms. In some places X-ray examination of the breast is performed routinely. With adequate experience of the significance of the findings, it may be that progress will be made in the early detection of breast tumors also. Prophylactic X-ray examination of the stomach in the personnel of the restaurant industry specially at risk has achieved no results justifying its extension (GIMES, 1956; MORGAN, 1955). Routine proctoscopy, however, may uncover a remarkable number of pathological conditions (IHRE, 1953).

In the majority of malignant tumors the first symptom that brings the patient to the physician is pain. If the tumor is not in an advanced stage and presenting with textbook symptoms, the physician can suspect malignancy only on the basis of almost always uncharacteristic symptoms and his clinical findings. It is his duty and a test of his clinical skill to suspect malignant disease early. Diagnosis should follow with the aid of special examinations and be early. Unfortunately physicians often fail to suspect cancer. They are to blame for failure to be alert to the possibility, but they are not to blame when the limits of present diagnostic possibilities are the reason for failure in detection.

It is important that the patient should visit his physician at an early date and tell him about complaints and symptoms arousing suspicion of cancer, and the he should not, from ignorance or fear, put off having the diagnosis made at an early stage. This involves the task of enlightening the public about cancer. ROBBINS and his colleagues (1948) have studied the time intervals before the establishment of the diagnosis in patients in New York (Table 1). It is especially noticeable from

Table 1. *Frequency of Delay in Diagnosis of Cancer, in Five Groups (after* ROBBINS, CONTE, LEACH *and* McDONALD, *New York, 1948). From:* LINKE: *Früherkennung des Krebses, Stuttgart, 1962*

I   Superficial cancer group
II   Breast cancer group
III Group of cancer diagnosed by careful clinical examination
IV   Group of cancers diagnosed by special examinations
V   Summary of groups I—IV

Delay due to:	I per cent	II per cent	III per cent	IV per cent	V per cent
patient	45,1	36,4	26,5	22,7	31,2
patient and physician	14,3	7,8	14,3	13,4	12,9
physician	20,0	8,4	24,8	34,7	23,4
No delay	20,6	47,4	34,4	29,2	32,5

Table 2. *Delay in Diagnosis of rectal Carcinoma due to Patient (University Surgical Clinic, Tübingen);* W. DICK *(personal communication)*

	Number of patients	up to 3 months	up to 6 months	up to 9 months	up to 12 months
1944—1949	152	49,3%	20,4%	6,6%	5,3%
1950—1954	114	58,8%	23,7%	3,5%	0,9%
1955—1959	184	74,4%	16,8%	2,2%	1,6%
1960—1965	224	69,2%	15,6%	6,3%	4,0%
Total	674	64,4%	18,4%	4,7%	3,1%

the table that group I cancers, which present the fewest difficulties of diagnosis, show the longest periods of delay. Cancer of the breast, the signs and symptoms of which are widely known in the population, shows the best result. DICK has studied the delay in diagnosis over four five-year periods in patients at the University of Tübingen surgical clinic: delay due to the patient is shown in Table 2, that due to the family physician in Table 3. From these tables it is apparent that in recent years

Table 3. *Delay in Diagnosis of rectal Carcinoma due to Physician (University Surgical Clinic, Tübingen); W. Dick (personal communication)*

	less than one month	2 months	3 months	4 — 6 months	6 months more than	no data
1944—1949	55,9%	9,2%	5,9%	9,9%	12,5%	6,6%
1950—1954	43,9%	10,5%	5,3%	12,3%	25,4%	2,6%
1955—1959	34,2%	14,7%	7,1%	13,6%	29,3%	1,1%
1960—1965	44,2%	9,8%	7,1%	15,2%	20,5%	3,1%
Total	44,0%	11,1%	6,5%	13,1%	22,1%	3,3%

the patient has begun to visit his doctor sooner, but that the correct diagnosis is unfortunately not being established any sooner by the doctor. Individual symptoms were treated: in 14.4 % hemorrhoids, in 9.3 % diarrhea, in 6.7 % constipation, and in 2.2 % hemorrhoids and constipation. Nevertheless, 75,3 % of the 674 rectal tumors were palpable and 68.4 % of the tumors were localized within a distance of 10 cm, 31.6 % above 10 cm.

1. Methods of Early Detection

The early detection of cancer lies for the most part in the hands of the general practitioner. Most patients come to him with the first uncharacteristic symptoms for consultation. He has only simple diagnostic tools at his disposal but, together with his medical knowledge and his experience, they should suffice to make him think soon enough of the possibility of cancer and to confirm or dismiss his suspicion by means of further examinations. Suspicion of the existence of cancer receives support from knowledge and observations of various kinds.

In countries as far apart as Japan, the USA, and England the age distribution for cancer of all types shows an abrupt and astonishingly regular, almost straight, rise from age of 30 years to the oldest age groups (Fig. 1). Only the curve for the male sex is shown in the graph; the curve for females is very similar, but with a somewhat more gradual rise. Thus with increasing age the likelihood of cancer occurring is greater. People talk of the "cancer age" and usually mean over 40 years of age in women and over 50 in men. The regularity of the curve shows that this division is very arbitrary. Cancer may occur at any age; only its frequency and type vary.

In the younger age groups sarcomas and tumors of the central nervous system and the hemopoietic system (Fig. 2) are relatively more frequent, while in later age groups carcinoma predominates. The absolute frequencies of all tumors reach a peak at an advanced age. The exceptions are a few rare tumors (Ewing's sarcoma, Wilm's tumor, etc.), and uterine carcinomas, which reach their peak incidence at the end of the reproductive period (cancer of the cervix at 45—50 years or soon thereafter; cancer of the corpus uteri at around 55 years). Breast, stomach, and skin cancers continue to increase in frequency up to old age.

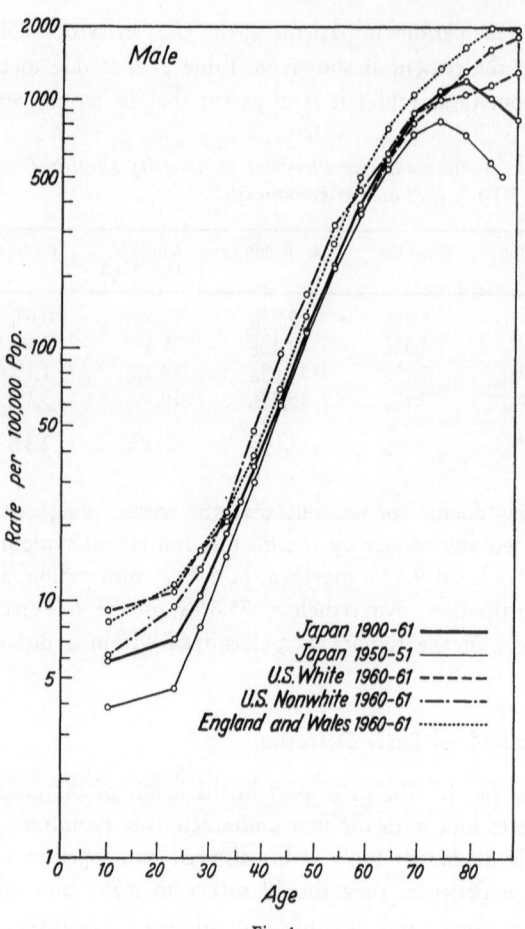

Male

Rate per 100,000 Pop.

Japan 1900-61 ————
Japan 1950-51 ————
U.S. White 1960-61 – – – –
U.S. Nonwhite 1960-61 –·–·–
England and Wales 1960-61 ············

Age

Fig. 1

Fig. 1. Age-specific death rates for cancer of all sites (male) in Japan, U.S.A., and England and Wales. From M. SEGI: Cancer Mortality in Japan, Sendai 1965

Fig. 2. Histological classification of malignant tumors to age 30. (563 cases at the University Surgical Clinic, Heidelberg.) From K. H. BAUER and G. OTT: Über die Krebsgefährdung des heutigen Menschen. Materia Medica Nordmark XVII/7, 1965

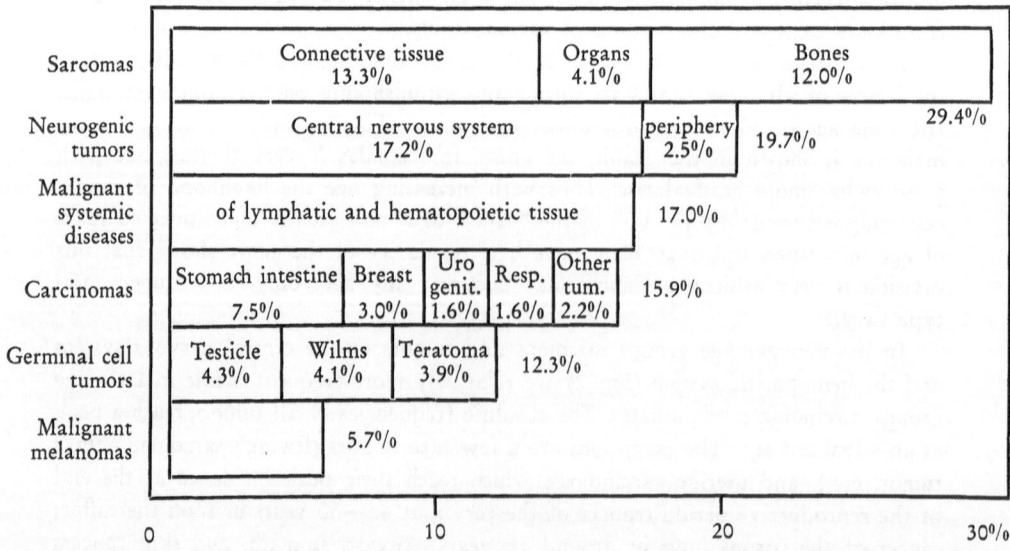

Sarcomas	Connective tissue 13.3%		Organs 4.1%	Bones 12.0%		29.4%
Neurogenic tumors	Central nervous system 17.2%			periphery 2.5%	19.7%	
Malignant systemic diseases	of lymphatic and hematopoietic tissue			17.0%		
Carcinomas	Stomach intestine 7.5%	Breast 3.0%	Uro genit. 1.6% / Resp. 1.6% / Other tum. 2.2%	15.9%		
Germinal cell tumors	Testicle 4.3%	Wilms 4.1%	Teratoma 3.9%	12.3%		
Malignant melanomas	5.7%					

0   10   20   30%

Fig. 2

The causes of the sharply rising frequency of lung cancer, with its peak at middle age, are the subject of much controversy.

The considerable differences in the incidence of cancer in individual organs are clearly seen in Fig. 3. It is the tumors of definite organ systems that constitute the

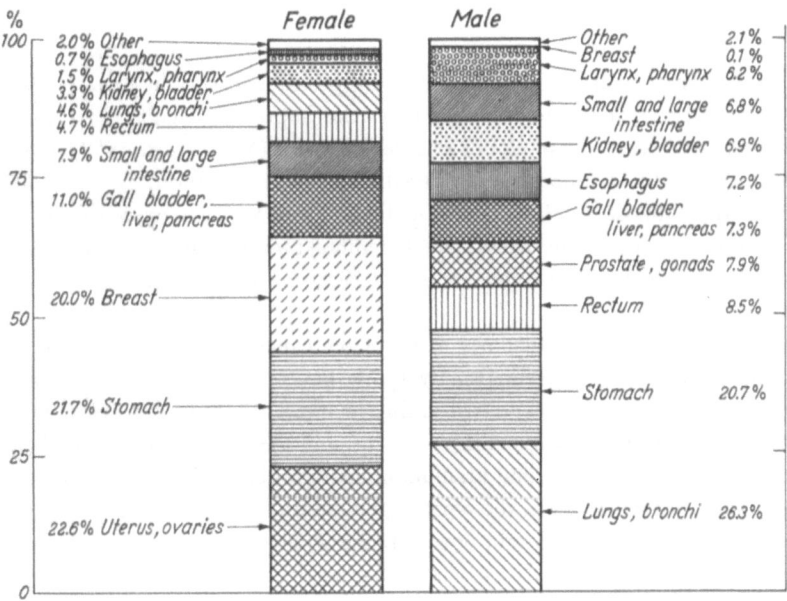

Fig. 3. Distribution of particular organ tumors per 100 deaths due to cancer (Canton of Basel-Stadt 1954). From J. BREITNER: Mkurse ärztl. Fortbild. 2, 100 (1964)

greater part of cancer, though with a considerable difference between the sexes. In a survey in Basel, tumors of the genital tract, stomach, and breast constituted more than 64.3 % of the total number of tumor cases in women; in men, tumors of the lung, stomach, rectum, and prostate constituted 62.9 %. In the geographical differences in frequency of particular organ manifestations of cancer, as well as genetic

Table 4. *Frequency of Gastrointestinal Cancer in Various Countries per Year per Million Population (Death Rates 1958/1959) from* E. HAFTER: *Mkurse ärztl. Fortbild.* 2, 90 (1964)

	Esophagus	Stomach	Colon
Germany	49	653	138
Austria	31	744	179
Switzerland	125	541	206
France	131	403	231
Japan	91	1077	56
USA white population	42	192	268

factors, harmful ways of living or conditions of life play an obvious part. HAFTER has listed these differences for three types of cancer of the intestinal tract (Table 4). The clearly demonstrable decline in stomach cancer in the USA as well as in Europe during the last 20 years suggests that external factors, perhaps carcinogenic agents, play an essential role in these differences. It is therefore all the more surprising that the total for all cancers in all countries remains almost constant. This has given rise to all kinds of speculations.

We should again like to emphasize that a knowledge of statistical probabilities only has value as an indication in the establishment of a diagnosis for the individual patient at a consultation. For the individual diagnosis such knowledge may never be of decisive importance.

A full past history of the patient also contributes greatly to the early detection of cancer. It can shed light on a hereditary disposition to certain diseases. Even if cancer constantly recurring in a family gives the impression that a hereditary disposition to cancer exists, the results of research on twins (VERSCHUER, 1959), however, have provided no firm support for a hereditary factor in cancer. A small number of diseases that almost regularly cause malignant tumors spontaneously or by the added action of carcinogenic agents are hereditary: retinoblastoma (an irregularly dominant factor), xeroderma pigmentosum (a recessive factor), and intestinal polyposis (single alleles).

Some occupations are particularly at risk from cancer, but this is to some extent only of historical interest nowadays. Everyone knows about the scrotal cancer of chimney sweeps, the bladder cancer of aniline workers, the skin cancers of tar workers, the arsenic cancers of workers in vineyards, and the lung cancer from inhalation of dust in the chrome, asbestos, and uranium industries. Leukemia seems to occur twice as often among physicians as in the normal population, perhaps because they receive heavier doses of X-rays. All in all, however, the number of cancers directly attributable to occupational causes is very small. If a particular frequency of stomach and lung cancer is found among workers in the restaurant industry, the chief part must be played by the whole way of life of this group of people.

Precancerous conditions deserve careful attention. There are diseases that favor the occurrence of cancer mostly because of chronic inflammatory irritation lasting over many years. At the head of the list are pernicious anemia (up to 30% of cases go on to stomach cancer), ulcerative colitis (about 30% go on to cancer within 10—20 years, with few symptoms), recurrent gastric ulcer (5—10% of all stomach cancers), duct papilloma (10% later go on to cancer), chronic cystic mastitis, Paget's bone disease (osteogenic sarcoma), neurofibromatosis, cryptorchidism, cirrhosis of the liver, and cholelithiasis. Diabetics are said to suffer with greater frequency than normal from cancer of the pancreas. The chronic bronchitis of smokers may also be mentioned here. Dermatomyositis and acanthosis nigricans are noteworthy; they are associated with malignant tumors in quite different sites with a frequency of 16% and 50% respectively.

Symptoms may be entirely lacking at the initial stage in cancer. At an early date, however, signs and symptoms of much significance can often be found: loss of vigour, constant fatigue, bodily weakness, nervous irritability, decline in appetite, and often, though not invariably, loss of weight. An attempt must be made by specific questioning to bring to light even subtler disturbances of function in particular organ systems. Awareness or impairment of swallowing, increased salivation (NISSEN), and regurgitation and vomiting of non-acidified food suggest disorder of the esophagus. Dislike for certain foods, especially meat, momentary pain with no relation to food intake, eructation, a feeling of fullness, abdominal distension, and painful peristalsis indicate a disturbance of the stomach or small or large intestine. Cancer of the large intestine is especially accompanied by a spontaneous change of bowel habit from constipation to diarrhea. If, in addition, there is an admixture of blood or mucus in the stools or involuntary defecation, these are alarming symptoms that call for further investigation. The esophagus, stomach, and intestine are easily accessible for X-ray examination. Examination of the small intestine is often omitted, for cancer of the small intestine is rare, but if it is present it is particularly lacking in symptoms in the early stages. The esophagus, stomach, and rectum are also accessible to direct observation endoscopically and biopsy specimens may be taken for histological and cytological study.

If in addition to the symptoms mentioned there are voluminous, foul-smelling stools, or a radiating, piercing, or girdle pain originating in the back that often subsides only when the patient adopts a crouching position, or thrombophlebitis migrans or perhaps transient jaundice, cancer of the pancreas or of the biliary tract should be suspected. Methods of X-ray examination for these organ systems are still limited (visualization of the duodenum and biliary tract, pneumoperitoneum and retropneumoperitoneum). New methods with radioisotopes will possibly bring diagnostic improvement. Peritoneoscopy is seldom rewarding. Enzyme examination of the blood, urine, and fluids secreted (obtained by suction) is open to different interpretations. Often only diagnostic laparotomy remains, and it usually reveals a cancer that is no longer in its early stages.

Persistent hoarseness, chronic bronchitis, thoracic pain, relapsing bronchial pneumonia, intense irritation from coughing, increased expectoration and sputum occasionally like raspberry jelly or sometimes with a stringy admixture of blood or associated with hemoptysis throw suspicion on the respiratory tract. X-ray examination, laryngoscopy, bronchoscopy, mediastinoscopy, and scalene node biopsy are methods of advancing the diagnosis.

In the urinary tract, macroscopic and microscopic hematuria are the main findings that arouse suspicion of cancer. The cause of bleeding must always be sought. The character of the hematuria gives a clue to the site of the bleeding. If a stream of urine is bloody in color, the site of the bleeding is in or above the bladder. If it is bloody only at the beginning of the stream, the blood is from the urinary tract. If it is bloody only at the end of the stream, the base of the bladder may be suspected as the source of bleeding, near the urethral opening. The cause may be papilloma of the bladder or urinary tract, or a hypernephroma. Cystoscopy, X-ray examination with a contrast medium, pyelography, or cytology may contribute further information.

Pain on passing urine is the chief symptom of carcinoma of the prostate bringing the patient to the physician. Of all enlargements of the prostate above 40 years of age 10—20 % are carcinomas, and in old age over half of all males have small foci of carcinoma cells in the prostate. The tumors often grow very slowly and are still capable of being influenced favorably by chemotherapy even in late metastasizing stages. The most important method of diagnosis, next to cystoscopy and exploratory puncture, is digital examination of the rectum.

Bleeding is also usually the first sign of cancer of the female genital tract. Bleeding between the menstrual periods and a bloody discharge or bleeding after intercourse are typical of cancer of the cervix uteri. Bleeding during the menopause arouses suspicion of cancer of the corpus uteri. Bleeding occurs when the cancer is no longer in the earliest stage. In spite of all efforts to inform the public about cancer, even today in over 75 % of women with the disease in Heidelberg, more than six weeks passed with definite symptoms present before they came under clinical treatment (Runge). The excellent opportunities for early detection of cancer afforded by regular examination and cytological check, particularly of the genital tract in women, make advanced stages of cancer avoidable. For the details of early diagnosis we refer the reader to specialized texts.

The early stages of breast cancer are generally not associated with any symptoms. Now and then someone complains of a dragging pain at the shoulder, but usually a hard lump is noticed by chance in the breast. In the early stages a firm diagnosis is established primarily by excision and histological examination.

Bone pain can be caused by metastases from a very small unrecognized carcinoma of the prostate or even a bronchial carcinoma. Plasmocytoma and leukemia can also cause this pain, or an osteogenic sarcoma can manifest itself with pain and swelling of the surrounding soft tissue.

Tumors of the central nervous system may remain without symptoms for a long time, depending upon their site. Often an isolated convulsion is the first symptom. Minor neurologic defects may long remain concealed from the patient himself — examples are deterioration of hearing on one side, limitation of the field of vision, latent pareses or sensory disturbances.

Localized headaches, unilateral dizzy phases, or paresis of the eye muscles may be noticed early. These signs and symptoms may be caused not only by neurogenic tumors but also by distant metastases, of, for example, bronchial carcinoma, as well as by a peripheral polyneuropathy, as a result especially of stomach or lung cancer. This can be a marked early symptom, but unfortunately it gives no clue to the site of the primary cancer concerned. The search for a diagnosis may be pursued with a careful evaluation of the findings, cytological and chemical examination of the cerebrospinal fluid, electroencephalography, electromyography, arteriography, and air and radioisotope encephalography.

It is often impossible to detect cancer from early symptoms; nor can every gap in diagnosis be promptly filled by complicated additional examinations. If the diagnosis remains unclear, it is the duty of the physician to continue to have further tests carried out at regular intervals to ascertain whether any new signs or symptoms have become manifest. Only in this way will the progression of cancer, so much a characteristic of the disease, become apparent and render a firm diagnosis possible while help can still be given in time.

Examination by inspection and palpation is of decisive importance for the early detection of all tumors of the skin and accessible mucosal surfaces of the body. Only by a thorough examination can the often small ulcerations of the eyelid, ear, lip, and tongue and the precancerous conditions of the nipple and penis be detected. The removal of all potential melanosarcomas is hardly possible. Tumors of the frontal bone and maxillary sinus, the alveolar margin, and the extremities may be revealed by swelling of the skin. Disturbance of innervation may provide further clues. Clubbing of the fingers and toes with watch-glass fingernails may indicate pulmonary disease. In addition, treatment-resistant polyarthritis may occur with hypertrophy of the upper and lower extremity, periosteal tags, and sometimes gynecomastia — the Marie-Bamberger syndrome (hypertrophic pulmonary osteoarthropathy). This is said to lead to bronchial cancer after a long interval. An increase in diffuse pigmentation may also occur with tumors of the stomach and intestine and also in bronchial carcinoma. In people with cancer the hair on the head may often become heavily pigmented, appearing from time to time as darker patches in hair that is already grey. Bluish-red striations, obesity, moon-face, and acne are characteristic of the cortical hyperfunction found in tumors of the adrenal cortex or pituitary. Some bronchial carcinomas also release hormonally active substances with glucocorticoid effects. Obesity may also occur with islet-cell tumors of the pancreas. In the early stages of some cancers such as stomach cancer the complexion may be extremely florid, and with hypernephroma be attributable to polycythemia. There may be suspicion of a carcinoid tumor if a patient suffers from hot flushes and diarrhea and his heart reveals irregularities on auscultation after he has eaten walnuts, tomatoes, or bananas (which are rich in tryptamine). Sudden pallor, outbreaks of sweating, headaches, and a rise in blood pressure may indicate a pheochromocytoma. General pallor of the skin and mucosae may indicate anemia. Petechial bleeding may indicate a hemoblastosis.

Hard glands in the region of the angle of the jaw, along the carotids, in the neck, or in the axilla always arouse suspicion of cancer. The metastases of an undetected primary carcinoma may be involved, or they may also signify the beginning of Hodgkin's disease, a reticulosarcoma, or leukemia. Supraclavicular glands, especially on the left (Virchow's node) may be linked with the metastases of cancer of the stomach or of the abdominal or thoracic cavity.

A hard or painful swollen thyroid gland may be the beginning of a carcinoma of the thyroid.

The mammary glands should be examined for lumps by careful palpation.

Auscultation of the lungs produces few results in the early stages of cancer. At most, signs of bronchopneumonia may be found in an area of the lung poorly ventilated because of constriction. Pleural effusions are not early signs of cancer. Abdominal distension and increased intestinal peristalsis may be observed. Diffuse pain on pressure may indicate a diseased abdominal organ. A tumor enlarged by congestion and surrounding irritation can seldom be palpated when it is operable, but is most likely to be palpable when in the region of the large intestine. Obstructive jaundice due to a papillary cancer or a cancer of the head of the pancreas may make the congested gall bladder palpable (COURVOISIER's sign).

Digital examination of the rectum should never be neglected in looking for a tumor. With the patient standing, the intestine lies lower, giving a larger area for palpation. As well as enabling the rectal mucosa and the size, consistency, and boundaries of the prostate to be assessed, the pouch of Douglas can be examined.

Fever is seldom a symptom at the early stage of cancer. High fever as the only symptom, and an early one, suggests Hodgkin's disease or hypernephroma. Cancer of the stomach may also cause fever, and bronchial carcinoma can do the same relatively early because of associated bronchopneumonia.

Only hormonally active tumors can be diagnosed in the laboratory — carcinoid by 5-hydroxytryptamine; pheochromocytoma by adrenaline and noradrenaline; islet-cell carcinoma of the pancreas by insulin; chorionepithelioma by gonadotrophin, etc. Up to the present no cancer-specific reaction has been discovered. All that can be done is to evaluate the results of the laboratory investigations along with the clinical picture. Much effort has been expended in looking for cancer-specific tests. As a rule only the first workers to describe a test have been convinced of its accuracy. Later confirmatory tests have always provided a high percentage of false positive findings, i. e., undoubtedly healthy persons have been declared to be suffering from cancer. The converse has also been true: there has been a high percentage of false negative findings, the reaction failing to occur in patients in whom cancer has been established.

The term "early stage" of a tumor means that the tumor is in contact with its surroundings and with the total organism at only a few points. Naturally therefore no marked changes in laboratory tests of body fluids can be expected. In individual cases cytology can be helpful, but this is not a subject for detailed discussion here.

Changes in the blood picture may be absent. It is important to recognize that anemia, even of moderate degree, may be caused by very early minor bleeding, especially from cancer of the stomach and intestinal tract. It could also be due to a lack of iron from increased absorption of iron by the reticuloendothelial system. In this connexion, determination of the serum iron and copper content and iron-combining capacity, transferrin content, and haptoglobin may yield further information. A shortening of the life-span of the erythrocyte (BÖTTNER and SCHLEGEL, 1960) is a further very valuable but likewise non-specific sign of cancer or of its recurrence. Macrocytic and megalocytic hyperchromic anemias may occur, especially with stomach cancer. More often there is moderate leukocytosis, occasionally with a shift to the left but more commonly with a shift to the right and, quite early, lymphopenia. In three-quarters of all persons suffering from cancer a reduction in the absolute lymphocyte count is demonstrable. Marked monocytosis and eosinophilia have been reported as occurring in metastasizing cancers.

The blood sedimentation rate may remain normal for a long period, but if it rises it needs investigation. In this connexion, the greatest effect is exerted by the fibrinogen content which is increased in many cancers. Associated conditions in a tumor, such as inflammation with bronchial carcinoma or a change in the serum albumin with a plasmocytoma, may affect the sedimentation rate more than the cancer itself. The albumin complexes elucidated by WUHRMANN and WUNDERLY (1957) for tumors — reduction in albumin and increase in the alpha-2 globulin fraction, and, at a later stage, in the gamma globulin fraction — are based on the same associated conditions. A positive result in various albumin lability tests is also based on similar changes; in themselves they do not permit a diagnosis, but observation of their course may be of great value. Nor is the early diagnosis of cancer achieved by determination of substrate-specific enzyme activity (lactate dehydrogenase, aldolase, glutamine oxalacetic acid transaminase, glutamine pyruvate transaminase, alkaline phosphatase, cholinesterase, lipase, leucine aminopeptidase, amylase, etc.) (HAUSS and RITTER). The great importance of these methods lies in their value for differential diagnosis. The division into isoenzymes makes it possible to narrow the field to specific organs. A marked rise in the lactate dehydrogenase level arouses suspicion of tumor metastases in the liver, if other causes of a rise such as hemolysis can be excluded. High alkaline phosphatase values point to the possibility of liver or bone metastases. A rise in acid phosphatase levels is specific for carcinoma of the prostate and is positive in about 45 % of all carcinomas of the prostate.

In looking for a tumor, urinanalysis is important for evidence of microscopic hematuria. In individual cases cytological examination for tumor cells may help in the diagnosis. Evidence of blood in the stools should not be overlooked. They should be tested on several successive days after the patient has been on a meatless diet for at least three days.

Examination of the gastric fluid, the bile, and the pancreatic fluid may, if, for example, achylia or pancreatic insufficiency is found, arouse suspicion of cancer. It should not be forgotten, however, that even normal findings do not exclude cancer; in stomach cancer approximately 11 % of patients have normal acidity and 6 % hyperacidity. In individual cases cancer has been diagnosed early on the basis of cytological examination of these secretions.

2. Successes in Early Detection

That a tumor has been diagnosed early and promptly on the basis of the first symptoms in no way implies that it is at a localized stage. Even small tumors may already have metastases in the regional lymph nodes, as well as distant ones. DAR-GENT (1964) has collected the data on cancers of two organs characterized by an abundance of symptoms — cancer of the tongue (Table 5) and cancer of the cervix uteri (Table 6). The data show that the cancers can attain advanced stages in a short

Table 5. *Distribution of Cancers by Stages in Relation to Duration of Development Before Diagnosis. 504 Cancers of the Tongue. From* M. DARGENT: *Pratique cancérologique, Paris 1965*

Delay	Number of cases	Stage I	Stage II	Stage III
up to 1 month	24	5	10	19
1—6 months	342	42	149	151
6—12 months	70	5	32	33
1—2 years	51	3	24	24
more than 2 years	17	6	3	8

Table 6. *Distribution of Cancers by Stages in Relation to Duration of Development Before Diagnosis (after* RUSS). *399 Cancers of the Cervix Uteri. From* M. DARGENT: *Pratique cancérologique, Paris 1965*

Duration	Stage I	Stage II	Stage III	Stage IV
1—3 months	23	40	28	8
3—6 months	18	41	31	10
6—12 months	21	43	30	6
more than 12 months	16	38	32	14

time, while they may still be at localized stages even after a long time. Additional criteria are thus necessary for the prognosis in cancer: the growth characteristics of the cancer cell, the powers of resistance of the host organ and, to a certain extent, environmental factors. FOULDS (1958) mentions as growth characteristics the degree of differentiation of the cancer cell, the rate of growth, the invasion potential, the tendency to metastasize, and the hormone requirements. According to SUTHERLAND

(1960) the resistance of the organism is represented by various cellular reactions such as lymphocytic infiltration of the tumor, nodal hyperplasia, and histiocytosis. The prognosis is determined by the rate of progress of the tumor, which may change during the course of the disease.

On the basis of practical experience it remains true that the smaller the tumor, the better the prognosis. If the primary tumor is of high or low malignancy, however, its size is of no real importance (SUTHERLAND, 1960). This explains the statistical finding that the survival period may be longer for tumors that come to treatment after a very long delay than for those detected and treated early.

In this age of active therapy longer periods of survival are readily attributed to the effectiveness of treatment. Data compiled by LAZARUS-BARLOW and LEEMING (1924) show how widely different the survival periods for untreated cancer patients can be (Table 7).

Table 7. *Natural Duration from Onset of Symptoms* (LAZARUS-BARLOW *and* LEEMING, *1924; from* R. SUTHERLAND: *Cancer, the significance of delay. London 1960*)

Site	Range of natural duration (in months)	Site	Range of natural duration (in months)
Lip (male)	7—42	Larynx (male)	3— 40
Tongue and mouth (male)	3—75	Larynx (female)	4— 37
Tongue and mouth (female)	6—37	Cervix uteri (female)	3—126
Pharynx (male)	3—26	Breast (female)	2—210
Pharynx (female)	7—34	Skin (male and female)	2— 39

Table 8. *The Possibilities of Surgical Procedures in Rectal Carcinoma in Various 5-year Periods (University Surgical Clinic, Tübingen).* W. DICK *(personal communication)*

	Radical	Palliative	By-pass operations	Inoperable	Operation refused	No data
1944—1949	37,5%	4,6%	48,6%	2,0%	6,6%	0,7%
1950—1954	42,1%	0,9%	44,8%	6,1%	6,1%	—
1955—1959	71,3%	1,6%	27,7%	2,7%	2,7%	—
1960—1965	61,6%	8,9%	24,6%	3,6%	1,3%	—
Total	55,6%	4,6%	32,6%	3,4%	3,7%	0,1%

The treatment of cancer must be adapted to the stage of the cancer found to be present. A cancer detected early and readily mobilized can be given radical treatment. Whether all the cancer cells have been eliminated from the organism thereby can only be shown by the subsequent course of events. If the cancer is more extensive and has already burst outside the confines of the organ, only palliative procedures are still possible; that is, parts of the tumor must be left at operation or radiation treatment must be limited because of the risk of injury to other organs. The prognosis for the patient is therefore markedly worse. Palliative surgery, e. g., colostomy, can bring some relief of pain only if the tumor is already far advanced. Table 8 shows that in recent years radical surgical procedures have become possible for cancer of the rectum owing to earlier detection of the cancer (compare with Table 2) and that the prognosis has been improved thereby. Fig. 4 shows the five-year survival rates for bronchial carcinoma, which were almost twice as good when the tumor was still so localized that a lobectomy was sufficient for extirpation of the tumor.

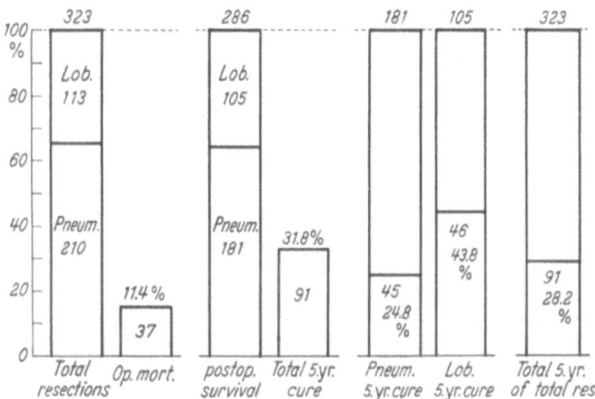

Fig. 4. Results of 323 cases of resection of bronchial carcinoma (Surgical Clinic of the Free University of Berlin 1952—1958). From F. Linder: Regensburger Jb. ärztl. Fortbild. XII/3, 188

The National Cancer Institute, Bethesda, USA has inaugurated the collection on a vast scale of the results of therapy for numerous cancer sites. At a symposium in 1963 the end results of cancer therapy in Denmark, England, Finland, France, Norway, Sweden, and the USA were presented. Fig. 5 has been prepared from the data submitted. The five-year survival rates from this uniquely large area of observation no longer leave any doubt that cancer can be treated successfully. But

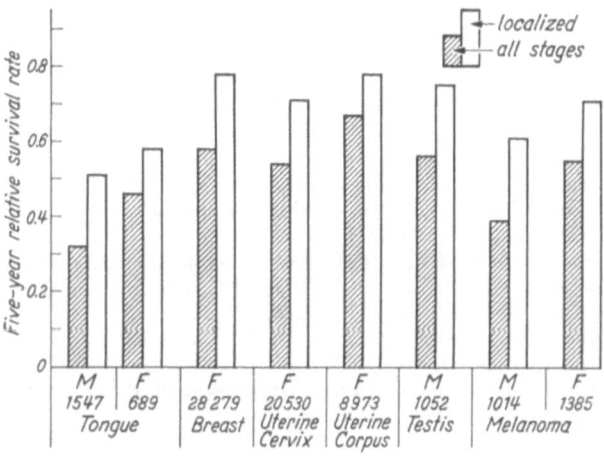

Fig. 5 a

Fig. 5 a and b. Comparison of 5-year survival rates for all tumor stages with those of still localized tumors. a. Tumors with good diagnostic accessibility. b. Tumors with poor diagnostic accessibility. According to statistics of the International Symposium on End Results of Cancer Therapy 1963 for histologically confirmed tumor diseases in the years 1950—1954 in Denmark, England, Finland, France, Norway, Sweden, and the U.S.A. (compiled by authors)

it is also clear that the prospects of cure for cancer of whatever site would be much better still if treatment were started earlier. The most successful step in treatment in the continuing struggle against cancer is early diagnosis.

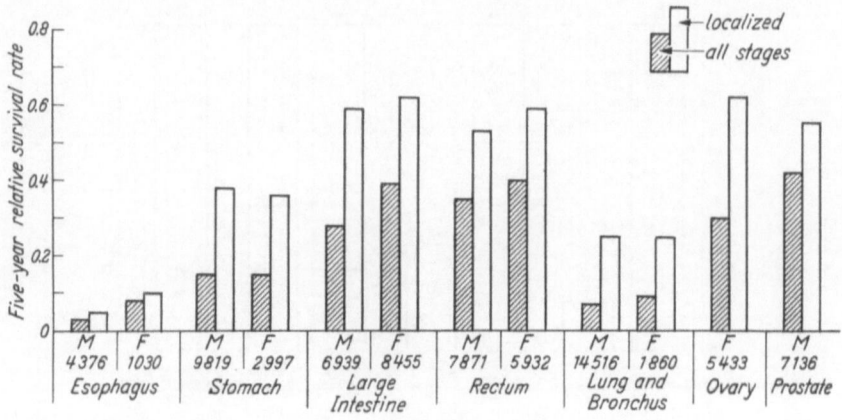

Fig. 5 b

References

BARTELHEIMER, H., und H. J. MAURER: Diagnostik der Geschwulstkrankheiten. Stuttgart: Thieme 1962.

BAUER, K. H., und G. OTT: Über die Krebsgefährdung des heutigen Menschen. Materia Medica Nordmark XVII/7 (1965).

BÖTTNER, H., und B. SCHLEGEL: Die Lebensdauer der Erythrozyten. In Hdbuch der gesamten Hämatologie, II.2.315. München-Berlin: Urban und Schwarzenberg 1960.

BREITNER, J.: Mkurse ärztl. Fortbild. 2, 100 (1964).

DARGENT, M.: Pratique cancérologique. L'éxpansion scientifique française. Paris: 1964.

DICK, W.: Dtsch. med. J. 17, 283 (1966).

FOULDS, L.: The biological characteristics of neoplasia. In Cancer, vol. 2. London: Butterworth 1958.

FRANKE, H.: Frühdiagnostik des Carcinoms in der Inneren Medizin. Berlin: Walter de Gruyter 1953.

GIMES, B.: Radiol. clin. 25, 26 (1956).

HAFTER, E.: Mkurse ärztl. Fortbild. 2, 90 (1964).

IHRE, B. J. E.: Routine sigmoidoscopy for the early detection of rectal carcinoma. Gastroenterologia (Basel) 79, 347—354 (1953).

International Symposium on End Results of Cancer Therapy, Bethesda, Maryland: US Dept. of Health, Education and Welfare 1964 (National Cancer Institute Monograph No. 15).

LINDER, F.: Regensburg. Jb. ärztl. Fortb. XII/3, 188 (1964).

LINKE, A.: Früherkennung des Krebses. Stuttgart: Schattauer 1962.

MORGAN, R. H.: J. chron. Dis. 2, 461 (1955).

SEGI, M.: Cancer mortality in Japan. Sendai: Department of Public Health, Tohoku University School of Medicine (1965).

SUTHERLAND, R.: Cancer, the significance of delay. London: Butterworth 1960.

VERSCHUER, U.: Genetik des Menschen. München-Berlin: Urban und Schwarzenberg 1959.

WUHRMANN, F., und C. WUNDERLY: Die Bluteiweißkörper des Menschen. Basel-Stuttgart: Benno Schwabe 1957.

Treatment of Precancerous Lesions

Marcel Dargent

With 3 Figures

The treatment of invasive cancer is still disappointing. Such being the case, any prospects of treatment for precancerous states will seem a definite step forward in cancer therapy.

Before considering such treatment, it is desirable to define the meaning of precancerous lesions.

Problems of Definition

Precancerous lesions can be defined in the following ways:

1. By Cytology and Pathology

A reference to the work of Foulds (1958) will show that in the cell the *initiation* phase has no morphological expression. Lesions become apparent only during the phases of *promotion* and then of *progression*.

The phases characteristic of the precancerous state in the cell are in principle manifested by abnormalities of volume, staining preferences, and nuclear morphology, or by cytoplasmic abnormalities. Merely on this basis, the commonly accepted criteria seem very flimsy. Some reversible states of cell proliferation may be manifested by cell lesions with aspects of malignity; this may, for example, happen in the thyroid cell of adolescent goitre or in the junction nevus at the same time of life, or in some postmenopausal endometrial hyperplastic states. This leads naturally to the question of the real nature of the so-called carcinoma in situ, as described in certain covering tissues. The following conclusions may be drawn from the innumerable controversies this lesion has given rise to.

a) The *etiological* arguments (based on the average age of the patients) and the *clinical* arguments (based on watching the course of the lesion over several years) support the view that carcinoma in situ is an intermediate stage in certain cases between dysplasia and metaplasia and invasive cancer.

b) On the other hand, the same arguments, especially the clinical arguments, prove that a certain number of these conditions are reversible. Pedersen (1958) and Lange (1960), after following up cases of so-called pre-invasive conditions of the uterine cervix for more than five years, have shown that more than two thirds regressed. It is therefore understandable that some authors question the very existence of the condition of carcinoma in situ; it may merely be a condition mimicking cancer. In any case, periods of 10—15 years or more may be needed to be sure that invasive cancer will never appear.

c) Some cancers — which according to pathologists and statistical estimates are very variable in their frequency — do not go through, or go very rapidly through, the pre-invasive stage and are invasive at once.

Cell examination, it is to be hoped on the basis of the work of Wied (1964) and others, will make it possible to determine whether the abnormalities encountered are characteristic of the pre-invasive type of lesion with a good prognosis or of the invasive type that is malignant from the beginning.

From the point of view of the tissues, the definition of a precancerous condition is based on the "enclosed" character of the lesion, the most certain sign of which is the integrity of the basement membrane where there is a Malpighian layer. This character is much more difficult to establish in lesions of glandular structures or connective tissue. The presence of an actual fibrous capsule suffices in principle to establish without any reservation that the lesion is benign. It is considered as potentially malignant if there is a false capsule caused by the progressive compression of the neighbouring tissues or adaptation of the new stroma (unless it considered straightaway as a carcinoma, as for example a parotid epithelioma or a thyroid adenocarcinoma, or as a sarcoma, as for example the recurrent tumours of connective tissue).

Another characteristic that some workers claim to have identified by colposcopy in the study of the cervix uteri is a change in the grouping of the capillaries at the time of transformation (MIKOLAS, STAFL and LINHARTOVA, 1962).

One of the most important characteristics of the precancerous condition is that it has several centers, whether it consists of predisposing congenital lesions or of

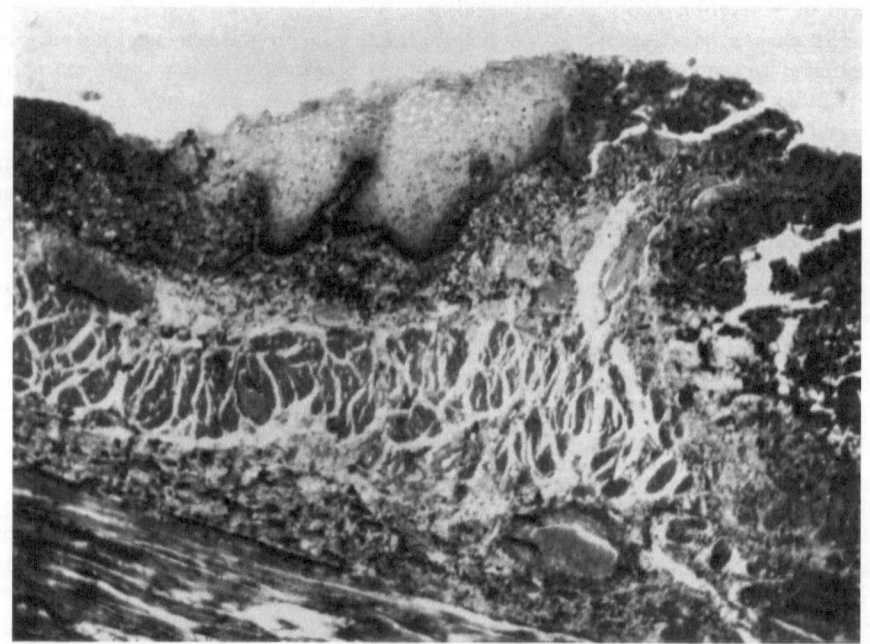

Fig. 1. Cancer of the esophagus. On the left the lesions of pre-invasive cancer. On the right an infiltrating cancer. Healthy mucosa elsewhere. (Léon Bérard Centre Collection. Esophagectomy surgical specimen.)

lesions induced by a cancerogenic factor. This characteristic is not confined to the covering tissues only but appears in glandular tissue (the mammary gland, for example) and even in new formations of connective-tissue derivatives (such as osteogenic exostoses).

Thus, whether cancer appears in foci of rectal polyposis, xeroderma pigmentosum, or papillomatosis of the bladder caused by bilharziasis or cancerogenic amines, the essential thing to remember is that the malignant transformation occurs *in stages* and may appear successively in many foci over a very long period of time. This explains why there are recurrences after operations that were believed to be carried out in time and to be effective. In 100 specimens of esophageal cancer, SUN SHAO CHIEN (1962) and WU SHIA found 20 with focal areas of epithelioma in situ in the esophageal mucosa, at distances as great as 7 cm from the lesion. We have confirmed this finding (Fig. 1).

2. By the Biochemical Characteristics

The passage from the precancerous state to cancer has been considered (NEIMANN, 1964) to be the transformation of a non-specific, possibly reversible, process caused by a chemical, physical, or biological agent into a specific, irreversible process characterized by a special kind of biosynthesis of nucleoproteins in a cell endowed with the capacity of reproducing itself in daughter cells. Enzymological research seems indeed to show that there are significant differences in the activity of precancerous and cancerous tissues; this is being more and more established, for example, for cancer of the cervix uteri, where there is depression of glycogen and the phosphoamylases (GODLEVSKI, 1964) or of 6-phosphogluconate dehydrogenase (WILSON, J. — personal communication) at the time of the malignant transformation.

It is also accepted in studies of experimental induction of cancer that the antigenic power of a cell that has become malignant is variable, as too are the numbers of such cells and especially the defensive capacities of the immunologically competent cells. The so-called precancerous condition corresponds by definition to one of an equilibrium between the host tissue and the groupings of malignant cells, an equilibrium that stands in the way of the *diffusion* of the malignant cell. This, however, is more a concept or a research hypothesis than an actual fact; while some evidence favours it, other evidence renders it doubtful — such as enlargement of the cervical, axillary, or inguinal lymph nodes indicating a malignant primary lesion still at a subclinical stage or even in situ and so theoretically precancerous, which will only become manifest long afterwards. More generally, the precancerous state could thus be defined as a state in which the defensive mechanisms — local, nodal, or visceral — are still effective, even though the malignant cell or group of cells is already capable of migrating into the lymph channels or capillaries.

The reason why the treatment of states considered as precancerous is sometimes followed by disappointing results is no doubt that we still cannot gauge exactly the effectiveness of the defense processes in the host-tumor relationship.

Practical Problems

Clinical Aspects

It is impossible to give a complete list of all precancerous conditions. If the very controversial problems of precancerous conditions in bone, hematopoietic, and nervous tissue are set aside, the following observations are the only ones that may be made from the clinical point of view:

1. There are clinically benign lesions that are practically never precancerous conditions. Examples of these are breast adenofibromas, thyroid adenomas, and small single polyps of the colon or rectum.

2. There are clinically benign lesions that are already cancerous conditions.

Examples of these are the "enclosed" cancers of the breast and thyroid. In the view of the pathologist, they are not encapsulated, but deserve the clinician's term of enclosed or circumscribed. The term "adenomorphic carcinoma" suits them very well. The same is true for the mixed epitheliomas with a stroma of the salivary glands and for the cylindromas, as well as for sarcomas of mesenchymal tissues in their initial stage (liposarcomas, fibrosarcomas, myosarcomas). It is also true for certain lesions of the mucosa and of covering tissues. Cancer of the stomach may for several years be ulceriform in type, and it is extremely probable that the symptomatic ulceration is malignant from the outset, especially if it is accompanied by atrophic gastritis. Erythroplasia of the mucosa of the penis is a papillary cancer. An established and apparently stable melanoma of the skin is often a cancer in the adult from the beginning. On the other hand, an apparently developing melanoma in adolescents may be a benign lesion.

3. Genuinely precancerous states exist whose potentialities for malignancy are very difficult to define.

a) This is so for leukoplakia of any mucosa. Leukoplakia of the mouth when of type I (a mere thickening of the mucosa) practically never degenerates, whereas as soon as keratinization occurs (type II), whether associated or not with hyperplasia (type III) or abnormalities of the structure of the epidermis and dermis (type IV), it indicates malignant degeneration. In all, 10 % of cases of leukoplakia are precancerous, but 34.5 % of cases of type IV are already cancerous (MORGENROTH, 1964). Leukoplakia of the cervix uteri is rarely precancerous.

b) The malignancy of polyposis is also difficult to determine. While diffuse congenital recto-colic polyposis is universally considered to be an undoubtedly precancerous condition, degenerating in successive centers, this is not so for adenomatous polyps of the rectum and colon, for which the risk of degenerating does not, according to ACKERMANN (1964), exceed one in 40. According to this author and to most others, cancers of the rectum or colon, even when very limited, have not passed through a pre-invasive phase. The same is probably true of gastric polyposis.

While laryngeal polyposis in the child is a reversible condition and practically never precancerous, in the adult, especially with hyperkeratosis, it is almost always so (CACHIN, 1959). So too, while polyposis of the bladder is undoubtedly a precancerous condition in workmen exposed to dyes, and is characterized by successively degenerating centers and especially areas of infiltration, it seems that the cystitis caused by bilharziasis, even when there is squamous metaplasia, is not a precancerous condition (ABDUL NASR AL et al., 1962).

c) Precancerous conditions of the skin are very well known. Xeroderma pigmentosum in the child always becomes transformed into cancer and, as Oberling has said, only a life permanently sheltered from the sunlight would prevent this from happening. This is also the case for senile keratosis.

Melanoma of the skin may be considered as a precancerous condition, especially if the ectodermal contribution is greater than the neural contribution in its structure; but the blue melanoma is much less dangerous than the domed nevus (DUPERAT,

1962). Considering the frequency of benign melanin-pigmented spots in the human species, the malignant transformation of a congenital nevus may be regarded as exceptional.

d) Scars are traditionally considered as precancerous conditions, but it is a misuse of terminology to call them so. The scar of an appendicectomy, for example, is practically never a precancerous condition. The scars that are precancerous are pathological, chronically ulcerated, like those observed after some burns, some varicose ulcers, or some tropical ulcers in black races. In these scars the cancerous process seems to have begun from the very outset (JOSSERAND, DARGENT and PINET, 1957). The same is probably true of some infarct scars or chronically inflamed scars in the pulmonary parenchyma (RAEBURN and SPENCER, 1957; GALY et al., 1958).

e) The precancerous states of glandular parenchyma, especially that of the mammary gland, deserve special mention. From the experimental findings it appears that while the mammary adenofibroma should not be considered as a precarcinomatous but perhaps as a presarcomatous condition, cystic mastitis and duct papillomatous conditions are precancerous. According to the statistics, however, the risk of their becoming cancerous varies from 1% to 80%. Most authors agree that breast cancer is a little more frequent in women with cystic mastitis after the age of 40 years, but the most established fact is that cancer of the breast is associated with this form of endocrine disturbance. In most cases it can be considered more as a lesion associated with cancer than as a precancerous condition.

4. Finally, asymptomatic precancerous conditions exist that are discovered by systematic examination.

Routine cytological examination of certain mucosal surfaces — especially the cervix uteri and the bronchial mucosa — has familiarized medical opinion with the concept of epithelioma in situ (or pre-invasive, or stage 0). It is accepted that the exfoliated cells may come from an epidermal centre, which may be the site of considerable hypertrophy or hyperplasia (of the Bowen type) without breach of the basal layer. Is this really a precancerous condition, or a benign condition of indefinite duration mimicking carcinoma, or a condition that even completely regresses, like those observed in the postpartum period?

Investigation by tests such as fluorescent staining or, for the cervix uteri, SCHILLER'S test has enabled biopsy specimens to be taken from the suspect zones and led to the discovery of zones of dysplasia, or of carcinoma in situ, or of undoubted invasive cancer, or of mixed zones of both carcinoma in situ and of invasive cancer. This raises the question whether the pre- invasive lesion is a precancerous condition or one associated with cancer. In cancer of the esophagus, for example, areas of epithelioma in situ are found alongside and even well away from cancerous areas. Are they incipient recurrences or are they associated conditions with no potentiality for malignancy? We do not know.

The only irrefutable arguments in favour of these conditions being precancerous are as follows. It is universally admitted that the age of patients with dysplasia and the so-called carcinoma in situ of the cervix uteri, as shown by all the statistics, is more than 10 years less than that of patients with invasive cancer. Again, the statistics obtained after several years of experience with mass campaigns for the detection of cancer of the cervix uteri (QUINSENBERRY, 1964, at Hawaii; FIDLER and BOYES, 1960, in British Colombia; GROSS, 1964, in Czechoslovakia) all seem to prove that detection and systematic treatment of pre-invasive cancer reduce year by year the frequency of invasive cancer.

From the clinical point of view the chief difficulties are as follows:

a) The absence or commonplace character of the signs (simple leukorrhoea for the cervix uteri, bronchorrhoea in heavy smokers, bladder pain in precancerous conditions of the bladder, etc.).

b) The rarity of cancer as detected by cytology alone (between 1 and 7 per 1000 women examined, for example). Thus there would have to be a large mass of the population involved for treatment of precancerous conditions to be considered effective.

c) The uncertainty, in even the most thorough investigation, that the malignant area will be detected — an uncertainty complicated by the fact that the lesions can be multicentric either spatially or in time.

Given the existence of all these pitfalls in the relatively accessible fields of gynecology, bronchology, and urology alone, it is understandable that the efforts made to detect precancerous conditions in the stomach, pancreas, esophagus, and kidney may by considered so far as experimental trials of very little practical value.

This general survey of some conditions considered as precancerous needs to be completed by a few words on one of the least known of the problems involved, that of the dynamics of these lesions. While some of them appear to be reversible or indefinitely benign and should therefore be left out of consideration in this study, others do in fact precede cancer or co-exist with it in an adjacent zone on its appearance. How much time is needed for a lesion of this kind to become dangerous? It is fairly well known empirically that about 10 years are needed in general for a carcinoma in situ to become invasive, and that often more than 15 years are needed for a burn scar, a radiation dermatitis, or a chronic ulcer to become malignant. These are only approximations. In a follow-up of a series of 150 cases of lesions of the buccal mucosa, two tongue lesions were considered to be precancerous leukoplakia and were followed up every three months, cytological examinations being carried out repeatedly. After seven and 22 years respectively they were succeeded by infiltrating cancers that arose in some weeks (DARGENT, 1964). These were undoubtedly immediately invasive cancers, appearing in the neighbourhood of the precancerous areas already treated. Similar observations have been made for the cervix uteri, the bronchi, and the bladder.

Because precancer appears in more than one site in the mucosa and in the covering tissues of the body, attention has had to be paid to the lasting risk involved if the treatment is directed to only one site detected during an examination.

Methods of Assessing the Development Potentialities of a Precancerous Condition

Methods of assessing the development potentialities of a precancerous condition are very many, and very inaccurate. Among them may be mentioned:

a) The past history of the case. The condition may be considered as a congenital precancerous condition or there may have been repeated exposure to known cancerogenic agents. Unfortunately, alongside the causes known for cancerous states, there are innumerable unknown or poorly defined ones.

b) The clinical aspect. There may be a change in the morphological appearance, volume, form, or limits of the lesion considered to be precancerous. There is the obvious risk of treating many benign lesions that would never have become malignant. This however is but a minor drawback. The chief danger is that of leaving untouched apparently healthy tissue where there is a risk of directly invasive cancer developing. Among the best known examples of this kind of failure of treatment of a condition presumed to be precancerous are breast cancer appearing in a woman operated on for cystic disease and thyroid cancer occurring in a thyroid remnant after thyroidectomy for benign goiter.

c) Radiological tests. Such tests may be of value for certain localizations. A rectal polyp, for example, that doubles in size in a year should be regarded as very suspicious.

d) Endoscopy. This is not always possible, and when it is it is badly tolerated by the patient if it has to be repeated for, e. g., the bronchi or the esophagus. For polyps coloscopy (DEDDISH) is not without danger.

e) Cytological examination by impression, direct smear, or puncture, or of the washings obtained from lavage of the maxillary sinus, stomach, or colon. This is considered to be the classic method of detection of the precancerous condition and the best means of following it up. The reasons for its defects are known, especially when puncture material is used; most often it brings to light an already invasive cancer.

f) Pathological examination, either of exfoliated mucosal fragments or of directly taken tissue. This provides very accurate information, but it is valid only for the fragment examined. Tests like that of Schiller or fluorescent staining make it possible to choose suitable sites to take tissue when the mucosa is easily accessible.

g) Paraclinical tests like the thermodifferential test. Some of these appear to have made it possible to distinguish a benign nevus from a malignant one or a cutaneous nevus-like metastasis, or to differentiate between a benign condition and a breast cancer. They are methods of making a differential diagnosis, not of diagnosing a precancerous condition.

The same is true of investigation by radioactive isotopes. Scintillation scanning does not differentiate between a benign tumor or a chronic inflammatory and a precancerous or even cancerous condition in the thyroid, kidney, or liver.

All the uncertainties in the evaluation of the risks of malignancy make the problems of treatment especially difficult.

If the essential principle that a precancerous condition is neither radiosensitive nor drug-sensitive is taken as the starting-point, only two forms of treatment are conceivable:

1. Surgical extirpation.
2. Treatment designed to prevent transformation of the condition into cancer.

1. Surgical Extirpation

General Rules

The surgical extirpation of a precancerous condition (in the widest sense, as defined by the clinical appearance) should in principle require the extirpation of all the area that might become cancerous. The risk of the operation should also be sufficiently small to justify the protection afforded against invasive cancer. RHOADS (1957) has defined a method of assessing the value of surgery for so-called precancerous conditions (with the considerable number of benign tumors included within this category). He postulates the relationship:

$$\frac{\text{on the credit side}}{\text{on the debit site}}$$

On the credit side appears a number defined by: C: the rate of cancerous lesions in the series; S-1: the survival rate five years after preventive surgery; and S-2: the survival rate five years after surgery for invasive cancer. On the debit side appear: M: the operative mortality rate; and I: the rate of the lesions definitively shown to be benign and in no way dangerous removed by these surgical procedures.

The ratio $\frac{C (S-1 - S-2)}{MI}$ should be greater than 1 to the farthest possible extent.

An example can be taken from gastrectomy for suspicious lesions and gives the following figures:

$$\frac{10\,(40-8)}{2 \times 70} = \frac{16}{7}$$

This is greater than 2 and therefore very acceptable. For the surgery of the thyroid as looked at from this point of view the ratio is even more acceptable.

Systematic surgery for congenital melanoma of the skin would not be acceptable, since a) the risk of the condition becoming malignant is not more than 1/10 000, b) surgery would not prevent an established malignant melanoma from developing, and c) in spite of a negligible mortality comparable to the risk of malignancy (0.001) the ratio is probably very much less than 1. In the same way, as long as total esophagectomy has an operative mortality of some 15 %—20 % even in the best series, this operation, proposed as a systematic procedure for all leukoplakias of the esophagus (many of which do not become transformed into cancer), would be absurd.

If the operative risk is to be the main preoccupation, however, two other aspects of the problem need to be considered.

a) Surgery for precancerous conditions should protect the patient completely from the development of cancer.

b) Surgery should not mutilate or lead to distressing sequelae. That is why surgery should be employed for all the area liable to become cancerous. But while in theory this idea is unchallengeable, in practice it is much more difficult to put into effect.

1. There are organs and areas where it can be carried out completely. For example, wide excision followed by a skin graft can be employed for an old burn scar that is very dystrophic or a radiation dermatitis subsequent to irradiation for lupus. A less good example is wide excision with or without thermocoagulation of an area in which an incipient malignant melanoma is developing, for this, unfortunately, can be already an invasive cancer of grave import. Other examples are the wide excision of the skin of the back of the hand followed by skin grafts in workers handling mineral oils and presenting hyperkeratoses in the course of transformation into cancer (Fig. 2); and total vulvectomy for atrophic vulvitis or kraurosis also

followed by skin graft. In a quite different field, the wide excision of congenital exostoses, which can become sarcomatous, is a very satisfactory operation.

In these cases surgery has in fact protected a whole area of the body from the risk of cancer and left the patient in a reasonable condition. If lymph-node enlarge-

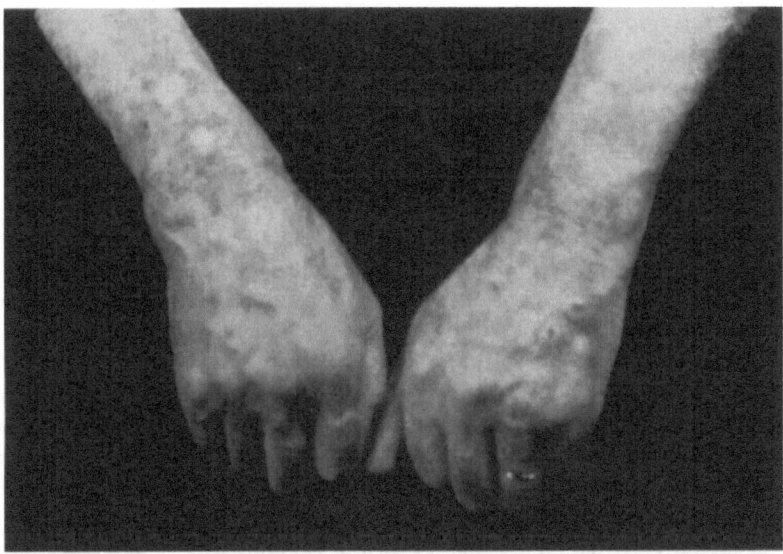

Fig. 2. Precancerous condition of the skin of the hands of a latheworker. The skin of the right hand has been totally excised because of multiple warty lesions and skin taken from the thigh has been grafted on. This operation, performed twelve years previously, has protected the skin from malignant changes. On the left hand, the lesions occurred later than those on the right because less exposed to risk, but are starting to degenerate

ment or a distant metastasis should occur, it proves that this was already more than a precancerous condition and that an area of invasive cancer lay outside the field of operation. For lesions of the mucosa some surgeons also carry out in addition a prophylactic removal of the lymph nodes, to counter this risk, which is purely hypothetical.

2. The present radical surgery for certain organs is completely acceptable. It more often extirpates frankly benign lesions or, by contrast, authentic but still circumscribed cancers than the so-called precancerous conditions. This is the case for subtotal thyroidectomy for thyroid nodules, two-thirds gastrectomy for a suspicious chronic ulcerous lesion, and rectosigmoid amputation or resection for a localized villous tumor or polyposis.

Radical surgery undoubtedly fulfils its preventive role best in cancer of the cervix uteri. It ranges from conization to amputation of the cervix and hysterectomy according to whether the lesion (or the cytological picture alone) is considered to be that of a pre-invasive or already an invasive cancer.

3. Radical organ surgery is difficult to accept if it should involve sequelae or mutilation disproportionate to the risk. Thus systematic mastectomy for cystic mastitis is unacceptable if it is bilateral, but is acceptable if one of the breasts has cancer, since the risk for the other if mastitis is present is at least of the order of 25 %—30 %. Total gastrectomy for gastric polyposis or for gastritis that appears

suspicious on cytological examination exposes the patient to an operative risk and to the danger of later anemia from achylia that make the operation unacceptable if the risks are compared with the small risk of cancer prevented thereby.

This brings us to other lesions rightly considered as typically precancerous in which at present the surgeon has to face an extremely knotty problem. There are at least three: papillomatosis of the larynx with hyperkeratosis, which should call for total laryngectomy; papillomatosis of the bladder, which should call for total extirpation of the bladder; and diffuse polyposis of the rectum and colon, which should call for total colectomy from the ileum to the anus. These three examples lead to the consideration of compromise solutions.

2. Compromise Solutions

Since it is rarely possible to extirpate radically an area or organ threatened with cancer, the solutions reached are a compromise.

One of the most interesting demonstrations of the effectiveness of a solution of this kind is furnished by total parotidectomy with conservation of the facial nerve for a mixed tumor of the parotid. Although the pathologists maintain that this lesion is to be considered rather as a cancer *ab initio* than as a precancerous condition, the very long clinical and apparently benign course before the cancer becomes manifest justifies its being regarded as a "potential" cancer that if extirpated might be prevented from becoming malignant. If untreated this tumor takes on the average 13.6 years before it becomes an infiltrating and spreading carcinoma, and it may in special cases take more than 50 (which explains why some people die with this tumor without its ever reaching that stage). If is operated on as a benign tumor, i. e., by enucleation, it is almost certain to recur, which shows that its so-called capsule does not exist and that it is already malignant. The correct surgical procedure would therefore be ablation of the entire gland in one piece, i. e., removal of the facial nerve, which would entail definitive paralysis of the area served by the nerve or a repair operation of doubtful effect. Many surgeons refuse to agree for the sake of a principle to sacrifice this perfectly intact nerve, and have adopted the solution of total parotidectomy (or excision of as much as possible of the gland) but conservation of the nerve by careful dissection. The mere fact that the tissues and generally the tumor itself are roughly handled to carry out the dissection successfully is a negation of the principles of cancer surgery; the operation is one of mere dissection and therefore blameworthy. But, judging from the statistics of all the surgeons trained to this technique of conserving the nerve, the long-term results are excellent, the number of patients without a recurrence and without facial paralysis practically reaching 100 %. Thus a compromise solution running counter to surgical principles has been attended with complete and almost constant success.

The frequency of recurrences after simple enucleation is explicable because fragments are left in the area of the false capsule and even, if some pathologists are to be believed, minute foci at a distance in the surrounding parotid tissues. Repeated operations for these recurrences are followed by still more recurrences, until eventually total parotidectomy with conservation of the facial nerve is proposed. Whereas, however, such an operation is attended with almost 100 % success when it is carried out on a parotid area untouched by operation, it is followed by at least 15 %—20 % recurrences in the five years after the operation when there have been

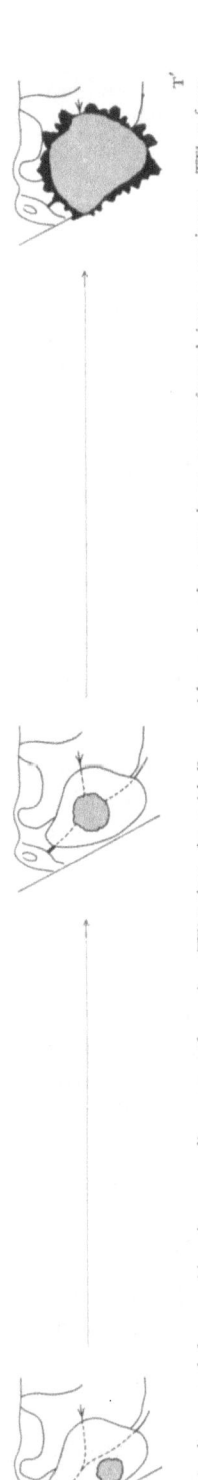

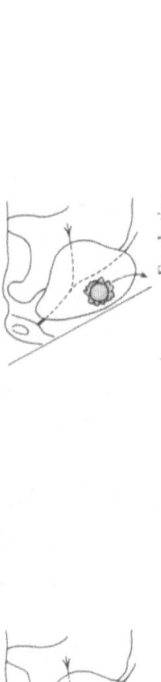
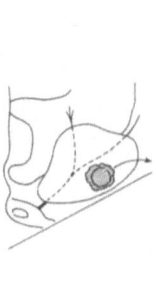
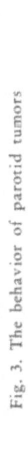
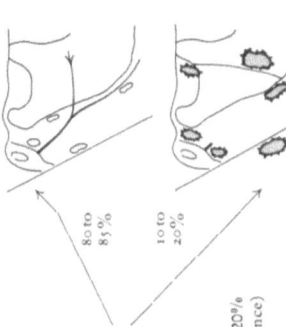
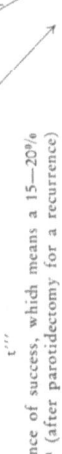
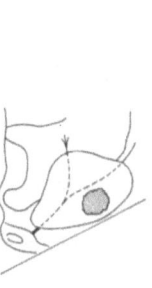

a) A mixed tumor of the parotid undergoes malignant transformation. TT' = time. An epithelioma with an altered stroma becomes transformed into a carcinoma. TT¹ = from several months to 40—50 years.

(diagram 1).

b) A mixed tumor extirpated by parotidectomy with conservation of the facial nerve to the greatest extent possible practically ensures that the cure is definitive.

c) Enucleation exposes the patient to repeated recurrences, but cancer does not appear any more rapidly. $t + t' + t'' + t''' + t^n = TT'$

d) Total or as nearly as possible total parotidectomy for relapse after enucleation gives an 80—85% chance of success, which means a 15—20% risk of recurrence in the parotid bed of foci that will become malignant. $t + t' + t'' + t''' + t^n$ (after parotidectomy for a recurrence)

Fig. 3. The behavior of parotid tumors

80 to 85%

10 to 20%

previous recurrences. The recurrences are not in the parotid area since the gland has been removed but in the skin, the masseter muscle, the scar, or the auditory meatus. To the extent that these operations have the validity of an experiment it can be said that:

a) the rough handling during the excision of the tumor has been of no importance and has not favored the recurrences, undoubtedly because the greatest part of the host tissue has been excised; and

b) the repeated trauma of limited operations conserving the host tissue has enabled the remaining fragments or the minute foci at a distance to acquire a special aptitude for multiplication to the extent that multiplication becomes possible in other tissues when the host tissue has finally been excised.

It has also been established that transformation of this tumor into an infiltrating invasive carcinoma is not hastened by these multiple recurrences. In our series the average time before this occurs is 15 years, whereas the "natural" time for transformation is 13.6 years (DARGENT, 1964).

These observations on the behavior of mixed parotid tumors considered as precancerous conditions (at least in a clinical sense) lead us to the opinion that transformation into an invasive carcinoma is a predetermined phenomenon independent of our therapeutic errors, but that our errors may make it possible for local recurrences to became more and more virulent, as if the host tissue, whether or not containing foci of cells capable of becoming cancerous, were behaving exactly like a more and more enriched culture medium (Fig. 3).

Diffuse polyposis of the colon and rectum is also treated by adopting a compromise solution. Total colectomy is such a serious operation because of the sequelae that are linked with a definitive ileostomy that total colectomy with conservation of the rectum is accepted. The rectal polyps are treated by electrocoagulation or even, if there is an area degenerating, by contact radiotherapy as needed.

In certain cases compromise solutions lead to the advocating of limited treatment in accordance with need during periods of continuous surveillance of the patients over several years. This is the practice adopted by most urologists for papilloma of the bladder and by laryngologists for papilloma of the larynx in the adult. Radical surgery is indicated only at the first histological sign of malignancy in one of the suspicious papillomas. In no case is penetrating radiotherapy indicated, although it might help improve certain functional disturbances and reduce the size of the lesions. It is certain that even the smallest amount of radiation may hasten the transformation to an invasive cancer.

Preventive Treatment for Malignant Transformation

Only too often the only possible attitude is preventive treatment for a malignant transformation, either as a measure during treatment or as a measure after treatment.

1. Value of Preventive Measures

Preventive measures are valuable only in so far as the lesions are still reversible.

I. Effective prevention is sometimes achieved by withdrawing the threatened tissue from a recognized cancerogenic stimulus, as the skin of workers exposed to mineral oils or the vesical mucosa of workers in the dyeing industry. This may also be true of circumcision for chronic balanitis, although the only effective circumcision is that carried out in the first week of life.

II. When the precancerous state is conditioned by a congenital lesion (diffuse polyposis of the colon or xeroderma), the situation is like fate in "FATUM" of ancient tragedy, dreaded but impossible to avoid.

III. When a habit is involved that can be "corrected", persuasion may be used to have it abandoned. This is especially so with lung cancer and the habit of smoking cigarettes. As it seems to be a vain task to try to educate a whole population from childhood on, there seems at least to be some interest in pursuing such a study as that of AUERBACH et al. (1964). The cytological study of the bronchial secretions of heavy smokers, ex-heavy smokers, and non-smokers shows considerable differences in the frequency of atypical nuclei and even of the signs of cancer in situ between the first and the third group, but the second group also has fewer disturbing cytological appearances. Surveillance of the bronchial mucosa, leading to no therapeutic action until the cytological warning is corroborated by radiological or endoscopical indications, may at least have the advantage that it tells the heavy smoker that he has reached the danger threshold when metaplasia, dysplasia, or even in situ appearances are seen. It is still perhaps not too late to give up smoking.

IV. Finally, there are conditions in which it is possible to wait and see, in a state of armed alert. Among them are the benign melanomas of the skin, which should be extirpated only if they are subjected to irritation. There are also the states of diffuse leukoplakia of the buccal cavity, which respond poorly to vitamin treatment or to electrocoagulation of the foci, since other foci appear later. The only thing required is to know when to remove the plaques of leukoplakia in time when they become suspect. Finally, the same attitude is desirable for cystic mastitis, for which a waiting policy and symptomatic treatment are preferable, especially after the age of 40 years, to hormone treatment even on a moderate scale, since the effect of the latter may be to stimulate a slow-growing cancer and bring it into the phase of malignant development.

2. Post-therapeutic Measures

Post-therapeutic measures are necessary, since by definition a precancerous condition is often multicentric. They generally become necessary after treatment of invasive cancer considered to be early. Precancerous conditions of the bronchi are certainly disseminated; LE GAL and BAUER (1961), found four fresh cancers in 63 patients (6.4%) 30 months after resection for lung cancer. A conclusion to be drawn from this finding is that lobectomies should be done as far as possible. Single or multiple polyps of the colon in association with cancer of the rectum should be regarded as undoubted precancerous conditions, to be very carefully watched. A patient treated for malignant melanoma who has multiple congenital melanomas should also be examined frequently, as should one who has multiple hereditary exostoses when one has become malignant and been treated. Yet another subject to be watched is the individual exposed to the sun who has dyskeratosis of the skin of the face or lip, a patch of which has already become malignant.

The same post-therapeutic precautions must be taken and are equally important in relation to mucosal surfaces elsewhere than those treated, since the same cancerogenic stimulus may affect them. A heavy smoker operated on for cancer of the larynx should have his bronchi and lungs specially watched.

Conclusions

There are tissues (generally covering tissues) in which precancerous conditions can be progressively better defined and are more and more accessible. The extirpation of suspect sites usually detected by cytological investigations should make it possible to reduce the frequency of invasive cancer. But there are still many organs and tissues in which the multicentricity of the precancerous areas and the fact that they become malignant at different periods in time make surgical treatment, which should be radical, impracticable or too mutilating. It is then necessary to adopt compromise solutions, among which often the only possible ones are prevention or a policy of wait and see. A last point is that cancer does not always begin with at least morphologically detectable precancerous condition; it may begin in an apparently healthy tissue or in the neighbourhood of a so-called precancerous site. That is the reason why the treatment of precancerous conditions can still only be applied in very limited fields. It would be utopian to consider it as an effective method of preventing all cancers.

References

ABDUL NASR AL, F. EL GAZAYERLIM, and I. EL SIBAI: Symposium on cancer of the bladder, Cairo, March, 1961. Acta Un. int. Cancr. 18, 528 (1962).

ACKERMAN, L. V., H. J. SPJUT, and J. S. SPRATT: The biological characteristics of colonic and rectal neoplasms with refutation of the concept that adenomatous polyps are highly malignant tumors. Acta Un. int. Cancr. 20, 716 (1964).

AUERBACH, O., A. P. STOUT, D. C. HAMMOND, and L. GARFINKEL: Changes in bronchial epithelium in relation to smoking habits. Acta Un. int. Cancr. 20, 732 (1964).

CACHIN, Y.: Les papillomes du larynx. Ann. Oto-laryng. (Paris) 76, 744 (1959).

DARGENT, M.: Réflexions sur la valeur du dépistage précoce en cancérologie. Presse méd. 72, 1951 (1964).

DUPERRAT, B.: Les tumeurs noires de la peau. In Duperat, B. (ed.): Expansion scientifique française, POULY, R., et Cl. ROMIEU (1962).

FIDLER, H. K., and D. A. BOYES: Proceedings of the First International Congress of Exfoliative Cytology, Vienna. Philadelphia: Lippincott 1960.

FOULDS, L.: The natural history of cancer. T. chron. Dis. 8, 1 (1958).

GALY, P., et al.: Cancers broncho-pulmonaires sous-pleurax développés sur cicatrice. Un aspect de l'adéno-carcinome pulmonaire péripherique. J. franç. Méd. Chir. thor. 12, 518 (1958).

GODLEVSKI, H. G.: Histochemical studies of phosphoamylases in cancerous and precancerous lesions in the uterine cervix and mammary gland. Acta Un. int. Cancr. 20, 706 (1964).

GROSS, K.: Cancer detection. Acta Un. int. Cancr. 20, 785 (1964).

JOSSERAND, A., M. DARGENT, and F. PINET: Les cancers des brûlures. Presse méd. 66, 1479 (1957).

LANGE, P.: Clinical and histological studies on cervical carcinoma. Precancerous early metastases and tubular structures in the lymph nodes. Acta path. microbiol. scand., 143 (Supp.) (1960).

LE GAL, Y., and W. C. BAUER: Second primary bronchogenic carcinoma. J. thorac. cardiorasc. Surg. 41, 114 (1961).

MIKOLAS, V., A. STAFL, und A. LINHARTOV: Das terminale Gefäßbild der Portio vaginalis uteri bei Schwangeren. Zbl. Gynäk. 84, 524 (1962).

MORGENROTH, K.: Precancerous changes in the oral cavity. Acta Un. int. Cancr. 20, 713 (1964).

NEIMAN, J. M.: About the biological nature of precancer. Acta Un. int. Cancr. 20, 697 (1964).

PEDERSEN, O.: Precancerous changes of the cervical epithelium in relation to manifest cervical carcinoma. Copenhagen: Danish Science Press 1958.

QUINSENBERRY, W. B.: Exfoliative cytology laboratory service in a cancer control program. Acta Un. int. Cancr. 20, 795 (1964).

RAEBURN, C., and C. SPENCER: Lung scar cancer. Brit. J. Tuberc. 51, 237 (1957).

RHOADS, J. E.: Development of preventive surgery in the field of cancer. Ann. Surg. 146, 782 (1957).

SUN SHAO CHIEN: Investigation on early carcinomatous changes of the epithelium adjacent to the principal lesion in squamous cell carcinoma of the oesophagus. In Selected papers on cancer research. Shanghai: Shanghai Scientific and Technical Publishers 1962.

WIED, G. L.: The use of cytology in the detection of precancerous lesions. Acta Un. int. Cancr. 20, 669 (1964).

Cancer Chemotherapy

L. F. LARIONOV

1. Brief Historical Outline

Development of antitumor drugs. Modern cancer chemotherapy dates from 1946, when the first clinical reports were published by HADDOW *et al.* on the therapeutic effect of urethane in myeloid leukemia and on nitrogen mustard in Hodgkin's disease, chronic leukemia, and lymphoreticulosarcoma (GILMAN and PHILIPS, 1946; GOODMAN *et al.*, 1946; RHOADS, 1946). Hormone treatment [1] was started at about the same time (HUGGINS and HODGES, 1941).

Twenty years have elapsed since then, a short period in the history of medicine. However, nearly 30 anticancer drugs that are used with some effect in many forms of malignant tumors have been developed during this period.

The existing agents may be divided into the following main groups: (1) alkylating agents; (2) antimetabolites; (3) antibiotic-type substances; (4) substances of plant origin; (5) hormones and related compounds; and (6) miscellaneous substances. Agents in all these groups have been developed simultaneously. Thus in 1948, two years after the introduction of nitrogen mustards and urethane, the therapeutic properties of the first antimetabolite were discovered. This was an analogue of folic acid, aminopterin (FARBER *et al.*, 1948). Somewhat later methotrexate (Amethophthin) was discovered.

The clinical effectiveness of two new alkylating agents — chloronaphthin and tretamine (TEM) — was established in 1950; it turned out that these agents could be used orally. The year 1952 was marked by studies of the therapeutic properties of the first antitumor antibiotic — actinomycin C — and the alkaloid colchamine (demecolcine). In 1953 nitrogen mustard-N-oxide (nitromin) and a new antimetabolite — 6-mercaptopurine — were added.

Many new agents were developed and their effectiveness was established in 1954—1955. They included chloroethylamines — chlorambucil, dopan, sarcolysin, and degranol; ethyleneimines — E-39 and thiophosphoramide; sulfonoxy com-

---

[1] Since the hormone treatment of cancer of the breast and prostate is dealt with in other chapters, it is not considered here.

Table 1. *Drugs Commonly used in*

Drugs	Tumor types	Hodgkins' disease	Lympho-reticulosarcoma	Acute leukemia	Chronic lymphatic leukemia	Chronic myeloid leukemia	Multiple myeloma	Bone reticulosarcoma, Ewing's tumor	Lung cancer	Skin cancer	Cancer of esophagus	Cancer of stomach
Chlorethyl-amines	Chlormethine	++	+		+	+			±[1]			
	Novembichin	++	+		+							
	Chlormethine oxide	++	+		+	+			+[2]			
	Chlorambucil	++	+		+							
	Dopan and Uracil mustard	++	+									
	Degranol	++	+		+							
	Cyclophosphamide	++	+	+	+		+	+	±			
	Sarcolysin (Melphalan)		+				++	++			S,+[3]	S[3]
Ethyleneimines	Tretamine (TEM)	+	+		+							
	E 39 and Trenimon	+	+		+	+			±			
	Thiotepa				+				S			
	Benzotepa								S			
	Dipin and Thiodipin				+							
	Azetepa	+	+						±			
	AB 100, AB 103								±			
Methane sulphonyloxy compounds	Myleran					++						
Antimetabolites	Methotrexate			+[8]					+			
	6-Mercaptopurine			++								
	5-Fluorouracil								+[6]		±[6]	+
Plant products	Colchamine (Demecolcine)									++	S,+[3]	
	Vinblastine	+		+								
	Vincristine	+		+								
Antibiotics	Actinomycin C	+										
	Actinomycin D	+										
	Mitomycin C											
	Mithramycin											
	Streptonigrin			+					±			
Miscellaneous	Methylhydrazine	+	±									
	Hydroxyurea											
Hormones	Androgens											
	Estrogens											
	Corticosteroids			+	+							

S   Symptomatic effect

±   Objective effect in individual patients, for the most part incomplete or brief

+   Immediate (in less than half the patients) but marked objective effect with different degrees of tumor regression and duration of "remission". "Long-term" results are not achieved or are as yet unknown.

++   Regression of tumors (remission) in more than half the patients with a possibility of producing long-term results (3—5 years).

Cancer Treatment and their Effects

Cancer of pancreas	Cancer of liver	Cancer of colon and rectum	Mammary cancer	Prostatic cancer	Cancer of corpus uteri	Cancer of cervix uteri	Ovarian cancer	Seminoma	Choriocarcinoma	Melanoma	Osteogenic sarcoma	Wilm's tumor	Bladder cancer	Hypernephroma	Brain tumors	Neuroblastoma	Retinoblastoma
							±										
					±		++	+		±						+[4]	
	+	+[3]					+	++		+[5]			+[6]				
			+		±		++										
							+										
														±			
					±	±											
						+[9]			++								
									±								
+	+	+	+		±		+						±	+			
													±				
			+												+		
									+			+[6]					
		±	+								±				+		
											+				±		
			±			+[5]											
										±							
			++														
			++	++													
			+														

[1] Effect on lymph node metastases
[2] When administered after surgical removal of the cancer
[3] In combination with colchamine at an early stage
[4] In combination with vincristine
[5] On perfusion
[6] In combination with radiation treatment   [7] On intracavitary administration
[8] In combination with mercaptopurine and steroids   [9] On intra-arterial infusion

pounds — myleran; and antibiotics — actinomycin D. The years 1957 and 1958 were also marked by successful experimental and clinical studies of a number of compounds, namely, antimetabolites — 5-fluorouracil; chloroethylamines — endoxan and sarcolysin peptides; new ethyleneimines — ethymidine, benzotepa and dipin; a myleran homologue — nonane; and antibiotics — mitomycin C. The effectiveness of vinblastine, an alkaloid isolated from *Vinca rosea* L, and the alkylating agents trenimon and AB 100 and 103 was established in the tumor clinic. The literature is reviewed by LARIONOV (1965).

A number of new substances have been proposed and studied clinically and experimentally in the last five or six years; some of them are listed below. [2]

Alkylating agents: myleran homologues and analogues, mannitol-myleran, etc.; degranol derivatives — zytophenton (degranolheparinate), etc.; cyclophosphamide derivatives — mitarson, etc.; sarcolysin isomers — ortho- and metasarcolysin; chloro-ethylamine derivatives of lysine (lysepsin), tyrosine (phenthyrine) and tryptophan (tryptophan mustard), a number of sarcolysin and melphalan peptides, particularly asaline (ethyl ester of N-acetyl-sarcolysyl-D, L-valine), etc., phenesterin (cholesterol ester of p-di-(2-chloroethyl)aminophenylacetic acid), spirazidine (N^1, N^4-β, β'-(di-chloroethyl)-N^2, N^3-dispirotripiperazinium), BCNU (1,3 bis (2-chloroethyl)-1-nitro-sourea), imiphos (marcophan, 2-methyl-thiazolidino-3-diethylene-phosphoramide) azetepa (N, N'-diethylene-N''-ethyl-N''-1,3, 4-thiazole (2-yl-phosphoramide), epo-dyl-(triethyleneglycol diglycidil ester).

Antimetabolites — 6-azauridine and its triacetyl derivative; drugs of plant origin — vincristine, SPI (podophyllinic acid ethyl hydrazide), SPG (glucoside of podo-phyllotoxin); antibiotics — mithramycin (olivomycin), streptonigrin, daunomycin, etc.

Moreover, new compounds which do not belong to the aforesaid group have been studied clinically. They include 1,6-dibrommannitol, natulan (methylhydrazine) -N-isopropyl-α-(methylhydrazino) p-toluamide hydrochloride, methyl-GAG (methyl-glyoxal-bisguanylhydrazone), hydroxyurea, terephthalanilides, particularly NSC-60339 (2-chloro-4', 4''-di(2-imidazoline-2-yl) terephthalanilide), ambunol (chlor-hydrate-4-oxy-3,5-di(tert.) butyl-N,N'-beta oxyethylbenzylamine), 1-amino-cyclo-pentacarboxylic acid, etc.

Not all these compounds have proved clinically effective. Some of them produced a clinical effect but showed no differences from or advantages over compounds previously studied. Some of the new compounds, however, proved effective with a large number of patients, and their effectiveness has been confirmed by several investigators. They are listed in the table.

Inclusion of various forms of malignant tumors in the sphere of chemotherapy. The possibility of treating hormone-dependent tumors, i. e., prostatic and breast cancer, with estrogens and androgens was the first to be established, before 1946. For a period of almost 10 years, beginning with 1946, chemotherapy was applied mainly to malignant diseases of the hemopoietic system: Hodgkin's disease, acute leukemias, chronic lymphatic and myeloid leukemia, erythremia, lympho- and reti-culosarcoma (alkylating agents, Amethopterin, 6-mercaptopurine). Some effect was

---

[2] For the literature, see Cancer Chemotherapy Abstracts, Cumulative Author and Subject Indexes, 1961—1965, Cancer Chemotherapy National Service Center, Bethesda, Md., USA.

also noted in lung cancer (nitrogen mustard, TEM) and cancer of the ovaries (TEM and chlorambucil).

Data on the effects of treatment of a number of special forms of tumors began to appear in 1955. These included seminomas, multiple myelomas (treated with sarcolysin), cancer of the ovary and breast cancer (thiotepa), and skin cancer (colchamine ointment).

Lastly, from 1958 on, the effectiveness of chemotherapy was established in carcinomas of the gastrointestinal tract — the colon and rectum, stomach, pancreas, liver (5-fluorouracil), and esophagus (5-fluorouracil with irradiation, sarcolysin with colchamine). The possibility was being explored of producing regression of lung cancer by combining 5-fluorouracil with radiotherapy, of metastases of Wilm's tumor by combining radiotherapy with actinomycin D, of metastases of chorionepithelioma by administration of methotrexate, actinomycin D, vinblastine, and their combinations, of melanoblastomas by perfusing the extremities with sarcolysin, and of some tumors of the head and neck and metastases of cancer of the cervix uteri by intra-arterial infusion of methotrexate.

Thus in the last five years chemotherapy has begun to be used with some effect for most malignant tumors. Table 1 sums up the data on the effectiveness of modern antitumor drugs in various forms of malignant tumors.

Most of the agents are characterized by a rather marked affinity for certain forms of cancer. Fluorouracil, cyclophosphamide, sarcolysin, and methotrexate possess the broadest spectrum of antitumor action. The other compounds have a narrower spectrum, but are very effective in certain forms of tumor. For example, myleran is effective in myeloid leukemia, mercaptopurine in acute leukemia, and estrogens in prostatic cancer.

2. Variation of the Effect of Chemotherapy in Various Malignant Tumors

The effect produced by chemotherapy varies very widely. In some patients it is subjective only, i. e., the patients merely feel better. In other patients the effect may be characterized as symptomatic. It consists of an actual diminution or disappearance of pain (so that less analgesia is required), reduction or cessation of cough, improvement of appetite, improved passage of food through the esophagus and other parts of the gastrointestinal tract, and decrease of other symptoms. At the same time the size of the tumor, as established by palpation, measurement, or X-ray examination, or the picture of the blood and bone marrow (in leukemia) remains unchanged. A symptomatic effect may be accompanied by increased activity of the patient.

A regression of the tumor (or a return to normal of the blood and bone marrow picture in leukemia) is designated as an objective effect. It may vary in: (1) the extent of reproducibility, i. e., the percentage of patients with the given form of tumor in whom the effect produced; (2) the degree of regression of the tumor, i. e., from slight diminution to complete disappearance; and (3) the extent to which it remains constant from the end of the treatment to the beginning of the relapse. The period of objective improvement or asymptomatic period, sometimes called the remission, may be short (1—3 months) or averagely long (6—12 months), or may even last 3—5 years without relapse (positive long-term results).

An incomplete regression is usually brief. Complete regression and resultant remission may in some cases be brief and in others prolonged and stable, but of different reproducibility in different patients of the same group. An attempt is made in Table 1 to designate the effect with one mark (number of pluses). It is often difficult to do this, and these designations should be considered as very provisional. However, it is useful to give them so as to afford a general, even if approximate, idea of the present state of the chemotherapy of malignant tumors. The table shows not all, but the more commonly used, agents studied in a comparatively large number of patients, provided that the data furnished by authors have been confirmed by others. The designations refer to primary tumors or metastases, depending on which are more sensitive to the given compound. Most of the data given in the table refer to very advanced stages of the disease.

3. Possibility of Clinical Cure

During the first years of its development it was thought that cancer chemotherapy could produce only a palliative effect. This opinion was due to the facts that, first, chemotherapy was used mainly in malignant diseases of the hemopoietic system that were to an extraordinary degree inclined to relapse, and, second, it was administered to patients for whom the possibilities of another method of treatment (radiation) had been exhausted. These patients, in addition to being at a very advanced stage of the disease, suffered from functional insufficiency of the hemopoietic system and exhaustion of the compensatory powers of the organism. They could be given only an insufficient dose of the drug, and no considerable effect could be expected.

However, it was very soon established that, if the treatment of Hodgkin's disease with chlormethine (HN2) and novembichin was started at a relatively early stage, it was possible to produce complete regression of the affected nodes with a stable effect for three and five years (LARIONOV, 1956). These observations were later confirmed when dopan was used (IVANOVA, 1964). Data began to be accumulated also on the possibility of producing a stable therapeutic effect for three to five years and longer (without a relapse) in the treatment of other, including solid, tumors. This was established in sarcolysin treatment of seminoma metastases (CHEBOTAREVA, 1964), multiple myeloma (MERKULOVA, 1964), and bone reticulosarcomas with inclusion of Ewing's sarcoma (PEREVODCHIKOVA, 1965). The corresponding figures are shown in Table 2 for patients beginning treatment in 1954—1960 (PEREVODCHIKOVA, 1965).

Table 2. *Long-term Results of the Use of Sarcolysin*

Type of tumor	Total number of patients treated	Effect produced in	Remained alive 3 years later	Remained alive 5 years later	without a relapse
Seminoma	30	21	17	10	6 (20%)
Multiple myeloma	22	14	9	4	3 (14%)
Bone reticulosarcoma and Ewing's sarcoma	20	10	4	4	4 (20%)

HERTZ et al. (1958) published important data on the five-year results of methotrexate treatment of chorionepithelioma metastases in the lungs, positive for 25% of the patients treated. Administration of colchamine ointment in the treatment of the initial stage of skin cancer produced a cure with an absence of relapses for a period of 10 years in 89 % of patients (Movsesyan, 1965). Burchenal (1964 a) collected and analysed 101 cases of remission in acute leukemia patients lasting five years and longer after treatment with methotrexate, mercaptopurine, and corticosteroids.

Lastly, there are reports of single cases of complete regression without relapse for three to five years or longer in the treatment of esophageal carcinoma (Larionov and Chudakova, 1963) and of carcinoma of the large intestine in a very advanced stage with a combination of sarcolysin and colchamine (Larionov, 1965).

The results of treatment of malignant tumors by surgical and radiological methods with an absence of relapses and symptoms of the disease for a period of five years are conventionally designated as clinical cure. We deem it possible to use this term in chemotherapy, although it is well known that even a longer period, whatever the method of treatment, is no guarantee of absolute cure.

It has been demonstrated that chemotherapy is not only a palliative method of treating malignant tumors but that in certain conditions it may, like other methods, lead to clinical cure. At present clinical cure is rarely observed. However, in this connexion the following circumstances must be taken into consideration:

1. In the early stages of malignant tumors, when it is easiest to produce clinical cure, chemotherapy is extremely rarely used, other methods being preferred.

2. In various forms of tumor (multiple myeloma, choriocarcinoma, acute leukemia) positive long-term results may be produced by chemotherapy even in very advanced stages of the disease when other methods completely fail.

3. In comparing the number of patients cured by chemotherapy on the one hand, and by surgical and radiation treatment on the other, it is necessary that the comparison should be under similar conditions. Obviously, if we compare the percentage of patients cured by operation in early stages of cancer with the percentage cured by chemotherapy in all (but usually advanced) stages of cancer, the comparison will be in favour of the surgical method. But if the patients cured by surgical treatment (those, for example, with stomach, esophageal, or lung cancer) are considered in relation to all patients diagnosed with those forms of cancer, we get much the same figures as those shown in Table 2 (i. e., 15—20 % or even lower).

It may be objected that this argument applies to forms of cancer in which chemotherapy does not help at all. That is true but, on the other hand, chemotherapy has as yet not been used at the early stage when operation is feasible and a conclusion can be drawn only when this is done. We can nevertheless say that the possibility, in some patients with very advanced stomach cancer, of restoring the radiological picture to normal by means of 5-fluorouracil (Blokhina, 1965) and the cure of two patients with esophageal cancer at an early stage by sarcolysin and colchamine (Larionov and Chudakova, 1963) indicate the prospects of and provide a justification for such studies in, for example, patients for whom operation at an early stage is contraindicated for other reasons or who refuse to submit to it.

4. General Principles of Cancer Chemotherapy

From the large number of data furnished by experimental and clinical chemotherapy some general principles may be drawn. They will help both to prescribe adequate treatment and to explain the results achieved.

1. *The effect of chemotherapy is, as a rule, inversely proportional to the size of the tumor mass.* The greater the mass, the less the effect, and vice versa. The reason is that the therapeutic effect of chemotherapeutic agents is based on their chemical interaction with the cell constituents of importance to its vital activities. Thus alkylating agents enter into covalent bonds with DNA, RNA, proteins, and lipids. The most important for the therapeutic effect is apparently the alkylation of DNA, which after several stages leads to fragmentation of the high polymeric molecule.

Antimetabolites enter into easily or hardly reversible complexes with active centres of the enzymes, blocking at some stage the reaction catalysed by the enzymes. With a good imitation of the substrate, the antimetabolite may also be incorporated into the products of the reaction. Antibiotics may also function as antimetabolites. It follows that, as long as chemotherapy implies chemical interaction, the final effect will depend on the relative amounts of reacting substances.

The activity of the agents on a molar basis varies greatly and depends either on the chemical reactivity of the alkylating group under physiological conditions or on the degree of affinity of the antimetabolite with the enzyme. But, regardless of this, the end result corresponds to the percentage of damaged DNA or enzyme molecules. Naturally, when the mass of tumor tissue is large some of the DNA or enzyme molecules fail to react with the agent, and as a result the amount of damage and percentage of damaged cells are lower and the end effect is less pronounced.

On the other hand, the mass of normal tissue involved in the side reaction with the agent is fairly constant, so that the total dose of the agent cannot be increased beyond the amount that damages normal tissue cells within acceptable limits. It follows that the maximum tolerable dose of the agent is a relatively constant value. In practice it may vary in different patients, depending on such attendant circumstances as the absorption and destruction of the agent in the gastrointestinal tract and the extent to which the hemopoietic tissue is intact as a result of previous treatment and the patient's condition.

The following conclusions may be drawn:

1. If the mass of neoplastic tissue is large no great effect can be expected from the use of chemotherapy — not complete regression of the tumors (except the most sensitive ones).

2. To produce the maximum effect, chemotherapy must be initiated at earlier stages, or the amount of tumor tissue reduced beforehand by non-radical surgical intervention, or the treatment administered in several successive courses, thereby systematically diminishing the mass of neoplastic tissue.

3. In judging the results of chemotherapy, it is necessary to take into account the total size of the tumor mass.

Another conclusion could also be drawn, namely, that the effect of chemotherapy must be greatest on disseminated tumor cells remaining among normal tissues near the site of a tumor that has been removed or carried away by the circulation during the operation. According to some investigators (COSTACHEL — personal communication), disseminated tumor cells are less sensitive to antitumor agents than the lymph nodes, which have their own vascular network. If this is actually the case, administration of these agents directly after a so-called radical operation may prove insufficiently effective. This question requires further investigation.

2. *Other things being equal, the effect of chemotherapy with a given compound depends on whether it is administered for the primary tumor or for metastases and on the localization of the latter.* Primary tumors are less sensitive than metastases to some agents. For example, primary lung and stomach cancers are insensitive to alkylating agents, whereas their metastases in lymph nodes may regress. On the other hand, primary stomach carcinomas (and their relapses) are apparently more sensitive to 5-fluorouracil than their metastases (BLOKHINA, 1964).

The effect of chemotherapy on metastases also depends on the organ in which they are localized. Thus seminoma metastases in lymph nodes are very sensitive to sarcolysin, whereas metastases of the same tumor in the lungs are practically unaffected by this agent (CHEBOTAREVA, 1962, 1964). In prescribing chemotherapy and evaluating its results these facts should be taken into account. In fine, the effectiveness of compounds should be appraised separately in relation to primary tumors and to metastases.

3. *The effect of chemotherapy depends on the histological structure and bio-chemical characteristics of the tumor.* Different effects produced by the same agent may be observed not only in tumors of different organs but also in tumors of the same organ of different histological structure. For example, cholangiocellular primary cancer of the liver is sensitive to sarcolysin, while hepatocellular cancer is not. Epidermoid lung carcinoma is not sensitive either to alkylating agents or to fluorouracil, but undifferentiated lung carcinoma is more sensitive to alkylating agents and adenocarcinomas to fluorouracil. Observations of this kind must be accumulated and systematized for the purpose of compiling indications for chemotherapy and evaluating its results.

But even in tumors of the same histological structure sensitivity to any given compound may differ, owing apparently to biochemical peculiarities. Thus, for example, what seemingly are histologically similar melanoblastomas may be both sensitive and insensitive to sarcolysin. This question has hardly been studied at all.

5. Dependence of Results on Techniques of Treatment

The effect of chemotherapy on malignant tumors depends in very large measure on the method of treatment, the adequacy of which is often overlooked. It must be remembered that the *selectivity* of antitumor action, i. e., the ratio of the therapeutic influence on the tumor to the side effects is in most modern chemotherapeutic agents comparatively low. A considerable clinical effect may therefore usually be produced only by doses that produce certain side effects. Alkylating agents cause nausea and vomiting and, especially, depression of leuko- and thrombocytopoiesis, while anti-metabolites and antibiotics in addition cause gastrointestinal disturbances (stomatitis, diarrhea, etc.).

Maximum acceptable dose. Experimental chemotherapy shows that the maximum effect can, as a rule, be produced only by the maximum dose of the drug that can be tolerated. An increase in the dose kills the animals, whereas a decrease, even slight, leads to a sharp drop in effect. The concept of the maximum acceptable dose has therefore been adopted clinically. It implies a dose of a drug that produces certain toxic effects in the organism which, however, are at a "permissible" level. This level is interpreted variously. Thus some authors discontinue treatment when the leukocyte count falls below 5000 (WRIGHT, 1958, HARRIS *et al.*, 1964), i. e., even when it is, say, 4500. But clinical experience shows that such doses are not the maximum acceptable ones and that higher doses causing the number of leukocytes and thrombocytes to fall still further are tolerated quite satisfactorily.

The most generally accepted opinion is that at the end of the course the lowest permissible leukocyte count may be 3000 and the thrombocyte count 100 000. At the present stage of cancer chemotherapy, when this method of treatment has not been mastered everywhere and by everybody, *this level of depression of leukocytopoiesis and thrombocytopoiesis should be accepted, for the purpose of international standardization, as determining the value of the maximum acceptable dose of the drug to be used in treatment.*

However, just as a highly qualified surgeon may venture upon an occasional extremely radical operation, so an experienced chemotherapist may go beyond this limit for the purpose of producing a maximum effect and under certain conditions may use a dose causing the number of leukocytes to fall at the very end or even after the end of the course to 2000 and even 1500, and the thrombocytes to 50 000, i. e., to 25 % of their normal count. Numerous experiments conducted in our and in other laboratories show that a decrease in neutrophils to 25 % of the initial count is easily and rapidly reversible. Clinical experience similarly indicates that a brief leukopenia of 1500 leukocytes, when not accompanied by a decrease in thrombocytes to below 50 000 and in hemoglobin to below 60 units, not only fails to be felt by the patient himself (with minor exceptions) but, firstly, is quite reversible even without any special measures and, secondly, does not result in such weakening of the organism's immunological state as to lead to secondary infection and other undesirable phenomena.

But the chemotherapist must know when he can and when it is expedient to use doses at the limit of tolerance. First, there must be a reason for such action, i. e., it must be known or established at the beginning of the treatment that the tumor is in some measure sensitive to the given agent. If the tumor is very sensitive, complete regression of the tumor tissue may be attempted by the use of large doses. If the tumor is moderately sensitive the maximum possible regression in one course of treatment must be striven for. There is clearly no point in using large doses if the tumor is insensitive.

Second, it is necessary that the patient's hemopoietic system should not be exhausted by the disease itself, for example in abdominal and generalized forms of Hodgkin's disease or multiple myeloma, or by previous treatment, especially by the use of large doses of ionizing radiation in the region of the pelvis or the chest. In such patients, even if small doses are used, a sudden sharp drop in the leukocyte and thrombocyte counts and poor regeneration of the bone marrow may be observed. Greater depression of hemopoiesis may also be observed during repeated courses of chemotherapy, especially if such agents as thiotepa are used at short intervals.

Large doses must, of course, be used cautiously, a leukocyte and thrombocyte count being made before each administration of the drug and the properties of the latter being taken into consideration, with particular attention to the fact that with some drugs a delayed effect on hemopoiesis may be observed. Thus, for example, when thiotepa and degranol are used, for 5—10 days immediately following cessation of the treatment (when the leukocyte count may be 3000 and the thrombocyte count

100 000) a further decrease to 2000 for the leukocytes and 50 000 for the thrombocytes, and sometimes even more, may be observed.

A decrease in the leukocyte count below 1000 and the thrombocyte count below
50 000 should be considered absolutely inadmissible. At this level immunity against
infection noticeably decreases and the bone marrow is wasted to such an extent that
its regeneration is impeded. The non-specific resistance of the organism to the growth
of tumors and the development of metastases may apparently also weaken, and this
may lead to earlier relapses and metastases.

Thus we must consider as the maximum acceptable dose of an antitumor drug
one that at the end of the treatment or several days after leads to a decrease in the
leukocyte count to 3000 and in the thrombocyte count to 100 000 or, when antimetabolites and antibiotics are used, to incipient stomatitis and diarrhea. In patients
with an adequate hemopoietic system, when the tumor is of moderate sensitivity to
certain drugs, an experienced chemotherapist may, to produce the maximum therapeutic effect, cautiously increase the dose beyond the indicated limit, but not to such
an extent as to reduce the count to below 1500 leukocytes and 50 000 thrombocytes.

Correspondence between the extent of the side effects and the therapeutic effect.
Experimental pharmacological studies clearly show interdependence between the size
of the dose and the extent of both the therapeutic effects and the side effects. By
mathematical treatment of the mean figures this interdependence can be expressed
in terms of various curves and equations (DRUCKREY, 1959; EMMANUEL, 1964). But
an analysis of all the data of an experiment often shows that in some animals the
side effects and/or the therapeutic effects are considerably more marked than in
others and even that there is some disparity, for example, between the degree of
hemopoietic depression and the regression of the tumor. And this may be observed
despite the genetic homogeneity of the animals and the equality of the other conditions of the experiment.

Of course, when antitumor agents are administered to patients who have great
individual differences in regard to their preceding life, the treatment they have
received, the state of their organism, particularly the adequacy of hemopoiesis, and
the stage, size, histological and biochemical characteristics, etc. of their tumors, the
correlation between the extent of the side effects and the therapeutic effect may
vary greatly. Nevertheless, under certain conditions, as for example, when a particular agent is administered to relatively similar patients, a satisfactory correspondence
between the values under consideration may be observed.

Thus, according to data furnished by Japanese authors and analysed by FRANK
and OSTERBERG (1960), when mitomycin C was used in a total dose of 40 mg and
less, a decrease in the leukocyte count was observed in 35 % of the patients and
a clinical effect (in different forms of tumor) in 25 %. With the dose of mitomycin
between 60 and 80 mg, depression of leukopoiesis and thrombocytopoiesis was observed in 80 % of patients, while a clinical effect was produced in 50 %. Thus, with
a double dose of the drug, the frequency of the hemopoietic depression and of the
clinical effect also doubled.

But if a large group of patients with various tumors of varying sensitivity to
drugs is treated with different compounds, the resulting data may not show a correspondence between the manifestation of side effects and the therapeutic effect, and
this may lead to wrong conclusions. This is precisely the case with the work of

BROSS (1965) on the use of five different agents — 5-fluorouracil, AB-132, mitomycin C, chlorambucil, and 6-mercaptopurine — on 956 patients with most diverse tumors. The patients were divided into those in whom the treatment had a positive effect (responders — 208 patients) and those in whom it had no effect (non-responders — 748 patients). The former included patients whose tumors diminished at least 50 %. Considerable leukopenia (below 2000) was observed in 17 % of the responders and in 18 % of the non-responders. Thrombocytopenia (below 100 000) occurred in 41 % of patients of the first group and in 32 % of patients of the second group. According to the author, "These data suggest that patients manifesting toxicity do not respond more frequently than patients without toxicity". But the author tried to work out an equation with many unknown quantities by using a number of agents for different tumors with different sensitivity to these agents and, of course, with different states of hemopoiesis. Moreover, he failed to consider the different degrees of therapeutic effect, dividing the patients into only two groups according to the "all or none" principle.

The correspondence between the side effects and the therapeutic effect is determined primarily by two factors: (1) the sensitivity of the given tumor to the agent used, and (2) the sensitivity of the patient (and especially of his hemopoietic system and gastrointestinal tract) to the agent. If the tumor is entirely insensitive to the given agent, not even the highest dose (with all its toxicity) will help to produce a therapeutic effect and, of course, there will be no correlation between the toxicity and the effect. If the tumor is highly sensitive to the compound, a therapeutic effect, especially a moderate effect (such as a decrease of the tumor to half its size) may be produced with weak or even with no side effects. But here, too, no simple correlation is observed, although there may be a correlation between the degree of toxicity and the extent of the effect. If the tumor is characterized by moderate sensitivity to the drug and the hemopoietic system is exhausted by the disease and previous radiation treatment, hemopoietic depression may occur when the dose is as yet insufficient to produce a therapeutic effect, and again there will be no correlation. In addition to these two main factors there may be many others, e. g., the stage of the disease, the age of the patient, or the individual characteristics of the organism. It goes without saying that, if all these differences are mixed together in one group of patients, as, for example, in non-responders, it will be impossible to deduce any general principles.

It would be ideal if we could produce complete regression of a tumor without any side effects. Although very rare, cases of this are observed when the tumor is highly sensitive (as, for instance, metastases of seminoma in lymph nodes are to sarcolysin) and the hemopoietic system of the given patient is stable. But at the present stage of cancer chemotherapy the tumors are in most cases moderately sensitive to certain drugs, and the maximum effect may be produced only by administering the maximum acceptable dose as determined by the extent of the side effects. Otherwise, when a smaller dose is used and the toxicity is lower, there is no assurance that the full possibilities of the drug will have been explored. The main correlations between the extent of the side effects and the therapeutic effect are set out in Table 3.

The work of BROSS (1965) is vitiated by the fact that the author summed up results obtained by various investigators with different agents.

The aforesaid data warrant the conclusion that *the principle of using the maximum acceptable dose and of determining it by "titration" according to the side effects was and still is the first principle of present-day chemotherapy.*

Table 3. *Correlation between Side Effects and Therapeutic Effects in the Chemotherapy of Cancer*

Therapeutic effect	Side effects	Notes
Complete	None or weak	Ideal of chemotherapy (so far exceptionally rarely achieved)
Considerable	Considerable, but within permissible limits	Maximum acceptable dose (MAD) used, tumor sensitive to the agent
None	Considerable, but within permissible limits	MAD used, tumor insensitive
Differing in extent	Very strongly pronounced (beyond permissible limits)	Overdosage or inadequate hemopoietic system
Incomplete	None or weak	Dose smaller than MAD used, no assurance that full possibilities of the agent were explored
None	None	No judgment can be passed because the dose may have been below that productive of an effect

At the same time, *there can be no doubt that the maximum acceptable dose should not be exceeded, and that everything must be done to avoid overdosing.* Exceeding the maximum acceptable dose not only directly harms the patient by virtue of the pronounced side effects; the correlation between the dose and the effect also changes, and in the end the effect may diminish, despite the increase in the dose. The resistance of the organism greatly diminishes and this may lead to an increase in the metastases and in the malignancy of the tumor. That is why, in systemic chemotherapy, both undertreatment and overtreatment must be avoided. The art of correct treatment is mastered only by experience, which once more emphasizes the necessity for oncologists to specialize not only in surgical and radiological methods of treatment but also in chemotherapy.

It is necessary to deal with these questions in detail because they are very important. A correct understanding of them is needed to produce the maximum therapeutic effect with the available drugs at the minimum risk to the patient, as well as to achieve success for clinical trials of new compounds.

Repetition and prolongation of treatment. In surgical treatment the first act, the operation, is for the most part also the last act. Repeated operation is far from being the rule. In radiation treatment, attempts are also made to utilize the entire range during the very first course. Repeated courses of treatment are administered mostly in cases of relapse in systemic forms. Preventive irradiation is very rarely carried out.

In chemotherapy, however, *the first course is only the beginning of contact with the patient.* With one course of treatment, even when the maximum acceptable dose is administered, we cannot expect to achieve complete remission of systemic disease or complete regression of solid tumors with destruction of all their cells. However, this is sometimes achieved by repeated courses and subsequent maintenance and preventive treatment.

The second important difference in the management of patients with chemotherapy is that the chemotherapist must never await a relapse but must initiate the second course in a "planned" manner a short time after even seemingly complete remission or regression of the tumor. The essential aim in chemotherapy, besides administration of an individually acceptable maximum dose, should be to institute repeated courses of treatment *before* relapses set in so as to influence the practically always persisting tumor cells.

Between the first and second course of treatment a month to a month and a half (or rarely two months) should be considered the maximum interval. Where 5-fluorouracil is used the interval must not exceed one month, and in cases of alkylating agents one to one and a half months, when the depression of hemopoiesis usually disappears. If there is complete regression of the tumor the total dose of the second course may be reduced to three-fourths that of the first. In complete regression of a solid tumor it is very important to administer a third course of treatment. If the regression is incomplete, long maintenance treatment may be resorted to, with increased intervals between the doses, but as far as possible with the same single dose (because the treatment may prove ineffective if the latter is also reduced).

The third distinctive feature of chemotherapy is the use of "preventive" courses which, despite the absence of symptoms, are administered once or twice a year with a total dose of 50—75 % of the maximum acceptable dose established in the first course.

Continous treatment with small doses for a long period of time may serve instead of periodical courses. This is Golton's method of treating chronic myeloid leukemia with myleran. HESSE and KAMPEN (1957) described a case of complete regression of lung cancer after daily oral administration of 15—20 mg of E. 39 for a period of 9 months (amounting to the very large total dose of 4 g). We succeeded in curing an inoperable case of cancer of the large intestine (adenocarcinoma) by oral administration of 10—15 mg of sarcolysin and 4—5 mg of colchamine (demecolcine) 3 times a week for 6 months. During this period the patient received 750 mg of sarcolysin and 360 mg of colchamine. There were hardly any side effects, and the patient has been clinically well for three years.

Cyclic treatment as used in acute leukemia, with alternating periods of methotrexate, mercaptopurine, and corticosteroid administration, is another variant of the method. The cycles are then repeated.

Thus *the second most important principle of chemotherapy is persistent treatment by repeated therapeutic and preventive courses or even continuously over a period of several months.*

Administration of the maximum acceptable dose and repeated or continuous treatment are directed toward achieving the final aim — destruction of all the tumor cells.

6. Regional Chemotherapy

General remarks. Regional chemotherapy administered in two variants — intracavitary and intravascular — is a definite step forward in methods of chemotherapy. Its importance may be understood if we compare the antitumor effect of irradiation of the whole organism with local radiotherapy. Modern achievements with local irradiation are absolutely impossible with total irradiation, since the dose that is lethal for the organism in general irradiation is but a fraction (about 10 %) of the therapeutic dose for a tumor.

In its selectivity of antitumor action chemotherapy immediately greatly surpassed radiotherapy. The effect of treating Hodgkin's disease, for example, with nitrogen mustard proved from the very outset comparable with the effect of radiotherapy, despite the fact that the drug was administered intravenously (i. e., analogously to total irradiation) and often under less favourable conditions as regards the stage of the disease and the patient's condition. Subsequently this greater selectivity was repeatedly confirmed; for example, the effect of systemic administration of sarcolysin or endoxan was found to be equal to that of local radiotherapy in metastases of seminoma, solitary and multiple myelomas, and reticulosarcomas.

But if the selectivity of the antitumor action of systemically administered drugs is greater than that of total radiotherapy, still greater selectivity may be expected from regional chemotherapy. This was first clearly shown in the administration of melphalan or sarcolysin by the perfusion method for melanomas of the extremities (CREECH et al., 1958; STEHLIN et al., 1959; TRAPEZNIKOV and AVDEEVA, 1964). Whereas systemic administration of sarcolysin practically fails to affect malignant melanoblastomas and their metastases, partial and even complete regression is observed in a large percentage of cases when sarcolysin is administered by perfusion.

Prolonged continuous intra-arterial infusion of drugs has another advantage: the influence of the drug may be exerted on the most sensitive phase of the vital cycle of the tumor cell (phase S or G_2 or mitosis), which occurs at different times in different cells.

However, the increase in selectivity (and effectiveness) of chemotherapeutic agents in regional as compared with systemic administration is not so great as it is in radiotherapy. Indeed, regional chemotherapy has a number of limitations. Even in isolated perfusion with extracorporeal circulation a loss of part of the drug is observed, the loss being particularly great in perfusion of the pelvis and internal organs. In intra-arterial infusion, especially without ligation or constriction of the veins, a considerable part of the drug enters the general circulation, while only the smaller part (though it is larger than in intravenous administration) is retained in the region of the tumor. Thus strictly regional chemotherapy is actually impossible. In isolated perfusion the second limiting factor is the comparatively short period of action of the agent (about one hour) and the difficulty of repeating the procedure frequently. To this we may add that increase in concentration of the drug in perfusion or infusion is limited by the possibility of injuring the vessel walls.

Regional chemotherapy undoubtedly enhances the possibilities of systemic chemotherapy, though not to the same extent as strictly directed many-field local radiotherapy exceeds the action of total irradiation in effect and selectivity.

The technique of *regional perfusion* was developed in 1957—1958 by CREECH, KREMENTZ, STEHLIN and their associates and is described in their works (CREECH et al., 1958; STEHLIN et al., 1959). Of prime importance is perfusion of the extremities for melanomas and sarcomas with melphalan, sarcolysin and, to a lesser extent, nitrogen mustard and other drugs. Summing up their use of perfusion at Tulane University

(505 perfusions in 441 patients) KREMENTZ and CREECH (1964) arrived at the conclusion that the greatest effect in perfusion of the extremities with alkylating agents is produced in melanomas and sarcomas. Long-term positive results are also achieved. Thus, four years after perfusion (sometimes supplemented by excision of the remains of the tumor) there was no relapse in six of the nine patients with primary melanomas, in 11 of the 30 patients with secondary nodes, and in five of the 14 patients with multiple skin metastases on the extremities. Perfusion as a supplement to the excision of sarcomas of the extremities resulted in the absence of relapses for four years in five of the six patients.

Positive results were also produced in individual patients by perfusion of the pelvis with the antibiotic streptonigrin for tumors of the urinary bladder and the cervix uteri (HURLEY, 1964). Attempts at using the perfusion technique were also made for the treatment of tumors of other sites. Although the perfusion method holds out few prospects for further development, it can and should be used when certain indications exist.

Prolonged intra-arterial infusion with antitumor drugs has been developed since 1959, mainly by SULLIVAN et al. (1959, 1960, 1963, 1965), KISKEN et al. (1962), GOLOMB et al. (1964), and others. This method has achieved considerable results. Radio-opaque polyethylene catheters are used and fluoroscopic control is practised. The catheter is inserted into the femoral or other arteries and pushed into the internal iliac, superior mesenteric, splenic, hepatic, or renal arteries. It may also be introduced into the subclavian, carotid, internal mammary, bronchial, and other arteries.

With special apparatus, an infusion may be administered by the drip method continuously for a period of several days or weeks, not only to patients in hospitals but also to ambulant patients. A portable clock-driven chronometric infusion pump has been designed for the latter so that they can carry it along while working (WATKINS, 1963). Infusion may also be administered in fractional doses.

Methotrexate, 5-fluorouracil, 5-fluorodesoxyuridine, sarcolysin, streptonigrin, vincristine, and other agents have been used for prolonged continuous infusion. Intra-arterial infusion has been administered with some effect for various tumors, in particular: tumors of the head and neck (methotrexate — SULLIVAN, 1959; fluorouracil — FRECKMAN, 1963) carcinoma of the cervix uteri (methotrexate — SULLIVAN, 1959), liver metastases of carcinoma of the stomach and large intestine (fluorouracil and FUDR — SULLIVAN, 1965), breast cancer (sarcolysin — COSTACHEL, personal communication; streptonigrin — SULLIVAN, 1963), tumors of the tongue and jaws (sarcolysin — KAZANSKY, 1965; BRONSTEIN and KHODZHAEV, 1964); fluorouracil — JOHNSON et al., 1962), cancer of the urinary bladder (fluorouracil), hypernephroma relapses (fluorouracil — FRECKMAN, 1963), and tumors of the brain (vincristine — OWENS et al., 1964).

Prolonged intra-arterial infusion may sometimes prove effective when general chemotherapy does not, for example in liver metastases of cancer of the stomach and large intestine (SULLIVAN et al., 1965). The scope of this article does not make it possible to consider the indications for intra-arterial infusion of particular compounds, especially since they are still in the stage of investigation. It cannot be doubted, however, that the method of treating malignant tumors by prolonged intra-arterial infusion of drugs holds out great prospects and deserves intensive study.

7. Combined Chemotherapy

Several chemotherapeutic agents may be administered simultaneously (combined therapy proper) or successively, when one agent is replaced by another at the end of a course or in a relapse to avoid drug resistance. Simultaneous administration of two or more agents aims at utilizing compounds with different mechanisms of action and is justified if the effect produced by (usually reduced) doses of the agents exceeds the sum of effects of each of the agents used or the effect of one of the agents administered in its full dose. Such a combination is of clinical value if the toxic effect of the combination does not exceed that of their sum. But the purely additive effect of two compounds administered in reduced doses is also of clinical value if the toxicity is lower than when a full dose of one (or both) of the components is used. It is clear that these conditions are not easy to observe and it is very difficult to study them clinically since it is necessary to have several groups of patients.

In experimental studies combinations of drugs have been found to exist in which an additive therapeutic effect is accompanied by reduced toxicity. Potentiation of the therapeutic effect without increased toxicity has also been shown to occur (GOLDIN and MANTEL, 1952; BURCHENAL, 1964 a; SOROKINA, 1957).

During the first decade of cancer chemotherapy the combination of several agents was rarely attempted in clinical practice. An exception was the successive administration of antifolic compounds, mercaptopurine, and corticosteroids in acute leukemia. Today a number of combinations of compounds are used. It may be regarded as established that repeated administration of the three compounds mentioned in succession produces the highest percentage of complete 5-year remissions in acute leukemia (BURCHENAL, 1964 a). Vincristine has now been added to these three. FREIREICH et al. (1964) have tested a combination of all the four substances. Mercaptopurine and prednisone were administered daily, methotrexate once in four days, and vincristine once a week. An immediate complete hematological and clinical remission was produced in 14 out of 16 patients. Good results were also produced with this combination by KARON et al. (1966), not only in acute leukemia but also in the blastic phase of adult chronic myeloid leukemia. In combined chemotherapy of acute leukemia, HANANIAN et al. (1965) used, in addition to these agents, endoxan and BCNU (1,3-bis(2-chloroethyl)-1-nitrosourea) and produced a large percentage of prolonged remissions. BOIRON et al. (1965) made successful use of a combination of mercaptopurine and methyl-GAG (methylglyoxal-bis-guanylhydrazone).

The effectiveness of chemotherapy for choriocarcinoma was first established by administration of methotrexate (HERTZ et al., 1958). Complete regression of metastatic tumors and disappearance of chorionic gonadotropins in the urine was achieved in about 25 % of patients. In 1960 it was discovered that choriocarcinoma was sensitive to vinblastine (HERTZ et al., 1960); later it was found that it was also sensitive to actinomycin D (HERTZ et al., 1961) and to its variant chrysomalline (AINBINDER et al., 1964). It was shown that combined administration of methotrexate and actinomycin D or chrysomalline produced regression not only of the lung metastases but also of the primary tumor in the uterus. It now became possible to treat choriocarcinoma without surgical intervention.

The combination of methotrexate, actinomycin D, and chlorambucil is also apparently of established value (LI, 1961).

A combination of hormonal substances — androgens (or estrogens) — and thiotepa is often used in breast cancer. GREENSPAN (1964) used a combination of androgen, thiotepa, and methotrexate and brought about regression of cutaneous, subcutaneous, and pulmonary cancers in three-fourths of his patients. BRULÉ (1955) recently reported that a combination of fluorouracil and methylhydrazine was effective in lung cancer.

The scope of this article forbids enumeration of all the combinations of agents now in use. Combined chemotherapy may, however, it can be said, produce much greater effects than individual compounds and, what is more, without essentially increasing the toxicity. The trend towards greater use of combinations of drugs deserves the encouragement it is now receiving.

8. Combination of Chemotherapy and Radiotherapy

The relations between chemotherapy and radiotherapy were for a long time unhappy. During its first ten years drug treatment (not counting hormone therapy) was used mainly for Hodgkin's disease and the leukemias. The first chemotherapeutic agent, nitrogen mustard, and its derivatives were first tested on patients on whom the resources of radiotherapy had already been exhausted, the disease was generalized, and the hemopoietic system was depressed both by the disease itself and by repeated exposure to ionizing radiation. Although a dramatic effect was observed in individual patients even under these conditions, for obvious reasons it was always short-lived and failed to prolong life. For this reason, radiotherapists who had formerly enjoyed a monopoly in the treatment of Hodgkin's disease came to the opinion that chemotherapy produced only a temporary effect and could not be used in the early stages, in which radiotherapy could achieve prolonged remission. Hodgkin's disease consequently continued, as before, to be treated either only by radiation (as it is still in specialized radiological and other institutions) or by chemotherapy after the possibilities of radiation treatment had been exhausted.

In the meantime it was demonstrated that the drug treatment of Hodgkin's disease, if instituted at an early stage (without radiation treatment) and with a rational technique, produced even better long-term results (LARIONOV and ZIV, 1958). In my opinion, however, if properly combined, the two methods produce still better results. The treatment should be begun with chemotherapy and radiotherapy should be administered in addition, if necessary, to unresolved nodes or their remains. In this case fewer fields of irradiation and a smaller total dose are usually required, so that smaller areas of bone marrow are irreversibly changed. As a result, it is almost always possible to repeat the drugs with sufficiently large doses and to combine the two methods again.

A tempting prospect is to enhance the effectiveness of treatment by potentiation. The first positive result of this kind was described when synkavit (synthetic vitamin K) was reported to enhance the effect of radiation treatment of lung cancer (MITCHELL, 1954). The enhancement, however, proved to be insignificant.

Subsequently radiation was shown to be potentiated by the halogenated pyrimidines, 5-iodo- and 5-fluorouracil. Several papers have appeared asserting that 5-fluorouracil in a somewhat smaller than maximum dose enhances the effect produced by ionizing radiation administered in one-half or one-third of the regular dose, with the result that a similar or greater effect is produced than by radiation treatment alone (FOYE et al., 1960; ALLAIRE et al., 1961; and others). Enhancement of the effect of ionizing radiation by fluorouracil was observed in tumors where fluorouracil alone is ineffective, for example in epidermoid carcinoma of the lungs and the esophagus.

In a strictly controlled study, however, DEDERICK (1964) failed to enhance the effect of radiation in the treatment of tumors with 5-fluorouracil when using the full radiation dose. However, this result may have been due to the fact that fluorouracil, although administered for the long period of five weeks, was apparently given in a subthreshold dose — 5 mg/kg. It is known that the effectiveness of fluorouracil diminishes sharply when the optimum dose is reduced. This is also attested to by the diminished effectiveness of 5-fluorouracil when infused intravenously by the drip method. If, however, the addition of fluorouracil can make one-third or one-half of the therapeutic dose of ionizing radiation equal to the full dose with a diminution in toxic side effects, it is worth while using it.

First noticed on the skin, the potentiation of ionizing radiation has also been established for actinomycin D. According to FARBER (1961), by combining actinomycin D with radiation for metastases of Wilm's tumor in the lungs, it is possible to produce immediate and long-term results not achievable when only one form of treatment is used.

The possibilities of potentiating radiation treatment by other chemical substances are still being investigated. The problem of the combination of chemotherapy with radiation treatment is important and its study may yet yield new results.

9. Combination of Chemotherapy and Surgery

Chemotherapy may be combined with surgery by various methods. It may be used pre-operatively, in the same way as pre-operative radiotherapy. Attempts are made, for example, by chemotherapy to reduce the size and increase the mobility of inoperable tumors or get rid of ascites, in order to make operation feasible. This has in fact proved possible in a number of cases, for example, in pre-operative chemotherapy of large sarcomas (by means of alkylating agents) and cancer of the ovaries (thiotepa, etc.). In this case chemotherapy acts as surgery's helper by increasing the indications for it and making surgical intervention a more promising prospect.

Sometimes the roles may change, surgery becoming the helper of chemotherapy, as, for example, when the operation removes the larger part of the tumors, their size sharply diminishes, and subsequent chemotherapy becomes more effective. This is observed in cancer of the ovaries when it becomes evident during the operation that it is impossible to remove all of the tumor masses radically. Whereas before the introduction of chemotherapy partial removal was considered irrational, now the situation has changed; if the tumor is sensitive to antitumor agents, non-radical operations are carried out.

It may be noted that little change in the opinion of surgeons has as yet occurred. If inoperable metastases in lymph nodes are discovered before or at the beginning of an operation (for example, for cancer of the lungs, esophagus, or stomach), no resection is usually made. And yet in such cases chemotherapy can produce a regression of these metastases, which are reasonably sensitive to some alkylating agents.

In some cases chemotherapy combined with surgery may permit a minor ("sparing") operation without removing the entire organ. Thus, for example, according to KREMENTZ and CREECH (1964) a sparing excision of sarcomas of the extremities followed by perfusion with melphalan resulted in clinical cure in five out of six patients observed over a period of four years.

The succession of methods of treatment may also be reversed, i. e., a sparing surgical operation may supplement chemotherapy, for example after perfusion of the extremities with sarcolysin for malignant melanomas (KREMENTZ and CREECH, 1964, TRAPEZNIKOV et al., 1964).

A form of combining the two methods on which many hopes were pinned was chemotherapy following radical operation. Experiments on animals show good results when surgical removal of tumors is combined with chemotherapy (DRUCKREY et al., 1958; BROCK, 1959; MOLKOV, 1960; and others). However, it cannot as yet be considered definitely established clinically that postoperative chemotherapy produces useful results in preventing local relapses and late metastases, although there are some observations to that effect.

Extensive co-operative studies of postoperative chemotherapy were undertaken in the USA in 1958 with regard to the following tumors and agents: cancer of the lung (nitrogen mustard), cancer of the stomach (thiotepa), cancer of the colon and the rectum (thiotepa), breast cancer (thiotepa), and ovarian carcinoma (chlorambucil). These studies were very well organized as regards the number of patients and their selection according to prognostic categories, their division into groups (by the "blind" system), the administration of placebos, and the thorough statistical treatment of the material. Regrettably, several defects are discernable in the studies from the point of view of chemotherapy. First, it is hardly possible to expect results from the postoperative administration of thiotepa in carcinoma of the stomach and intestine, which is practically insensitive to this compound. True, at that time 5-fluorouracil, which is almost the only agent so far producing any effect on cancer of the gastrointestinal tract, was not available.

Second, the agents were administered only on the day of the operation and for the next two or three days. During this period, owing to the possibility of increasing postoperative complications, only a small dose of the agent could be administered. Thus the dose of thiotepa administered for cancer of the breast, stomach, and large intestine was in all 0.8 mg/kg, i. e., an average of 50 mg per patient. This is only 20—25 % of the average therapeutic dose for one course. It is difficult to expect a real effect from such a dose.

Third, no drugs were administered after the end of the postoperative period, although, a month or two after the operation, full doses of the agent could have been administered as repeated courses. One-fourth of the dose can hardly be expected to destroy both the cancer cells in the blood and those remaining in the parts of the organ not removed and in nodes appearing clinically to be unaffected.

Under these conditions, it is not surprising that the studies, though extensive, produced generally negative results. It is interesting that where the agent used was the most suitable for the given tumor a positive result was obtained, despite the very small doses. This was the case for thiotepa after operations for breast cancer. According to the report of the Roswell Park Institute, Buffalo, a year after operation premenopausal patients with more than three enlarged lymph nodes relapsed in

67 % of the cases in the control group and in 37 % only in the group receiving thiotepa. The average interval between operation and relapse increased from 13 to 22 months. These differences were statistically significant. Within 30 and 54 months the difference in the proportion of relapses was less.

It is probable that repeated courses of thiotepa would have enhanced the effect produced. This conclusion may be drawn not only as a presumption but also on the basis of co-operative studies organized by Austrian scientists (DENK et al., 1961). In this work first nitromin (mitomen) and then endoxan were used after operations for lung cancer. The number of patients surviving the operation served as a criterion of the effect. At the beginning of the studies the agents were administered only over a period of one year (two courses) after the postoperative period. The difference between the groups of patients to whom nitromin was or was not administered was small and in the second year disappeared. But when four courses of treatment with this compound were administered annually over a period of two years the difference became more noticeable and persisted for two more years. Of the patients who had received chemotherapy 50 % more survived than did among those who had not received it. This is the more significant since, firstly, the long-term results of surgical treatment of lung cancer are still poor and, secondly, not one of the existing agents, nitromin and endoxan included, is very effective in lung cancer — at best it may produce no more than partial regression of its metastases.

Thus the frequently expressed opinion that postoperative chemotherapy is ineffective is unfounded. On the contrary, the available data attest the possibility of producing successful results and indicate the necessity of continuing intensive studies on postoperative chemotherapy. Due regard must, however, be paid to the methodological errors committed in the past and appropriate consideration must be taken of the progress made in the arsenal of chemotherapeutic agents, of the spectrum of their action, and of the effectiveness of their use in combination.

10. Role and Position of Chemotherapy in Modern Methods of Cancer Treatment

We sometimes hear or read that today cancer chemotherapy is of no value by itself but is merely an "adjunct" to "radical" methods, i. e., to surgical and radiation treatment. This opinion is entirely mistaken and is mostly based on inadequate knowledge of the present situation and particularly of the results of the chemotherapy of malignant tumors. Thus the layman thinks that cancer generally is incurable, since he remembers that doctors refused to operate on either relative or friend because of advanced disease, or did operate on him but he died immediately after the operation or a little later as a result of a relapse. Moreover, the layman does not know and has never seen patients cured by a timely operation. Surgeons or radiotherapists, if they are not working in an institution where chemotherapy is administered in suitable conditions and are not in contact with patients greatly improved and even cured by drugs, also think that chemotherapy is ineffective. This is a misconception.

As an example, for neoplastic diseases of the hemopoietic system surgical treatment cannot, with but few exceptions, be used and radiotherapy not infrequently is of little effect. And yet, in acute leukemia, which invariably used to end fatally within several weeks or months, it is now possible by means of chemotherapy to produce complete clinical and hematological remission in a large percentage of patients and in some (not many as yet) a clinical cure for five years and longer. As new agents go on being introduced and methods of administration improve, the percentage and duration of remissions are increasing and will continue to increase. The chemotherapy of chronic myeloid leukemia produces better results than radiotherapy, and in Hodgkin's disease it may under equal conditions produce at least as good results. In multiple myeloma and erythremia radiation treatment does not produce such good results as chemotherapy; in a number of cases of the former disease drugs lead to amazing repair of bone.

In the field of cancer of the female genital tract, the treatment of cancer of the ovaries today is unthinkable without chemotherapy and, although it is usually combined with surgery, there is difficulty in deciding which of the two methods is more important. Without doubt, in the treatment of cancer of the ovaries long-term results — with three to five years of survival — can now be achieved by chemotherapy.

In chorionepithelioma most patients until very recently died of metastases in the lungs, despite the removal of the uterus and its adnexa. At first about one-fourth of these patients began to be saved by methotrexate therapy when combined with removal of the primary tumor. Then the percentage increased and of late, owing to combined chemotherapy (methotrexate, actinomycin D, vinblastine), it has been possible to produce regression of the primary tumor. A conference held in Manila in February 1965 arrived at the conclusion that it is not only possible to do without operation for primary chorionepithelioma of the uterus, but that in some cases an operation does not have to be performed at all because it is possible to save the uterus. Cases of normal births given by such cured women have been described. Can we say then that chemotherapy is only an adjunct of surgery?

It has also become possible to cure patients who have seminoma metastases with sarcolysin. At any rate, the effect of the treatment is not inferior to that of the most modern radiotherapy.

As regards breast cancer, in which surgical and radiation treatment is often insufficiently effective, hormone treatment and chemotherapy are the last resort for women who have developed local relapses and regional and distant metastases after surgery and radiation. And yet, in conditions more difficult than at the beginning of the disease, many lives are prolonged by means of drug treatment.

In the initial stage cancer of the skin can be cured with colchamine ointment just as well as with close-focus X-ray therapy.

It may be argued that, while all this is true, it is not so for the most frequent and important tumors, for example cancer of the lung, stomach, and esophagus. Chemotherapy can indeed as yet do very little in these cases. But then surgical treatment, which is administered to only a small number of these patients who have been diagnosed early, cures no more than 10—20 % of the patients seeking assistance. Thus there is nothing to boast of in surgery. And has anybody ever treated these forms of cancer in their early stages with drugs? The answer is no. Chemotherapists deal with patients who have been denied operation because of the advanced stage of their disease, or they attempt to prolong the life of patients after unsuccessful operation. Even in these much more difficult conditions it is sometimes possible to achieve results by chemotherapy.

By way of example, at the Institute of Experimental and Clinical Oncology of the USSR Academy of Medical Sciences an objective effect was produced with 5-fluorouracil in 50% of patients with stomach cancer at a very advanced stage (including relapses after surgical treatment) and in some cases the roentgenological picture became normal, the mucosal pattern returned, and peristalsis reappeared (BLOKHINA, 1965). Can we consider chemotherapy an adjunct of surgery if surgical methods successfully treat about one-tenth of stomach cancer patients, while chemotherapy can help (even if not appreciably as yet) the other nine-tenths, whether operated on or not?

Chemotherapy has clearly demonstrated its value as a new method of treating malignant tumors, since it can help in some cases, equal the two older methods in other cases, and, when the first two methods cannot be used or fail, replace them or produce some results.

11. Prospects for Cancer Chemotherapy

It may be assumed that surgery as a method of treating malignant tumors has already done about all it can do, that it is reaching the limit of its usefulness. Further progress depends on achievements in other branches of biology and medicine — on, for example, the solution of the problem of organ transplantation. As for radiation treatment of cancer, although progress is still possible it is limited by the fact that the radiotherapist always uses different variations of the one agent, with the same or a related mechanism of action.

Chemotherapy, on the other hand, is already using extremely diverse substances with absolutely different mechanisms of action, although it has been in use for only one-third of the time that radiotherapy has (20 years as against 60). Its main achievements still lie before it.

In fact, unlike the other two methods, there are no limits to the development of chemotherapy. As the biochemical differences between tumor cells and normal cells and the biochemical characteristics of the cells of different tumors are studied, we shall gain an increasingly deeper insight into them and they will suggest new ideas for developing antitumor agents. Again, chemical synthesis will also continuously improve, and it will be possible to synthesize new substances of an assigned structure and with the properties desired. The empirical search for antitumor substances, for example, so-called antibotics, may also continue indefinitely even after exhausting all the producers, in particular by artificial modification of their products by the addition of various ingredients to their nutrient media.

Thus there are no limits to the development of new antitumor agents, which will continue to appear indefinitely. There can be no doubt that, as new agents are developed, their selective antitumor activity will increase and they will be increasingly more adapted to curing specific tumors. The methods of administering drugs, as well as the different combinations of various compounds with each other and with surgical and radiation methods, will also improve.

References

AINBINDER, N. M., V. M. DILMAN, E. P. MUKHINA, I. D. NECHAEVA, and J. M. SHARKOVA: The use of the antibiotic 2703 in six cases of chorionepithelioma of the uterus. Vop. onkol. 10 (5), 103 (1964).

ALLAIRE, F. J., E. T. THIEME, and D. R. KORST: Cancer chemotherapy with 5-fluorouracil alone and in combination with X-ray therapy. Cancer Chemother. Rep. **14**, 59 (1961).

BLOKHINA, N. G.: The use of 5-fluorouracil in cancer patients. Vop. onkol. **10**, (11), 62 (1964).

— The treatment of cancer of the gastrointestinal tract by 5-fluorouracil. Diss. Moscow, 1965.

BOIRON, M., C. JACQUILLAT, M. WEIL, and J. BERNARD: Combination of methylglyoxal bis (guanylhydrazone) (NSC-32946) and 6-mercaptopurine in acute granulocytic leukemia. Cancer Chemother. Rep. **45**, 69 (1965).

BROCK, N.: Neue experimentelle Ergebnisse mit N-Lost-Phosphamidestern. Strahlentherapie **41**, 347 (1959).

BRONSTEIN, B. L., and V. G. KHODZHAEV: Regional intra-arterial chemotherapy in cancer of the maxillofacial area. Vop. onkol. **10** (4), 8 (1964).

BROSS, I. D. J.: Is toxicity necessary? Proc. Amer. Ass. Cancer Res. **6**, 8 (1965).

BRULÉ, G., J. R. SCHLUMBERGER, and C. GRISCELLI: N-isopropyl-α-2(-methyl-hydrazino)-p-toluamide hydrochloride in treatment of solid tumors. Cancer Chemother. Rep. **44**, 31 (1965).

BURCHENAL, J. H.: Recent advances and perspectives in the chemotherapy of acute leukemia. Fifth National Cancer Conference: Philadelphia, 1964 a.

— Improvement of cancer chemotherapy in man. Multiple drug therapy. Acta Un. int. Cancr. **20**, 48 (1964 b).

CHEBOTAREVA, L. I.: Long-term results in treatment of testicular seminoma with sarcolysin. In 8th International Cancer Congress: Moscow, Medgiz, 346 (1962); Acta Un. Int. Cancr. **20**, 380 (1964).

CREECH, O. jr., E. T. KREMENTZ, R. F. RYAN, and J. N. WINBLAD: Chemotherapy of cancer: regional perfusion utilizing an extracorporeal circuit. Ann. Surg. **148**, 616 (1958).

DAVIS, W., and L. F. LARIONOV: Progress in chemotherapy of cancer. Bull. Wld Hlth Org. **30**, 327 (1964).

DEDERICK, M. M.: Effect of actinomycin D and 5-fluorouracil in combination with X-ray in carcinoma of the lung. Proc. Amer. Ass. Cancer Res. **5**, 14 (1964).

DENK, W., K. KARRER, and P. WURNIG: Ueber den Wert und die Risiken einer postoperativen Chemotherapie maligner Tumoren. Arzneimittel-Forsch. **11** (2a), 233 (1961).

DRUCKREY, H.: Pharmacological tests in cancer chemotherapy. Acta Un. int. Cancr. **15** *bis*, 85 (1959).

—, B. T. KUK, D. SCHMAHL, and D. STEINHOFF: Kombination von Operation und Chemotherapie beim Krebs. Münch. med. Wschr. **100**, 1913 (1958).

EMMANUEL, N. M., L. M. DRONOVA, I. P. KONOVALOVA, Z. K. MAIZUS, and I. P. SKIBIDA: Antileukemic action of 2,6-di (tert.) butyl-4-methylchinol (Ionol Dokl). Akad. Nauk SSSR. Otd. Biokh. **152**, 481 (1963).

—, and L. P. LIPCHINA: Anti-tumor activity and the mechanism of action of radical reaction inhibitors. In 8th International Cancer Congress: Moscow, Medgiz, (1962); Acta Un. int. Cancr. **20** (1-2), 103 (1964).

FARBER, S.: Current clinical and experimental studies in cancer chemotherapy. Cancer Chemother. Rep. **13**, 154 (1961).

—, L. K. DIAMOND, R. D. MARKER, R. F. SYLVESTER, and J. A. WOLFF: Temporary remission in the acute leukemia in children produced by folic acid antagonist, 4-aminopteroyl-glutamic acid (aminopterin). New Engl. J. Med. **238**, 787 (1948).

FOYE, L. V. jr., F. M. WILLETT, B. HALL, and M. ROTH: The potentation of radiation effect with 5-fluorouracil. Cancer Chemother. Rep. **6**, 12 (1960).

FRANK, W., and A. R. OSTERBERG: Mitomicin C — an evaluation of the Japanese reports. Cancer Chemother. Rep. **9**, 144 (1960).

FRECKMAN, H. A.: Cancer chemotherapy: continuous intraarterial infusion. Cancer Chemother. Rep. **28**, 57 (1963).

FREIREICH, E. J., M. KARON, and E. FREI: Quadruple combination therapy (VAMP) for acute lymphocytic leukemia of childhood. Proc. Amer. Ass. Cancer Res. **5**, 20 (1964).

GILMAN, A., and F. S. PHILIPS: The biological actions and therapeutic applications of the β-chloroethyl-amines and sulfides. Science, **103**, 2675, 409 (1946).

GOLDIN, A., and N. MANTEL: The employment of combinations of drugs in the chemotherapy of neoplasia. Cancer. Res. **17**, 635 (1952).

GOLOMB, F. M., B. P. SAMMONS, and J. C. WRIGHT: A new technique of visceral artery catheterization for infusion cancer chemotherapy. Proc. Amer. Ass. Cancer Res. 5, 22 (1964).

GOODMAN, L. S., M. L. WINTROBE, N. DAMESHEK, M. I. GOODMAN, A. GILMAN, and M. T. McLENNAN: Nitrogen mustard therapy. Use of methyl-bis-(β-chloroethyl)-amine hydrochloride and tris-(β-chloroethyl)-amine hydrochloride for Hodgkin's disease, lymphosarcoma, leukemia and certain allied and miscellaneous diseases. Amer. Med. Ass. 132, 126 (1946).

GREENSPAN, E. M.: Combinations of methotrexate, thio-tepa and 5-fluorouracil in advanced breast carcinoma. Proc. Amer. Ass. Cancer Res. 5, 23 (1964).

HANANIAN, J., J. F. HOLLAND, and P. SHECHE: Intensive chemotherapy of acute lymphocytic leukemia in children. Proc. Amer. Ass. Cancer Res. 6, 26 (1965).

HARRIS, M. N., T. MEDREK, F. M. GOLOMB, S. L. GUMPORT, A. H. POSTEL, and J. C. WRIGHT: Chemotherapy with streptonigrin in advanced cancer. Proc. Amer. Ass. Cancer Res. 5, 25 (1964).

HERTZ, R., D. M. BERGENSTAL, M. B. LIPSETT, E. B. PRICE, and T. F. HILLEBISH: Chemotherapy of choriocarcinoma and related trophoblastic tumors in women. J. Amer. med. Ass. 168, 845 (1958).

—, J. L. LEWIS jr., and M. B. LIPSETT: Five years experience with chemotherapy of metastatic choriocarcinoma and related trophoblastic disease in women. Proc. Amer. Ass. Cancer Res. 3, 235 (1961).

—, and M. C. LI: Cited by Cancer Chemotherapy Abstr. 5, 73 (1964).

—, M. B. LIPSETT, and R. H. MOY: Effect of vincaleukoblastine on metastatic choriocarcinoma. Cancer Res. 20, 1050 (1960).

HESSE, F., and G. KAMPEN: Orale Dauermedikation von Bayer E-39. Krebsarzt 12, 150 (1957).

HUGGINS, C., and C. V. HODGES: The effect of castration, of oestrogen and androgen injection on serum phosphatases in metastatic carcinoma of the prostate. Cancer Res. 1, 293 (1941).

HURLEY, J. D.: Perfusion therapy with streptonigrin. Proc. Amer. Ass. Cancer Res. 5, 29 (1964).

IVANOVA, Ye. M.: Direct and long-term results of treatment of Hodgkin's disease with Dopan. In 8th International Cancer Congress: Moscow, Medgiz, 345 (1962); Acta Un. Int. Cancr. 20, 375 (1964).

JOHNSON, R. O., W. A. KISKEN, and A. R. CURRERI: The response of squamous cell carcinoma to intra-arterial infusion with 5-fluorouracil. Cancer Chemother. Rep. 24, 29 (1962).

JONES, A. C.: Thio-tepa in the treatment of tumours of the bladder. Lancet, 2, 615 (1961).

KARON, M., S. FREIREICH, and P. CARBONE: Effective combination therapy of adult leukemia. Proc. Amer. Ass. Cancer Res. 6, 34 (1966).

KARRER, K.: Zur kombinierten cytostatischen und operativen Behandlung des Carcinoms. Arzneimittel-Forsch. 14, 859 (1964).

KAZANSKY, D. A.: Regional chemotherapy of maxillary, lingual and pharyngeal tumors by the method of carotid perfusion and infusion. Vop. onkol. 11, 42 (1965).

KISKEN, W. A., R. O. JOHNSON, and A. R. CURRERI: A technique of intra-arterial infusion. Cancer chemotherapy Rep. 24, 27 (1962).

KREMENTZ, E. T., and O. CREECH jr.: Current evaluation of cancer chemotherapy by perfusion. Proc. Amer. Ass. Cancer Res. 5, 37 (1964).

LARIONOV, L. F.: Immediate and remote results of chloroethylamine treatment of Hodgkin's disease. Brit. med. J. 1, 252 (1956).

— Cancer chemotherapy, Moscow: Medgiz 1962 (English edition. London: Pergamon Press 1965).

— Ten years of experimental and clinical study and use of sarcolysin. Moscow: Medexport 1965.

—, and M. A. CHUDAKOVA: The treatment of esophageal carcinoma by sarcolysin with colchamine. Vop. onkol. 9 (12), 3 (1963).

—, and M. A. ZIV: Late results of chemotherapy of Hodgkin's disease. Vop. onkol. 4 (2), 161 (1958).

LI, M. Ch.: Management of choriocarcinoma and related tumors of uterus and testis. Med. Clin. N. Amer. 45, 661 (1961).

Merkulova, N. V.: Treatment of multiple myeloma with sarcolysin. In 8th International Cancer Congress, Moscow: Medgiz, 347 (1962); Acta Un. int. Cancr. 20, 389 (1964).
— Treatment of multiple myeloma with sarcolysin. Vop. onkol. 10 (3), 51 (1964).
Mitchell, J. S.: Clinical trials of tetrasodium 2-methyl-1:4-naphthohydroquinone diphosphate as a radiosensitiser. A. R. Brit. Emp. Cancer Campgn 34, 274 (1954).
Molkov, Yu. N.: Prevention by aurantin of recurrence and metastases after surgical removal of transplantable tumors. Vop. onkol. 6 (9), 19 (1960).
Movsesyan, A. Kh. Cited by Vermel, E. M.: The next tasks of cancer chemotherapy. Vop. onkol. 11 (6), 115 (1965).
Owens, G., R. Javid, and L. Belmusto: Intraarterial vincristine therapy of primary gliomas. Proc. Amer. Ass. Cancer Res. 5, 49 (1964).
Paterson, E., A. Haddow, J. A. Thomas, and J. M. Watkinson: Leukaemia treated with urethane combined with deep X-ray therapy. Lancet, 1, 677 (1946).
Perevodchikova, N. I.: The use of chloroethylamines in the oncological clinic. Inaugur. Diss.: Moscow (1965).
Rhoads, C. P.: Nitrogen mustard in the treatment of neoplastic diseases. J. Amer. med. Ass. 131, 656 (1946).
Sorokina, I. B.: The study of combined action of 6-mercaptopurine with some other drugs of chloroethylamino group on transplantable mouse tumors. Vop. Onkol. 3 (6), 683 (1957).
Stehlin, J. S. jr., R. L. Clark, E. C. White, and J. L. Smith: Adjuvant regional chemotherapy (perfusion) for malignant melanoma. Amer. Surg. 25, 595 (1959).
Sullivan, R. D., E. Miller, and M. P. Sykes: Antimetabolite-metabolite combination cancer chemotherapy: effects of intra-arterial methotrexate-intramuscular citrovorum factor therapy in human cancer. Cancer, 12, 1248 (1959).
—, C. W. Yung, E. Miller, N. Gladstein, B. Clarkson, and J. H. Burchenal: The clinical effect of the continuous administration of fluorinated pyrimidines. Cancer Chemother. Rep. 8, 77 (1960).
—, E. Miller, W. Z. Zurek, and F. R. Rodrigues: Clinical effects of prolonged infusion of streptonigrin (NSC-45383) in advanced cancer. Cancer Chemother. Rep. 33, 27 (1963).
—, E. Watkinson jr., W. Z. Zurek, and A. M. Kazei: Chemotherapy of liver cancer by prolonged ambulatory hepatic artery infusion. Proc. Amer. Ass. Cancer Res. 6, 63 (1965).
Trapeznikov, N. N., and I. A. Avdeeva: Preliminary data in regional chemotherapy of malignant tumors of the extremities by perfusion. In 8th International Cancer Congress, Moscow: Medgiz, 350 (1962); Acta Un. Int. Cancr. 20, 462 (1964).
Watkins, E. jr.: Chronometric infusor — an apparatus for protracted ambulatory infusion therapy. New Engl. J. Med. 269, 850 (1963).
Wright, J. C., F. M. Golomb, and S. Gumport: Summary of results with triethylene thiophosphoramide. Ann. N. Y. Acad. Sci. 68, 937 (1958).

Progress in Radiotherapy

M. Tubiana and D. Chassagne

Progress in radiotherapy over the past twenty years seems to be the most important factor in the overall improvement of results in the treatment of cancer. The progress has been both technical and in methods of treatment and these aspects will be analysed before considering the results in some forms of cancer. Finally, an attempt will be made to define the factors which appear to prevent further progress in radiotherapy.

Technical Progress

1. High-Energy Radiation

Conventional radiotherapy alone was used in cancer treatment before 1950. New apparatus has since then facilitated the use of high-energy radiation in radiotherapy. The relative biological efficiency (RBE) of high-energy photons with respect to conventional X-rays has been extensively studied and there is general agreement on a value of 0.85 (SINCLAIR, 1962). High-energy radiations have numerous advantages over conventional X-rays because of their physical properties, which have been intensively investigated (TUBIANA *et al.*, 1963). We summarize them briefly.

1. The attenuation of the high-energy beam in the tissues is low, thus the depth dose is superior to that of conventional X-rays. In the case of deeply seated tumors, the dose of radiation received by the tissues lying between the skin and the tumor is for this reason less in comparison with lower-energy X-rays, and the irradiation of healthy tissues surrounding the tumor is the factor limiting the dose that can be delivered to the tumor.

2. The skin dose is much lower than the dose received with conventional X-rays because, contrary to the last case, the maximal dose occurs subcutaneously at some depth within the body. Even after high doses the skin remains in good condition and cutaneous reactions do not interfere with the treatment. In addition, the good condition of the skin at the end of treatment facilitates surgical intervention through irradiated tissues. Because of the frequent association of radiotherapy and surgery, this has considerable advantages.

3. Bone absorption is lower than with conventional X-rays. Bone absorption was previously important for two reasons. Firstly, overdosage in bone and cartilage predisposes to serious radiation damage; bone and cartilage radionecrosis was a formidable complication of radiotherapy for head and neck cancer. With high-energy radiations, overdosage of bone no longer occurs and the risk of necrosis has diminished. In addition bone no longer shields tissue which lies behind it and the irradiation of tumors in such situations is greatly facilitated.

4. In the interaction of X-rays with tissue, scatter occurs, producing secondary rays of lower energy and altered direction. This results in the edges of the beam becoming less well defined at depth; thus the tissues lying outside the geometrically defined limits receive doses that are far from negligible. Scatter occurs less with higher-energy X-rays, and it has therefore become possible to treat tumors in the immediate vicinity of essential structures that might be affected by the irradiation. In addition, the reduction of scatter at higher energies helps to reduce harmful radiation to peritumoral healthy tissue.

The reduced importance of scatter facilitates the use of shielding to adapt the isodose distribution to the target volume. This technique of beam shaping, to which we will return later, has become extremely important in the past few years from the point of view of sparing healthy tissue to the greatest possible degree.

Using multiple fields or rotation therapy, it has become possible to deliver any given dose to any point within the organism. However, not all machines allow full exploitation of all the possibilities of high-energy radiation.

2. The Apparatus

Progress in the field of equipment is associated with both rapid increase in the number of installations and improvement of the apparatus used. In 1955, there were 120 telecobalt units in the world. They increased to 1100 in 1961 and 1500 in 1963, by which time there was one cobalt unit per 0.5—1 million population in western countries. There were then about 100 cesium units, 137 telecobalt units, 80 betatrons,

45 linear accelerators, and 35 Van de Graaf machines in the world. In Europe, the USA, and Japan, most high-energy radiotherapy of cancer is carried out on tele-cobalt units.

At the same time, the apparatus has been improved. Considerable differences exist between the earlier machines and those recently constructed.

Telecobalt Units have many advantages over other machines generating high-energy photons: low maintenance costs, a simple monitoring system, and assured reproducibility of treatment conditions. They are also easy to handle and do not necessitate any special electrical installation. This is particularly important in countries where the constancy of the voltage and frequency of the electrical supply cannot be guaranteed. The presence of a penumbra is the main inconvenience of these units, since this affects, firstly, the dose outside the limits of the beam at depth and, secondly, the homogeneity of the dose on a plane perpendicular to the axis of the beam. If the dose falls off gradually at the edge of the beam, the fields used to deliver a homogeneous dose to a tumor will be several centimeters larger than the field that would suffice if the penumbra was less. To reduce the penumbra it is necessary to improve both the characteristics of the source and the collimator.

To improve the characteristics of cobalt-60, sources of small diameter (1 cm) and high specific activity (for example 100—200 curies/g) can now be obtained. The cost of the source increases proportionally to the specific activity but recent comparative economic studies show that the cost of treatment remains competitive (ELLIS and OLIVER, 1961; ASHTON and CHESTER, 1962; FARMER, 1962; KELLER, 1963). Small-volume sources with a high specific activity mean that patients can be treated at a source-skin distance (SSD) of the order of 70—80 cm. This results in improved depth dose (the depth dose increases by 12 % at a depth of 10 cm for a 10 × 10 cm field when the SSD is increased from 50 to 80 cm).

As regards the collimator, the geometrical penumbra is reduced as the source-collimator distance is increased. Thus an attempt is made to put the collimator as near the skin as possible. The older apparatus in which the source-collimator distance was variable and the collimator-skin distance constant is, however, impracticable. In addition, in rotation therapy a collimator-skin distance of 25 cm is advantageous. In this case, it is useful to have secondary diaphragms or penumbra trimmers of tungsten or uranium which are placed near the patient on a telescopic mounting attached to the collimator (FARMER, 1962).

Part of the beam traverses a thin part of the inner edge of the collimator and is attenuated slightly. This physical penumbra can be reduced by reducing the thickness of the collimator diaphragm, which can be achieved by using tungsten or uranium and by constructing the collimator so that the inner surface of the diaphragm always remains tangential to the edge of the beam, regardless of the field size. This means in effect placing the plates of the collimator on a sphere which has the source at its centre (JOHNS).

By these means, the penumbra can be reduced to a few millimeters and penumbra conditions obtained which are comparable to generators with point sources such as the linear accelerator.

Telecesium units cannot compete with the telecobalt units, in spite of the lower cost of cesium and the longer half life (30 years as compared with 5.6 years for cobalt-60). The physical factors are less favorable: the depth dose is less and the penumbra more obvious because of the large source size, and the skin-sparing effect is less marked. Cesium-137 can, however, be useful for irradiation at a short SSD and may be substituted for conventional radiotherapy installations.

The betatron and linear accelerator have a few advantages over cobalt-60: a potential high-output point source and a good depth dose which enable treatment of even deeply seated tumors to be carried out using only two or three fields. Against this, the cost is higher and the maintenance more complicated. One of the most considerable advantages of this type of unit is the possibility of using it as an electron generator.

Electron therapy is one of the interesting new developments in radiotherapy in the past ten years. High-energy electrons have a limited track in the tissues, the length of which is proportional to the energy; for example, the track of a 20 MeV electron in tissue is about 10 cm. Because of the scattering and straggling of the electrons in a beam, the dose falls off slowly up to a certain depth, then to nothing at all at a depth greater than the maximal track length of the electron. The use of electron beams allows healthy tissue beyond the target to be spared.

Against this, the skin-sparing effect is much less than is obtained with high-energy photons. Skin reactions arising during treatment, however, are less than those occurring with conventional radiotherapy and the mucosal tolerance is very satisfactory.

Electron therapy appears to be particularly useful for certain forms of cancer such as epitheliomas closely related to the bony structures of the face.

Progress is limited by the difficulty of evaluating depth doses in heterogeneous tissue; it seems particularly difficult to obtain a homogeneous dose in the target volume. In addition, electron beams are clinically useful only if their energies are sufficiently high, at least 18—20 MeV but preferably 30—40 MeV.

3. Beam-Shaping Methods

Modern apparatus for radiotherapy at high energy allows for beam shaping. This can be achieved in several ways. Shielding introduced between the collimator and the skin of the patient allows critical areas to be protected and also geometrical fields of more or less complex shapes to be obtained to suit the region being treated. Either a two-cm thickness of tungsten (which reduces the primary beam to 10 %) or a five-cm thickness of lead (which reduces the primary beam to less than 2 %) is used. The shielding is held in the beam so that it is effective whatever the orientation of the beam; this should be ensured at the time of construction of the apparatus.

Wedge filters are filters of graduated thickness which cause a progressive decrease in intensity across the beam. They are increasingly employed to obtain satisfactory depth dose distributions using a small number of fields. In using them one can keep the advantages of skin sparing. A limited number of wedges offers the possibility of a large number of depth dose distributions. Mention should be made of compensating filters (ELLIS et al., 1959; SUNDBORN, 1964), which act in the same way as bolus does at conventional energies and which spare the skin.

The form of the filters can be calculated in the light of the contours of the patient and the composition of the tissue interposed between skin and tumor, so that the desired distribution is achieved within the patient's body.

4. Curietherapy

Interstitial and intracavitary therapy, which was previously restricted to radium and radon, has progressed considerably in the past few years, owing to the introduction of artificial isotopes. The principle of treatment is to place radioactive sources in contact with or actually within the tumor in order to deliver in a short time to the whole tumor and practically nothing else a tumoricidal dose. The indication for this is that the tumors should be easily accessible and of limited volume.

With this technique, the tissues are preserved and the results more esthetically pleasing.

Artificial radioactive isotopes enable older techniques to be replaced and the indications for curietherapy to be extended, for two reasons (PIERQUIN et al., 1964).

One is protection. Because of after-loading techniques for intracavitary radiotherapy in gynecology and interstitial radiotherapy, there is almost complete protection for the operator and his assistants. This means that the loading tubes that are not radioactive can be placed very carefully in position, their position checked radiologically, and the radioactive sources introduced. In addition, the use of radioactive sources with gamma energies lower than radium, for example cesium and iridium-192, reduces the problem of protection during manipulation and hospitalization as well as for storage. This means that the indications for curietherapy can be extended to include tumors of large volume, for example of the breast.

The other reason for curietherapy is that the easy management and the specific activity, which can be varied at will, mean that the material can be adapted to suit each case. Thus interstitial implantation can easily be carried out in situations considered inaccessible to radium such as epitheliomas at the base of the tongue (PIERQUIN et al., 1964). In this way, the dosimetric quality of implants is improved, the dose received by the operator is reduced, and the comfort of the patient is improved owing to better tolerance of the material.

5. Metabolic Radiotherapy

This was one of the first aspects of radiotherapy to benefit from the discovery of artificial radioactivity, and since 1939 the main principles of its application have been known.

There has been no spectacular progress in the past few years, but techniques and indications are being constantly improved, and, more importantly, the follow-up period is now sufficient for results to be assessed. The techniques were at first received over-enthusiastically, and the setbacks encountered resulted in over-severe criticism from some quarters. In cancer of the thyroid, for example, surgery has remained the main form of treatment and external radiotherapy, which allows selective irradiation of the tumor areas, should be used for cancers with local spread, except when the tumor is able to take up radioactive iodine. On the other hand, radioactive iodine is the most important treatment for metastases; many patients with pulmonary metastases are in remission with apparent cure more than 15 years after treatment.

Treatment Methods

1. Principles

The introduction of high-energy radiation into radiotherapy has meant that any desired dose can be delivered to a chosen tissue. The limitations imposed by skin reactions have largely been overcome. The general tolerance is improved because the integral dose, that is, the total dose received by the whole of the organism during irradiation of the tumor, is less. In particular, the hematological disturbances associated with radiation are less pronounced. Local or general intolerance, however, although troublesome, tended to protect the patient from overdosage. As it has become possible to deliver almost unlimited doses to the body, it has become necessary to measure with the greatest possible accuracy the quantity of radiation given; to establish the optimal dose for each tumor; and to deliver exactly this dose to the chosen tissue.

a) *Dosimetric accuracy.* The aim of dosimetry is to measure the quantity of radiation absorbed by the tumor and neighbouring tissues, especially tissues that are radiosensitive. In the past twenty years, there has been a great improvement in its accuracy, owing on the one hand to recognition by radiotherapists of the importance of the problem, and on the other to improvement in the methods used (International Commission on Radiological Units and Measurements, 1963). Finally, accuracy has been facilitated by the replacement of conventional radiotherapy by high-energy radiation.

The human body is not a simple volume with rectilinear contours like the phantoms in general use, and although isodose curves are calculated for beams perpendicular to the wall of the phantom and for geometrically simple sections they are often far from suited to actual cases. It is often necessary partly to ignore the complexity of the body in order to calculate the doses without excessively complicating the calculations, which need to be based on a routine. In addition, the introduction of correction factors is only useful if they are sufficiently well known to increase the accuracy of the calculation. The relative importance of scatter makes corrections complicated and of doubtful accuracy at conventional energies, so that the depth dose calculation of an obliquely entering conventional X-ray beam is too complicated to be carried out. It is relatively simple with high-energy radiation. In the same way, it is relatively easy to take account of the contour of the patient as well as the cross section of the beam when this is complex in form (International Commission on Radiological Units and Measurements, 1963). This was previously impossible.

The body is not made up solely of homogeneous soft tissues. Two heterogeneous tissues are bone, which is of high density, and air-containing cavities, of lower densities. The significance of bone is, as we have seen, less important with high-energy radiations. Air-containing cavities, especially the lungs, which attenuate X-rays much less than the surrounding soft tissue, introduce a variation in the dose distribution within the tissues which may be as much as 50 %. With high-energy radiation, this is less and, more importantly, the dose can be calculated accurately (International Commission on Radiological Units and Measurements, 1963).

The increased accuracy of dosimetry is a major factor in the progress of radiotherapy. Radiotherapists are increasingly helped by hospital physicists, who play an essential role in the radiotherapy department. In the near future, the general use of computers will mean that rapid calculations of doses received at any point in the body will be possible, including detailed calculations for interstitial and intracavitary therapy, which is practically impossible otherwise.

b) *Choice of dose — concept of the optimal dose.* If the highest tumor doses produced the best results, it would suffice in all cases to deliver the maximal dose.

In practice, some tumors are resistant even to very high radiation doses, and the incidence of secondary complications increases rapidly with the dose, even if the treatment itself seems well tolerated. Thus there is an optimal dose that gives the best long-term results, i. e., the maximum tumor sterilization with the minimum of serious complications. This is an old concept, and more recent observations have confirmed its validity for even the newer radiation techniques. Thus in advanced (stage III) carcinoma of the cervix treated by cobalt teletherapy alone to the whole pelvis, the highest percentage of survivals — 46 % of 52 patients — at three years has been obtained using between 6000 and 7000 rad. With higher doses, the results were less satisfactory, not one out of 16 patients treated with doses higher than 7000 rad surviving to the third year (Lalanne and Tubiana, 1964).

The margin for maneuver between underdosage and overdosage is often narrow and the optimal dose varies from one tumor to another. It can only be established by statistical methods using therapeutic trials. This is however a long and difficult investigation and one that requires the collaboration of numerous radiotherapy departments.

As a general rule, the smaller the volume treated the higher the dose that can be delivered. To reconcile the necessity of irradiating a large target volume, including the tumor and its possible extensions, with that of delivering a dose high enough to sterilize the tumor, which may contain anoxic and therefore radioresistant cells, the older technique of the Paris School is being increasingly adapted. This consists of reducing the size of the field towards the end of treatment when the dimensions of the tumor have diminished. In this way a high dose — sometimes up to 8000 R — can be given to the residual tumor, and as the volume is small it is tolerated (although such a dose given to the original volume would not have been tolerated).

Such a technique, which underlines the importance of close clinical observation, is easy to carry out when the tumor dimensions can be followed, but it can be adopted routinely, for example in carcinoma of the esophagus, by using a smaller field towards the end of the treatment. Treatment is started using a large field delivering a dose of 4500 R, then continued by irradiation of the residual tumor with smaller fields delivering an additional 3500 R to the reduced volume. Such techniques can be achieved only by a combination of accurate positioning and supervoltage therapy. In other situations, the augmented dose may also be achieved by interstitial therapy, which confines irradiation to a small volume of any shape.

c) *Planning treatment.* In addition to selecting the area to be treated and the dose to be given, it is necessary to ensure that the treatment is delivered accurately. The higher the dose given, the more potentially dangerous it becomes and the more it should be localized to the tumor area. To ensure this the treatment is planned to achieve:

(a) localization of the tumor;

(b) centering of the beams on the tumor and calculation of the dose distribution in the tissues by using schematic sections of the patient; and

(c) defining of reference points so that the patient can be placed in the same position for each treatment.

The main problem in the planning of treatment is orientation. As most tumors are not accessible to direct examination, it is necessary to relate them to reference points or, even better, to planes of reference, which can then be used in all the subsequent stages from tumor localization to the placing of the patient under the apparatus. Using a constant set of reference points is the best way of ensuring that planned radiation treatment is carried out accurately.

There are two types of treatment apparatus, those with fixed fields and those which rotate. Any preference for the latter type of machine is related not so much to rotation therapy itself as to the ease and precision with which patients can be placed for treatment. Whatever the type of apparatus, it should have the four following features so as to facilitate the planning of treatment:

1) A treatment table that can be moved in all three dimensions.

2) Reference points that allow the position of the radiation source relative to the table to be known at any given time.

3) Means of centering the beam such as light focusing, back pointer, and pin and arc.

4) Equipment enabling radiographs to be taken on the treatment table, to check that the beams are centered on the tumor. Either the same beam as is used for treatment (such as with telecobalt) or a radiodiagnostic tube incorporated within the apparatus will do.

The necessity to treat as many patients as possible and the high cost per treatment with expensive apparatus mean that treatment planning is often carried out outside the treatment room. In departments where several high-energy machines are in use, it is common practice to equip one or more rooms with radiodiagnostic equipment. Usually two sets for localizing the tumor at right angles to each other and an apparatus for tracing body contours are installed. Apparatus may also be installed for transverse tomography on sitting and lying patients. This is very useful in defining the relations of the tumor to surrounding tissues and therefore helps both treatment planning and the calculation of corrections for heterogeneity.

Beam simulators, i. e., radiodiagnostic sets that reproduce the geometry of the radiation beam, allow more time for beam selection and ensure that the treatment machine is not interrupted. A weak cobalt source can be incorporated to measure the effective thickness of the patient so as to facilitate calculation of the doses received by various tissues.

Finally, treatment planning would be useless if the patient was able to move during the treatment. Each time a patient is treated in the sitting position there is danger of slight alterations in his position. Moulds, corsets, etc. should be used to prevent this.

2. Radiotherapy and Surgery in Combination

The association of radiotherapy and surgery is one of the important factors in the progress of radiotherapy and cancer treatment in general. It has various aspects, but in all cases difficult human problems are involved because very close cooperation between radiotherapist and surgeon is necessary — especially coordination of action, which is difficult to achieve even when the two are used to working as a team. This is the most important argument for cancer treatment centres in which radiotherapists and surgeons become used to working together on the same patient in an atmosphere of cooperation and equality.

Four types of cooperation can be defined.

1) Shared treatment in cancer requiring the treatment of several regions, some by the radiotherapist and others by the surgeon. An example of this is Mc Whirter's technique (1955) for treatment of carcinoma of the breast: the treatment of the primary lesion is surgical (mastectomy), and the lymph nodes are treated with radiotherapy. In other cases, in particular for some pharyngolaryngeal cancers, the reverse occurs, the primary lesion being irradiated and surgical lymph node clearance being subsequently carried out. This type of association is useful when the volume of tissue to be treated is considerable and the least traumatic means can be chosen for each area.

2) Pre-operative radiotherapy can be carried out with two quite different aims. One is to facilitate surgery or to reduce the risk of dissemination by manipulation of the tumor at operation. Relatively low doses are sufficient — of the order of 2000, or sometimes 3000 rad, which means that only one cell in 10,000 or 100,000 will survive. Animal experiments have shown that these doses are adequate to reduce considerably the frequency of the metastases of certain types of tumors and post-operative recurrences. The low doses have the advantage of producing minimal reaction in surrounding tissues and therefore of not hindering surgery. They can be given in a week or less and do not delay surgery. At present there is a tendency more and more to extend the indications for pre-operative radiotherapy. This is a logical step for all types of cancer, even those that reputedly are radioresistant, when the diagnosis is certain and when local recurrence is an important factor in operative failure.

Conversely, when radiotherapy is the important element in treatment, high cancericidal doses are necessary (6000 R or more). Prolonged treatment is therefore necessary, and the surgeon must choose the most suitable time for operation after the end of radiotherapy. Surgical intervention in these cases is useful either to remove a persisting tumor, which may be particularly resistant, or as a toilet procedure. An example of this kind of treatment is rapidly growing cancer of the breast, which at Villejuif is treated by irradiating the breast with a high dose (as high as 6000—7000 rad in some cases) and then performing mastectomy.

3) Post-operative radiotherapy is often indicated after surgery when the surgeon feels that the excision has been incomplete. Radiotherapy is then carried out in poor conditions, on tissue whose vascularization has been disturbed by operation. It is therefore not reasonable to carry it out routinely, but it is nevertheless often very effective. An example is radiotherapy after a thyroidectomy in which incomplete clearance of an undifferentiated carcinoma of the thyroid has occurred. This type of association is only reasonable for cancers which are essentially surgical problems and in which excision is generally easy. In these cases, post-operative radiotherapy is relatively rarely indicated.

4) Extensive surgery may be required after unsuccessful radiotherapy or irradiation after failed surgery. This type of association is one of the most useful and one of the most important innovations in cancer treatment in the past twenty years. Irradiation for local recurrences of breast cancer, for instance, is well recognized, but it is necessary to stress the importance of extensive surgery after failed radiotherapy or for recurrences appearing several months or years after radiotherapy. Brunschwig, for example, has shown that extensive surgery is practicable in about half of the patients with recurrences of carcinoma of the cervix after radiotherapy.

The apparent cure rate at five years for such cases was more than 25%. Similarly, in recurrences of pharyngolaryngeal cancer after radiotherapy, extensive surgery produces comparable results. Although these are mutilating procedures, the results nevertheless justify their being considered routinely in all cases of failed radiotherapy.

3. Problems in Cancerology

Radiotherapy should not be considered in isolation but as part of the field of cancerology. Increase of knowledge in this field can contribute to the improvement of radiotherapy. A better understanding of the natural history of cancer would be of great value to the radiotherapist, since useless treatment could be avoided thereby. At Villejuif, for example, under the direction of Professor DENOIX, the frequency with which lymph nodes are involved in the various lymph node areas is being studied. In carcinoma of the outer quadrant of the breast, when the axillary nodes are clear or there is involvement of only one node, nodes in other areas, especially the internal mammary chain, are involved only exceptionally (ROUQUETTE et al., 1962). Moreover, in none of these cases has local recurrence been observed. It therefore appears useless in such cases to irradiate other lymph node areas after simple mastectomy and axillary clearance.

Although irradiation of areas in which the chances of involvement are slight can be avoided, it appears to be dangerous to carry out localized intensive irradiation if the cancer is already generalized. To establish whether or not this is the case is of fundamental importance. In this respect, lymphography represents considerable progress, since involvement of nodes that are not clinically apparent can be detected. This is especially useful in Hodgkin's disease and seminoma. The technique also enables the effect of radiation on the nodes to be followed.

It is all the more important to establish whether the cancer is localized or generalized since combined radiotherapy and chemotherapy may be more effective than radiotherapy alone.

If the growth potential, tendency to invade the lymph nodes, and host-tumor relationship characteristics could be established for a tumor, the choice of treatment for each clinical situation would be facilitated. Tests and classifications have been established with this in mind. C. HEROVICI (1962), for example, has divided cancer of the cervix into three classes according to the peritumoral connective tissue reaction. Of 126 stage-I cases studied, node involvement could not be demonstrated in the 45 cases where the stroma formed a barricade around the tumor. On the other hand, when such a stroma reaction was not present, node involvement occurred frequently and the survival time was shorter. In this last group, even for a tumor in stage I the volume of tissue treated should logically be enlarged. The third histological class is defined by the presence of pathological connective tissue, especially hyaline sclerosis. Survival in these cases is poor, being 0% after three years.

The long-term follow up of patients with cancer shows that, apart from definitive "cures", long-term remissions with stabilization of the neoplastic process can be achieved and a normal life resumed, possibly for many years. These results, often classed as palliative, are of great importance to the patient and demonstrate that in the treatment of cancer a defeatist attitude should be replaced by a more aggressive one. Aggressiveness is often effective, for example in Hodgkin's disease, to which we shall return later. We know already that apparently lasting cures can be obtained by radiotherapy of pulmonary metastases from seminoma testis, Wilms' tumor, or differentiated thyroid carcinomas, and it is probable that this list will be added to in the future.

Some Results of Radiotherapy

The effect of the introduction of new techniques and of changing concepts on treatment methods and results has varied from one tumor to another. Some cases such as skin carcinomas of small dimension could be satisfactorily treated using traditional methods and both the technique and the results have changed relatively little. Similarly, in tumors, such as carcinoma of the bronchus and esophagus, which were rarely cured by conventional methods of treatment, the end results have remained much the same. Between these two extremes, and for the majority of tumors treated by radiotherapy, there has been considerable progress, difficult, however, to express as a definite figure. In fact, better tolerance of treatment has meant that patients have been treated who would have previously been considered unsuitable because of the extent of the tumor, the rapidity of its growth, or their poor general condition. This broadening of the indications to include cases with a poorer prognosis in part counterbalances the better results obtained in other patients, and the overall results have therefore only improved a little. However, if an attempt is made retrospectively to assess the improvement, it is, depending on the type of tumor under consideration, about 10 %. The progress might seem small, but it should be remembered that:

a) among the hundreds of thousands of patients treated, a 5 % to 10 % improvement represents thousands of patients; and

b) the outcome in more than half of patients with cancer is already determined by the time treatment is undertaken because of the presence of occult metastases which become evident months or years later. In fact, a metastasis only becomes clinically or radiologically detectable when it contains about 1×10^9 cells, which represents about thirty cell cleavage times. The cell cleavage time lasts in human cancer from several days to several months. In osteogenic sarcoma of a limb, for example, in more than 90% of cases treatment is unsuccessful owing to the appearance in the subsequent year of pulmonary metastases (whether the treatment is surgery or radiotherapy). The metastases can be measured and from the rate of enlargement the time when they first appeared can be calculated. It has been shown that they are practically always present at the time of diagnosis. Conversely, 10—20 % of cancers are small, well defined, and easily cured, regardless of the type of local treatment used. The difference between mediocre and good treatment of the primary tumor and local nodes (and this applies to about 30 % of cancers) means a gain of 10 %, which is far from being negligible.

Carcinoma of the Cervix

When the extension of the tumor is limited the classical treatment method of combined radium and radiotherapy to the parametria produces good results. The percentage cure rate at five years as recorded in the literature equals or sometimes exceeds 90 % for stage I and 80 % for stage II. On the other hand, results obtained in cases where the tumor extension is considerable are less satisfactory. This latter group has occupied radiotherapists since 1950 (Fletcher et al., 1962).

The good results obtained in stages where the extension is minimal and where radium is the essential element of the treatment show that if conditions are good radium can deal with cervical and uterine lesions. Relatively few modifications have therefore been introduced. Replacement of the classical applicators by new apparatus has largely been to facilitate: a) after-loading and reduced irradiation of the operator (for similar reasons radium is often replaced by cesium, which emits less powerful γ rays and therefore requires less thickness of lead for protection); and b) more accurate dosimetry. The calculated dose is often verified by measuring the rectal dose at the time of insertion. Irradiation of the parametria and nodes is carried out using external radiotherapy, and particular attention has been directed towards improving this aspect of the treatment. Combined radium and high-dosage external radiotherapy can only be achieved without overdosage and with minimal risks of complications if the dose received from the radium is taken into account at the time of the external radiotherapy. This can be done either by limiting the size of the fields or by using a compensating filter to attenuate the beam in the areas which have received the highest doses during the radium insertion. This explains the necessity of accurate dosimetry, which will be greatly facilitated by the use of computers (FLETCHER et al., 1962; PIERQUIN et al., 1964).

The results of controlled clinical trial carried out by PATERSON and RUSSELL (1963) showed that for stages I and II there is no difference between those patients treated by radium alone and those treated by a combination of radium and external parametrial irradiation at a dose of about 3000 rad either by conventional radiotherapy or by high energy (kilovoltage 2500 rad X-ray at point B + 7000 R radium at point A; megavoltage 3000 rad X-ray + 7500 R radium at point A) (Table 1).

Table 1. *Carcinoma of the Cervix Uteri. Comparison of Two Series After Radium Therapy* [1]

	Stage I		Stage 2		Stage 1 and 2	
	Number treated	Survival rate per cent	Number treated	Survival rate per cent	Number treated	Survival rate per cent
No X-ray (1)	58	87.2	164	60.4	222	67.4
Kilovoltage (2)	38	91.4	69	54.5	107	70.4
Megavoltage (3)	40	80.9	74	58.1	122	67.8

(1) No X-ray: 8000 rad radium point A.
(2) Kilovoltage: Conventional X-ray 2500 rad point B + 7000 rad radium point A.
(3) Megavoltage: 3000 rad X-ray point B + 7500 rad radium point A.

[1] From: PATERSON, R., and M. H. RUSSELL: Clin. Radiol. 14, 17 (1963).

The interpretation of the trial is difficult because the dose to the parametria is relatively low. However it confirms the paramount importance of radium in these early cases.

The results obtained by FLETCHER (Table 2) comparing two series of cancer of the cervix (FLETCHER et al., 1962), one treated by orthovoltage and the other by supervoltage, show that the overall survival differs only slightly in patients treated by conventional radiotherapy (59% had a five-year survival with a tumor dose of about 3000 rad) and those treated by high energy (63% had a five-year survival with a tumor dose of 5000—6000 rad). But the overall results are deceptive. If the results are analysed taking the stage into account, it is seen that there is little difference between the early stages (I and IIa) and for the most advanced cases (stage IV) when the tumor has extended beyond the cervix and parametria. On the other

Table 2. *Treatment Results. All Patients Treated for Carcinoma of the Uterine Cervix* [1]
(August, 1948 — August, 1958)

Stage	Before Supervoltage 1948 — September, 1958		Supervoltage 1954 — September, 1958	
	No. treated	Per cent survived 5-years	No. treated	Per cent survived 5-years
	All squamous cell carcinomas on intact uteri			
I	64	90 ($\pm$ 3.6) (1)	117	93 ($\pm$ 2.4)
IIa	129	80 ($\pm$ 3.5)	106	83 ($\pm$ 3.9)
IIb	123	60 ($\pm$ 4.4)	114	73 ($\pm$ 4.2)
All stages II	252	70 ($\pm$ 2.9)	220	78 ($\pm$ 3.0)
IIIa	93	44 ($\pm$ 5.3)	130	56 ($\pm$ 4.7)
IIIb	87	31 ($\pm$ 4.9)	148	38 ($\pm$ 4.2)
All stages III (2)	180	37 ($\pm$ 3.6)	278	46 ($\pm$ 3.2)
IV	19	5 ($\pm$ 5.1)	37	14 ($\pm$ 6.4)
All stages	515	59 ($\pm$ 2.2)	652	63 ($\pm$ 2.0)

(1) Standard error. Prepared, according to Berkson-Gage method, by Mary C. Macdonald, biometrician in the section of radiotherapy.
(2) The greatest increase in survival rate is in the Stage III cases. The survival rates for Stage I, II a, and IV cases are relatively unchanged.
[1] From: Fletcher, G. H., F. N. Rutledge, and P. M. Chau: Amer. J. Roentgenol. 87, 6 (1962).

Table 3. *Results of 142 Pelvic Lymphadenectomies After Radiation Therapy for Cancer of the Cervix* [1]

Stage	No. of patients	No. of positive lymph nodes	Per cent
I (1)	39	1	3.3
IIA (1)	39	4	10.3
IIB (2)	25	5	20.0
IIIA (3)	23	4	17.4
IIIB (3)	25	2	8.0
Total	142	16	11.3

(1) Dose to the lymph nodes: 4000—6500 rad in overall time of 5 to 6 weeks.
(2) Dose to the lymph nodes: 4750—5200 rad in 5 to 6 weeks.
(3) Dose to the lymph nodes: 6000—7000 rad in 6 to 7 weeks.
[1] From: Rutledge, F. N., G. H. Fletcher, and E. J. Macdonald: Amer. J. Roentgenol. 93, 607 (1965).

hand, there is a considerable improvement in results for the intermediate stages (IIb and III) and in these cases infiltration of the lateral part of the parametria and node involvement determine the prognosis.

Can further improvement be expected? The problem is closely related to the determination of optimal doses. As has already been seen, large volumes treated with doses that are too high are dangerous; in patients treated with radiotherapy alone the results become worse if the dose to the whole pelvis exceeds 7000 rad (LALANNE and TUBIANA, 1964). On the other hand, it seems that a dose of 5000—6000 rad (8—17) should be given to deal adequately with involvement of the external iliac nodes. Thus RUTLEDGE *et al.* (1965) in 142 cases of lymphadenectomy after radiotherapy at 5000 to 6000 rad found that 11% of cases showed histological node involvement (Table 3). This figure is clearly lower than the usual percentage of patients with node involvement in stage III cancer of the cervix, but is far from being negligible.

Doses of this order to the whole of pelvis only increase slightly the incidence of intestinal and urological complications. LALANNE and FAJBISOWICZ (1965), who compared 189 cases treated by combined radium and conventional radiotherapy (3000 rad) and 129 cases treated by radium and telecobalt therapy (6000 rad), found that the percentage of complications only rose from 15 to 20% (Table 4). On the

Table 4. *Carcinoma of the Cervix. Complications after Radiation Therapy* [1]
(Comparison between conventional X-ray and cobalt therapy)

Treatment methods (1)	No. of patients	Bowel	Urinary	No. of complications Bone	Skin	Total	Per cent
Radium + 250 kV (2000—3000 rad in 4—6 weeks)	189	18	7	3	1	29	15.3
Radium + cobalt-60 (5000 rad in 6 weeks)	124	19	4	2	0	25	20

(1) Radium therapy was exactly the same in the two series.

[1] From: C. M. LALANNE, and S. FAJBISOWICZ: Ann. Radiol. 8, 697 (1965).

whole, it seems that the margin of safety between the effective dose and a dangerous dose is quite small (LALANNE and TUBIANA, 1964; FLETCHER, 1966). This underlines the necessity of accurate dosimetry, each case being taken into account individually.

Some radiotherapists think that for stages I and IIa intracavitary radiotherapy should be the main form of treatment and surgery and external radiotherapy should play a subsidiary role; while conversely, for stages IIb and III, external radiotherapy should be the essential form of treatment, intracavitary treatment supplementing the dose to the primary tumor. Others feel that intracavitary treatment should be used as the primary treatment in all cases, with doses similar to those used classically, but that the neighbouring tissues should be protected as much as possible by using beam-shaping methods in the subsequent external radiotherapy.

The main conclusion that emerges from the various trends in treatment is that better coordination between intracavitary and external irradiation would provide a basis for further progress.

Carcinoma of the Breast

The original work of BACLESSE had already shown that conventional radiotherapy alone could control carcinoma of the breast, but at the price of not inconsiderable cutaneous and subcutaneous sequelae. Mc WHIRTER's results (1955) have demonstrated the effectiveness of radiotherapy of the lymph nodes, after simple mastectomy. Recent work confirms the effectiveness of the radiotherapy of lymph node areas in an even more striking way. KAAE and JOHANSEN (1962) carried out a controlled clinical trial on 668 cases of breast carcinoma separated into two equal groups (Table 5). Group A were treated by simple mastectomy and postoperative radiotherapy by the Mc WHIRTER method and group B by extended radical mast-

Table 5. *Comparison of McWhirter's Method and Extended Radical Mastectomy* [1]

	Three-year follow-up			Five-year follow-up		
	No. of cases	Survival per cent	Recurrence-free survival per cent	No. of cases	Survival per cent	Recurrence-free survival per cent
Operable cases:						
McWhirter's method	192	78	68	124	66	55
Extended radical mastectomy	181	78	67	109	66	54
Clinical stage I cases:						
McWhirter's method	115	86	79	77	74	65
Extended radical mastectomy	115	87	77	68	77	63
Operable minus stage I cases:						
McWhirter's method	77	66	52	47	53	38
Extended radical mastectomy	66	62	50	41	49	39

[1] From: KAAE, S., and H. JOHANSEN: Breast cancer. Five year results: two random series of simple mastectomy with postoperative irradiation versus extended radical mastectomy. Amer. J. Roentgenol. 87, 82 (1962).

ectomy with dissection of the supraclavicular and internal mammary nodes from the second to the fourth intercostal space, according to the method of DAHL IVERSEN. The results after both three and five years are identical in the two groups.

R. G. GUTMANN (1966) has confirmed the effectiveness of the radiotherapy of nodes involved in breast cancer by irradiating all the lymph node areas with a minimal dose of 5000 R over 4—5 weeks in 168 patients in whom node involvement was verified histologically by the triple biopsy method. Of these patients, 123 developed a recurrence within five years, and 52% survived for that period. Most of the patients who came to autopsy showed no evidence of active tumor in the irradiated areas.

Can a mean cancericidal dose be determined for the treatment of carcinoma of the breast (Mc WHIRTER, 1964)? For the nodes, the minimal dose is 5000 rad over 4—5 weeks. It is possible that a dose of 6000 rad over 5—6 weeks increases the percentage sterilization, but there is no definite evidence for this. The minimal dose required is certainly higher for the primary tumor — of the order of 7000—8000 rad over 6—8 weeks. Such a dose can often be achieved by reducing the treatment volume above 5000 rad (LALANNE, 1965).

The combination of radiotherapy and surgery may be of two kinds. Both may be used as part of the same treatment, each for separate areas; an example is

Mc WHIRTER's technique of irradiation of the internal mammary and supraclavicular nodes after radical mastectomy. Radiotherapy and surgery, as has been seen, are equally effective, and in the choice the relative risks and subsequent skin damage are taken into consideration. Alternatively, radiotherapy and surgery may be used successively for the same area, e. g., for pre- and postoperative radiotherapy. In postoperative radiotherapy the aim is to deliver a dose of between 4000 and 5000 rad to the chest wall and axilla in an attempt to reduce local recurrences. In some centres this is routine practice, in others treatment is given only if surgery is thought to have been incomplete, untreated patients being closely followed up and treated if and when there is local recurrence.

The results of the clinical trial carried out by PATERSON and RUSSELL (1959) show that when excision has apparently been complete, the survival is the same whether postoperative radiotherapy is given routinely or only on local recurrence.

At the Institut Gustave Roussy (ROUQUETTE et al., 1962; LALANNE, 1965), postoperative radiotherapy is used routinely when there is histological evidence of axillary lymph node involvement (N+). When the nodes are clear (N—), the patients are not irradiated. This necessitates a particularly rigorous histological technique, that is, en bloc fixation of the material obtained at axillary clearance and serial sectioning. The results of CHU et al. (1966) appear to support this approach. They compared two series of patients (non-randomized), one of which was irradiated and the other not. No difference was found between N- cases, but a slight advantage was found for the N+ cases that were irradiated.

There is no agreement on the value of pre-operative radiotherapy. Some centres never use it, others feel that it is useful if the volume of the tumor or nodes is considerable or if the tumor, which may be small, is increasing rapidly in size (LALANNE, 1965).

Should the dose be moderate (2500 rad in 2 weeks), with the aim of reducing the risk of dissemination at operation, or should a higher dose (of the order of 5000—6000 rad) be given? At the moment there seems to be a trend in favor of the latter form of treatment; if high-energy radiation is used, subsequent surgery is not interfered with and may sometimes be less extensive. Some authorities favor even higher doses which, if delivered to a relatively small volume, do not interfere with subsequent simple mastectomy.

The final problem of combined radiotherapy and surgery is that of the optimal dose. LALANNE (1965) has compared the results obtained by conventional radiotherapy at moderate doses with cobalt therapy at higher doses. The results are identical for tumors of small volume and slow growth. For tumors of large volume or rapidly growing tumors, however, the survival rate after three years was 49 % for conventional treatment and 62 % for cobalt therapy. These results confirm the usefulness of radiotherapy in these cases and show that effectiveness is a function of dose. The increased survival time, however, is more marked in women under 50 years of age in whom routine castration has been carried out in the group treated with cobalt. Castration has probably contributed towards the improvement of results, as is suggested by the conclusions of the clinical trial carried out by PATERSON and RUSSELL (1959) on the value of castration. It may be noted at the same time that, in this respect, radiotherapeutic castration is as effective as surgery (LALANNE, 1965).

Carcinoma of the Bronchus and Esophagus

There were high hopes that high-energy radiation, which made it possible to deliver tumor doses of 6000 R or more in a short time to the whole mediastinum, would improve results in cancer of the bronchus and esophagus. Unfortunately this not been the case, the five-year survival figures not having changed appreciably. However, rapid palliation can be achieved and the survival time is longer after high-energy irradiation. The patient has also been made more comfortable with the shorter treatment.

At the Institut Gustave Roussy (PIERQUIN et al., 1965), the survival in cases of carcinoma of the bronchus with high-energy treatment was 33% at one year and 19% at two years, and with conventional radiotherapy at lower doses 22% at one year and 7% at two years. The three-year survival rate is the same in both groups. Increasing the dose does not therefore increase the long-term survival.

For carcinoma of the esophagus the situation is similar; the percentage survival, despite high doses, is mediocre. The results in carcinoma of the cervical and superior mediastinal esophagus are slightly less bleak (LEDERMAN, 1966). The possibility of pre-operative radiotherapy has been studied by some workers. NAKAYAMA et al. (1963) give 2000 rads over three days to the whole of the mediastinum several days before surgery. These results, if confirmed, seem encouraging.

The Lymphomas

In many centres the treatment of Hodgkin's disease and other malignant lymphomas had since 1945 become essentially chemotherapeutic. During the past few years it is becoming progressively more radiotherapeutic under the influence of two factors. First, the long-term results of chemotherapy are mediocre and show little improvement, in spite of the introduction of new drugs. Second, the long-term results of energetic irradiation in those centres in which it has remained the main form of treatment are remarkable encouraging; two symposia recently demonstrated this point (Symposium international, 1966).

EASSON, for example, has shown that in the localized forms of Hodgkin's disease (stages I and IIA) treated with doses of 3000 rad over three weeks to the areas involved the survival at 10 years was 44% and patients surviving more than 10 years had a life expectancy comparable to the normal subject of the same age and sex. These findings lead EASSON to use the word "cure" for Hodgkin's disease so treated.

V. PETERS of Toronto has obtained similar results. In addition, the results are better in the group of patients treated with a dose of more than 3000 rad + irradiation of adjacent lymph-node areas than in those treated with moderate doses (less than 2000 rad). Even in advanced stages (generalized disease with involvement of lymphatics above and below the diaphragm) it seems possible to obtain a 30% five-year survival rate and a 20% ten-year survival rate by using the more aggressive type of radiotherapy.

High-energy radiation should improve the results still more (H. S. KAPLAN). In fact, it makes it possible to irradiate extensive areas, including more or less all the lymphatics of the trunk, under good conditions.

There is now general agreement that radiotherapy is the treatment of choice for localized forms of Hodgkin's disease; 3500—4000 R should be given in 3—4 weeks.

Some authors irradiate only the areas involved with a surrounding margin of a few centimeters. Others (PETERS) routinely treat the adjacent lymphnode areas. A controlled clinical trial is at present in progress (KAPLAN) to determine which method is the more effective.

In generalized forms with involvement of nodes above and below the diaphragm (stage III), some workers prefer to give radiotherapy at a high dose to the areas involved, whereas others start with chemotherapy and follow with radiotherapy to the tumor persisting. Here also a controlled clinical trial is in progress.

In lymphosarcoma the results obtained were comparable to those obtained in Hodgkin's disease. In these cases also, an aggressive and energetic form of radiotherapy produces results that would have previously been considered impossible to achieve.

Epithelioma of the Head and Neck

The indications for either surgery or radiotherapy in treating epithelioma of the head and neck are not yet clearly defined. Some centres favor radiotherapy, others surgery. Between 1935 and 1950, radiotherapy tended to be abandoned in favor of surgery, but at present there is a movement in the opposite direction.

In centres where radiotherapy is the main form of treatment there has been an overall improvement in results since the introduction of high energy. Thus, at the

Table 6. *Results of Cobalt Therapy at Curie Foundation for Carcinomas of the Head and Neck* [1]

Localizations	3 years No. treated	3 years Alive	4 years No. treated	4 years Alive	5 years No. treated	5 years Alive
Nasopharynx	20	5	11	5	3	1
Tonsil region	127	57	88	38	46	18
Oropharynx	77	31	37	17	22	8
Hypopharynx	111	27	58	13	14	6
Supraglottic laryngeal region	52	30	32	18	17	10
Glottic and subglottic regions	41	20	32	14	23	7
	428	170	258	105	120	50

[1] From: ENNUYER, A., and P. BATAINI: Ann. Radiol. (1966).

Table 7. *Results of Conventional X-ray Therapy at Curie Foundation for Carcinomas of the Head and Neck* [1]

Localizations	No. treated	Alive	% alive
Nasopharynx	161	29	18
Tonsil region	293	39	13
Vallecula	389	39	10
Hypopharynx	525	35	6.5
Supraglottic region	154	29	19
Glottic and subglottic region	151	36	24

[1] From: ENNUYER, A., and P. BATAINI: Ann. Radiol. (1966).

Curie Foundation in Paris, BACLESSE and ENNUYER obtained a 12 % five-year survival rate (207 survivors out of 1693 cases) for epitheliomas of the pharynx and larynx in all three stages (Table 7). For tumors of the same site the percentage survival is now 40% at both three and five years (Table 6). This improvement could only have been achieved using radical treatment with doses of 6500 to 7500 rad to the tumor and often more to the nodes, over a period of 35—40 and sometimes 50 days (Ennuyer and Bataini, 1966). This means giving 1200—1400 rad per week, varying according to the site of the tumor. Such treatment necessitates a judicious choice of the volume to be irradiated, with small fields that should be reduced in size during the course of the treatment.

Whereas only 5000 rad in 8—10 weeks could be given using conventional irradiation, the newer techniques have meant in general that a higher dose can be given in a shorter time without meeting serious immediate, or eventual skin, bone, or cartilage complications.

Epitheliomas of the tonsillar region are particularly suited to retrospective study. The volume irradiated is the same for both conventional and cobalt teletherapy, two lateral opposed fields being used of about 8×6 cm, centered on the angle of the mandible and including the first node station in the submental fossa. The factors that differ are total dose and fractionation with 200 kV, 5000—6000 R. The tumor dose is given over 8—10 weeks with cobalt-60, and 7500 rad are given in five weeks. Using 200 kV, Ennuyer and Bataini (1966) obtained a 13% five-year cure rate (39 out of 293 cases), and with cobalt-60 a 40% five-year cure rate i. e., 8 out of 46 cases. Fletcher and Lindberg (1966) obtained similar results: 38 out of 104 cases at five years, i. e., 36%.

The same considerations apply to hypopharyngeal epitheliomas (piriform fossa). Tumors in this site have a poor prognosis and, using conventional radiotherapy, Ennuyer obtained a 6.5% five-year cure rate (35 out of 525 cases), often at the price of serious complications involving the laryngeal cartilages. With cobalt-60 the three-year cure rate was 24% (27 out of 111 cases) (Table 6).

After five years there were six survivals out of 14 cases. The use of new radiotherapeutic techniques such as high-energy electron therapy for epitheliomas of the mandibular and alveolar regions offers some hope of improving results in these sites, which carry a poor prognosis. At the same time, interstitial implantation using after loading techniques means that some cures can be obtained in previously hopeless situations such as advanced carcinoma of the tongue and floor of the mouth.

High-energy irradiation means that new radiotherapy-surgery combinations are possible, the skin being spared so that postoperative healing is not impaired. It now seems clearly established that a dose of 2000 to 4000 rad pre-operatively will not interfere with surgery or increase the incidence of pre- and postoperative complications. Is such a low pre-operative dose effective? There are no long-term results to commend the method, but on the other hand the immediate results of a controlled clinical trial carried out by Henschke et al. (1966) on two randomized series of radical neck dissections showed the incidence of local recurrence to be clearly reduced after pre-operative radiotherapy. In the series without irradiation the incidence of local recurrence at two years was 33%, and in the series receiving 2000 rad by electron therapy over one week pre-operatively, 20%.

As regards postoperative radiotherapy, 6000 rad in 4—5 weeks can be delivered to the operative region without increasing the risk of wound separation and without skin complications. For example, after an extended pharyngolaryngectomy for hypopharyngeal carcinoma, 6000 rad can be delivered to the whole of the scar from the tracheostomy inferiorly to the thyroid superiorly, using two lateral opposed fields and including the cervical lymph nodes.

After a cervical lymph-node clearance, irradiation can be started one week after surgery and 6000 rad can be given over five weeks to the whole of the scar from the mastoid superiorly to the retroclavicular region inferiorly. This can be given by a single tangential field without early or late skin reaction. Months after the irradiation the skin appears quite normal.

The possibility of surgery after failed radiotherapy with doses of up to 7000 rad must be stressed; 20—25 % of these cases can be salvaged. For example, Y. CACHIN has obtained a 20 % by an *en bloc* operation (radical neck commando) after failed radiotherapy of the tonsillar fossa.

The Future of Radiotherapy

In the past 20 years radiotherapy has made great progress, owing largely to improved treatment conditions: the replacement of conventional X-rays by higher energies, more precise irradiation techniques, and more accurate assessment of the doses received by the tissues.

It is possible that results will continue to improve in the next few years. The statistics now being published relate to patients treated at the latest in 1959, when the full potentiality of high-energy treatment had not been realized. However, it is unlikely that in the larger centres the progress achieved will be very considerable. Future progress probably does not lie in this direction but in one or more of the three following.

Education and diffusion of new methods. Even if in all countries radiotherapy is generally of excellent quality in the large centers, it is necessary to recognize that those standards are not maintained everywhere. There are many radiotherapists who are too timid or too routine, who continue to treat with low doses and do not take the measures necessary to ensure a precise technique; even if high-energy apparatus is available its full potentiality is not exploited. There are still too many departments where the radiotherapist works single-handed without the help of a physicist, without using the equipment necessary for tumor localization, for contour drawing, and for choice of the most satisfactory beam for selective irradiation of the tumor. The World Health Organization and the International Atomic Energy Agency have several times drawn attention to these problems. The International Commission on Radiological Units and Measurements has published reports describing the best methods of clinical dosimetry, but its recommendations would be more effective if each country made an effort to spread information on modern methods of radiotherapy. It cannot be too frequently stressed that even the best equipment is useless, even dangerous, unless operated by persons who are fully qualified to do so.

Radiobiology. This is the key to further progress in radiotherapy. Several lines of investigation seem promising.

a) *Oxygen effect.* Many investigations have demonstrated that anoxic cells are two to three times less radiosensitive than cells which are normally oxygenated.

Cancerous tissue is frequently poorly vascularized with a greater intercapillary distance than normal. At distances of more than 50 microns from a capillary the oxygen tension falls below 12 mm Hg and below this level cells become more radioresistant. The presence of a small proportion of anoxic cells (of the order of a few per cent) is enough to increase significantly the radioresistance of the whole tumor. For example, in a tumor composed of 10^{10} cells, the LD 90 of which is 400 rad, after a dose of 4800 rad there is only 1 chance in 100 that a viable cell will survive in the tumor. If 1/100 of the cells are anoxic the dose must be raised to 8000 rad to obtain the same effect. This is probably the reason why some tumors, especially large ones, are radioresistant while other apparently comparable tumors react quite differently. Because of the presence of these radioresistant cells high doses must be given to the residual tumor. The situation also provides a rational basis for fractionation of treatment, because as tumor regression occurs vascularization is improved at the same time. During the last part of the treatment the tumor is small and well vascularized with a considerably reduced proportion of anoxic cells.

Several methods are at the moment being developed with the aim of increasing the effectiveness of radiotherapy, either by reducing the radiosensitivity of healthy tissue or by increasing the radiosensitivity of tumor tissue. The radiosensitivity of healthy tissue can be reduced by rendering it anoxic while the poorly vascularized tumor tissue is not affected. All tissues are therefore brought to a minimal radiosensitivity, and it is possible to deliver doses two to three times higher than usual (12,000 to 14,000 rad). Because of the risk of cerebral anoxia, this method has only been used for the limbs, where some encouraging results have been obtained in treated sarcomas.

The opposite technique, the inhalation of oxygen during treatment, may be employed to increase the oxygenation of the tumor and thus increase its radiosensitivity. However, to achieve this in tissues which are widely separated from capillaries a high blood oxygen tension is required. Breathing oxygen at three times the pressure of the atmosphere produces adequate oxygenation in tissues 80 microns from the capillaries and reduces the amount of radioresistant tissue. Unfortunately with pressures as high as this the patients have to be treated in an oxygen tank. Results using this method are not yet conclusive but seem encouraging. At present many investigations on both human and experimental tumors are being undertaken to study this problem.

b) *Fractionation.* The ideal situation is that which produces the maximal effect on the tumor with the minimal effect on healthy tissue. Schedules which are used in general for all types of tumor, such as 6000 rad over six weeks with five treatments daily, have gradually grown up as a result of experience.

The ideal fractionation is probably not the same for all tumors; in establishing the best type of irradiation, radiobiological phenomena must be taken into consideration. The relation between the dose and the number of surviving cells capable of multiplying normally is described by a sigmoid curve. This means that the first few dozen rad given during one treatment session are less effective than those given at the end of the same session. For example, 100 rad at the beginning of the session will only kill about 10% of cells, but the same dose at the end of the session, when the cells have already received 300 rad, will kill 60% of the surviving cells. It seems as if irradiation only acts with full effectiveness on cells that have already received a sufficient dose, and that the initial lesions make the cells more susceptible to the effects of subsequent irradiation. This threshold dose, above which irradiation becomes fully effective, varies from one cell type to another. It can be estimated by taking the extrapolation number from the curve, which varies from 1.5 to 10 according to the cell type considered.

When the threshold dose in tumor tissue is higher than in normal tissue, higher doses per session (of the order of 300—500 rad) are preferable. If on the other hand the extrapolation number is lower in tumor tissue, smaller doses (50—100 rad) are desirable, as, for example, in chronic lymphatic leukaemia. Values for these various parameters are still largely unknown for tumor, as for normal, tissues. It is probable that they will be evaluated in the future and the choice of the optimal dose per treatment will become possible on a rational base.

In the few hours after irradiation the cells that remain viable repair their lesions and recover their normal radiosensitivity. However, the overall tissue radiosensitivity is modified for two reasons. One is that the radiosensitivity of a cell varies from one phase of its life cycle to another, being higher at some phases of the cycle than at others. After a single irradiation, many cells are blocked in the pre-mitotic phase. When the cell cycle starts again a considerable proportion of the cells remain semi-synchronized and pass together through the hyper- or hypo-sensitive phases. In situations where the time relations of these events vary between tissues an attempt can be made to exploit this difference and obtain the maximal effect on the tumor and the minimal effect on healthy tissue.

A second reason is that in growing tissues many cells have time to divide between each treatment. The total number of cells in this case depends on the interval between each session. If cell multiplication is slower in tumor tissue than in critical normal tissues it would be preferable to leave a relatively long interval; if the converse, a short interval would be indicated.

c) *Radiosensitivity and radioprotection.* Many chemical substances are capable of either increasing or decreasing the effect of radiation on cells. They are of interest from the therapeutic point of view only if they are preferentially taken up by either tumor or by normal tissue. Unfortunately it has not yet been possible to achieve this, and although some encouraging clinical results have been obtained methods of application have still to be investigated.

Controlled clinical trials. We have seen when discussing the basis of radiotherapy how difficult it is to assess progress due to the introduction of new methods and to choose the best technique when several are possible. Retrospective comparisons are always difficult and their results open to criticism. Comparisons between results obtained by treating two series of patients are valid only if the series are comparable and this is difficult to obtain because progress in radiotherapy has meant that the indications for treatment have been extended and patients have been irradiated who would previously not have received treatment. Thus a series of patients treated in 1948 is only rarely comparable with a series treated in 1954. The details of classification are insufficient for valid comparison because, apart from the stage, it is necessary to take into account the age and general condition of the patient and the rate of progress of the condition and two series of patients treated several years apart with the same controls may differ considerably in all these aspects.

To achieve valid results, the comparison must be made under satisfactory statistical conditions, which means that the treatment is randomized. Using this method, accurate results can be obtained for many medical problems. It is not however ethically possible to compare two treatments if one treatment is considered to be more effective than the other. This explains why, the immediate results of treatment at high energy being certainly better, no such comparison has been undertaken at any center. It is now too late to undertake such a comparison. The necessity is thus clear that in future statistical methods should be used when new treatment methods are introduced into radiotherapy.

A small apparent improvement in results such as 5—10 % is of great importance as it represents a large number of patients. Such an improvement can be demonstrated, firstly by considering a sufficiently large number of patients (e. g., about 500), so that treatment curing, say, 60 % of patients can be proved to be better than treatment curing 50 %. To collect this number of patients in a short time the collaboration of several treatment centers would be advantageous. Secondly, it is only by rigidly conforming to statistical principles that sources of error can be eliminated. The organization of such comparisons is certainly a difficult task but it represents one of the important tasks of radiotherapy.

Conclusions

More than 50 % of patients with cancer are treated at some stage of their disease with radiotherapy. The effectiveness of treatment methods and the patient's tolerance of them have increased considerably in the past 20 years, owing to improved techniques. This is particularly true for cancers that spread locally. However, the number of patients who die from local recurrences shows that radiotherapy has not yet developed sufficiently to be fully effective as treatment and that further progress is necessary. The two directions in which this could occur appear to be in the organization of clinical trials and in increased understanding of radiobiology.

References

Ashton, T., and A. E. Chester. Brit. J. Radiol. 35, 704 (1962).
Chu, F., J. C. Lucas, J. H. Farrow, and J. J. Nickson. Communication to the 48th Annual Meeting of the American Radium Society, 13 April, 1966.
Ellis, F., and R. Oliver. Brit. J. Radiol. 34, 720 (1961).
—, E. J. Hall, and R. Oliver. Brit. J. Radiol. 32, 421 (1959).
Ennuyer, A., and P. Bataini. Ann. Radiol. 9 (1966).
Farmer, B. T. Phys. in Med. Biol. 4, 5050 (1962).
Fletcher, G. H. J. Amer. med. Ass. 96, 574 (1966).
—, and R. D. Lindberg. Amer. J. Roentgenol. 96, 574 (1966).
—, F. N. Rutledge, and P. M. Chau. Amer. J. Roentgenol. 87, 6 (1962).
Guttmann, R. J. Amer. J. Roentgenol. 96, 550 (1966).
Henschke, U. K., E. L. Frazell, B. S. Hilaris, J. J. Nickson, H. R. Tollefsen, and E. W. Strong. Radiology 86, 450 (1966).
Herovici, C. Gynéc. et Obstét. 61, 623 (1962).
International Commission on Radiological Units and Measurements: Report 10 d, Clinical dosimetry. National Bureau of Standards Handbook 87 (1963).
Kaae, S., and H. Johansen. Amer. J. Roentgenol. 87, 82 (1962).
Keller, H. L. Acta Radiol. (Stockh.) 1, 369 (1963).
Lalanne, C. M. Communication to the 11th Congress of Radiology, Rome, September, 1965.
—, and S. Fajbisowicz. Ann. Radiol. 8, 697 (1965).
—, and M. Tubiana. Rev Inst. nac. Cancer. (Méx.), 419 (1964).
Lederman, M.: Brit. J. Radiol. 39, 193 (1966).
McWhirter, R.: Brit. J. Radiol. 28, 128 (1955).
— Amer. J. Roentgenol. 92, 3 (1964).

NAKAYAMA, K., et al. Arch. Surg. 87, 1003 (1963).
PATERSON, R., and M. H. RUSSELL. J. Fac. Rad. 10, 130 (1959).
— — J. Fac. Radiol. (Lond.) 10, 175 (1959).
— — Clin. Radiol. 14, 17 (1963).
PIERQUIN, B., D. CHASSAGNE, and R. PEREZ. Précis de Curiethérapie. Paris: Masson 1964.
—, P. GRAVIS, and X. GELLE. J. Radiol. Electrol. 45, 201 (1965).
ROUQUETTE, C., G. VOGT-HOERNER, J. LACOUR, and S. LELLOUCH. Acta Un. int. Cancr. 18, 6 (1962).
RUTLEDGE, F. N., G. H. FLETCHER, and E. J. MACDONALD. Amer. J. Roentgenol. 93, 607 (1965).
SINCLAIR, W. K. Radiol. Research. 16, 336 (1962).
SUNDBORN, L.: Acta Radiol. (Stockh.) 2, 189 (1964).
Symposium International. La Radiothérapie de la maladie de Hodgkin. Nouv. Rev. franç. Hémat. 6, 1—176 (1966).
TSIEN, K. C.: Vienna: International Atomic Energy Agency 1963.
TUBIANA, M., and B. PIERQUIN: Proceedings of IX International Congress of Radiology, 557 (1959).
—, J. DUTREIX, A. DUTREIX, and P. JOCKEY: Les Bases physiques de la Radiothérapie. Paris: Masson 1963.

The Surgical Treatment of Cancer

GEORGE T. PACK

With 15 Figures

1. The Rationale of Radical Surgical Treatment for Cancer

In the surgical treatment of cancer, it would seem that the limit has been reached in the extent of the body that can be dispensed with, with the continued maintenance of life. At times there has seemed to be more or less competition among surgeons as to how much of the human body could be removed surgically and leave a remnant compatible with living. The surgeon has to weigh these procedures carefully in the case of the individual patient. He must decide as to the prospect of palliative relief or the more remote possibility of cure. He should estimate the probable degree of relief in relation to the resultant disability; the temperamental make-up of the individuals concerned; their social and business obligations; and the risk of operative mortality. All these factors should enter into consideration when the surgeon is making his decision. He must take care that in deciding not to accept the risk of a major operative procedure he is not acting unjustly in deciding that the patient's cancer is too far advanced and the risk too great. He must not be influenced by his own fear of criticism from colleagues or the lay public. The surgeon faced with the challenge of an advanced cancer must be able to put himself in his patient's place. Very few surgeons ever close the chest or abdomen after a decision that they will not remove a certain cancer without experiencing a painful feeling of futility. They must weigh very carefully whether their decisions are based on an objective evaluation or whether they are influenced by their own state of mind and are looking for excuses not to put the patients through operations that are not only dangerous and of uncertain outcome but major ordeals for the surgeon as well.

The limit to the scope of surgical treatment for cancer seemingly depends upon the essentiality of the organ, i. e., whether life can be sustained without it. Improvements in anesthesia, the use of antibiotics, the recognition and correction of metabolic abnormalities after the sacrifice of important functional organs, and the maintenance of a proper water and electrolyte balance have made extensive operations feasible and relatively safe for the patient. A radical procedure should not be performed for its own sake. Rather, emphasis must be put on what should be considered *adequate* for a particular patient with a cancer of a given extent.

In their efforts to eradicate a cancer, and for want of something better to do, surgeons will continue to separate the patient from the multiple organs involved. No surgeon, however, has such a mechanistic attitude towards cancer and its spread as to believe that extirpative measures are the ultimate answer to the problems of cancer treatment. These extended and disabling operations will continue, however, even though surgeons know that they will afford cures for few. Many will be comforted, and, as Confucius said: "It is better to have a feeble light from a single candle than to live in utter darkness." "If every man would mend a man, how soon the world were mended."

The surgeon's attitude to the cancerous patient may be likened to that of the cardiologist confronted with patients with incurable heart disease. Treatment is not refused to such patients; they are kept alive, and complications are avoided by the institution of appropriate measures. This principle is adopted in the surgical treatment of cancer too. Even if the cancer is known to be incurable, still, if it can be excised without great hazard to the patient the operation may give him a period of relief, however short — usually less than the five-year survival period. If surgeons can add one, two, or three years of comfortable living, even without the ultimate achievement of a cure, or, for that matter, if the application of palliative efforts gives alleviation of suffering, their existence and practice would be justified. After all, many of the operations performed with the hope of cure, and which we optimistically classify initially as potentially curative, are ultimately only palliative measures. One cannot impugn the surgeon under these circumstances for his efforts to alleviate the patient's suffering.

The word "palliation" here, applicable not only to surgical treatment but to other disciplines of cancer therapy as well, does not mean prolongation of life with continued suffering. The mere prolongation of life is not the criterion of success, because palliation connotes a period of *comfortable* living that follows the application of therapeutic measures.

2. The Prevention of Metastases

Free cancer cells as contaminants have long been found (particularly at operation) in the peritoneal and pleural cavities, in the wounds of incisions and anastomoses, and in the washings of surgical gloves. The disconcerting discovery of cancer cells or their clusters in the blood stream causes intensified apprehension when their numbers increase manifold after certain resections of major cancers. Physical measures to lessen the iatrogenic dissemination of cancer by the surgeon are laudable and helpful; among them are preliminary ligation and severance of the efferent vessels of the organ, the use of tourniquets or occlusive vascular clamps, ligation of a cancerous segment of bowel above and below, and antiseptic irrigation of the lumen of the isolated segment prior to excision.

The vast majority of free cells fortunately perish in the blood stream owing to failure of implantation and growth in the various capillary beds.

The factor of host resistance or some indeterminate degree of immunity may have a role in the inability of cancer cell emboli to produce the localized deposits and growths known as metastases. Cures even become possible in spite of the presence of cancer cells in the blood stream — for example, in colonic cancer (ENGELL, 1959). SUMNER WOOD, jr., HOLYOKE and YARDLEY (1961) in their classic experiments on animals, clearly demonstrated that minute thrombi must incarcerate the embolic cancer cells in capillary beds to maintain their viability and successful invasion through the endothelial wall. Thrombosis, therefore, is the *sine qua non* for metastases to develop. It follows, as WOOD and others have shown, that measures lessening the tendency to thrombosis, such as the exhibition of heparin or fibrinolysin, will to a considerable degree prevent metastases, whereas agents such as cortisone and pituitary growth hormone will enhance the tendency. Clinical analogues of these experiments are: (1) reported instances of traumatic localization of metastases; (2) early and widely disseminated metastases after pancreatectomy or gastrectomy in patients showing concurrent evidence of thrombosis or phlebitis; (3) the appearance of nodular dermal metastases confined to the limits of the donor site when skin grafts have been taken in cancer operations. In due time, these facts may find application in the prevention of metastases in humans.

We have been sufficiently impressed by such experimental data to employ, in selected patients undergoing major surgery for cancers, such possible prophylactic measures as the administration of 250 mg of heparin every other day or 5 mg of Coumadin twice daily, while at the same time exercising close control over the prothrombin time.

3. Surgical Treatment of Cancer of the Gastrointestinal Tract

a) Cancer of the Esophagus

In earlier years, the opinion was held that cancer of the esophagus might be a highly curable neoplastic disease when once the technical difficulties of the operation and the complicating hazards were overcome. During recent years, in which esophagectomies have been done in considerable numbers at various centers, the removal of primary esophageal cancers has enabled patients to live long enough for the uncomplicated natural history of the cancer to become manifest. It is now realized that many esophageal cancers in the course of time — provided the patients do not die of esophageal obstruction, mediastinitis, hemorrhage, or something else — tend to become generalized, with visceral metastases. Furthermore, the tendency of esophageal cancer to extend intramurally far up and down the esophageal tube to remote lymph nodes in the neck superiorly and into the juxtacardiac and retroperitoneal regions under the diaphragm inferiorly, prevents simple segmental resection from being curative. Theoretically, for an operation intended for cure, it would be necessary to remove the entire esophagus, including the proximal segment of the stomach and the juxtacardiac lymph nodes inferiorly and the cervical esophagus up to the pharynx superiorly (Fig. 1 [a], [b]). The operation should also include mediastinal lymph-node dissection. The absence of a serosal coat on the esophagus

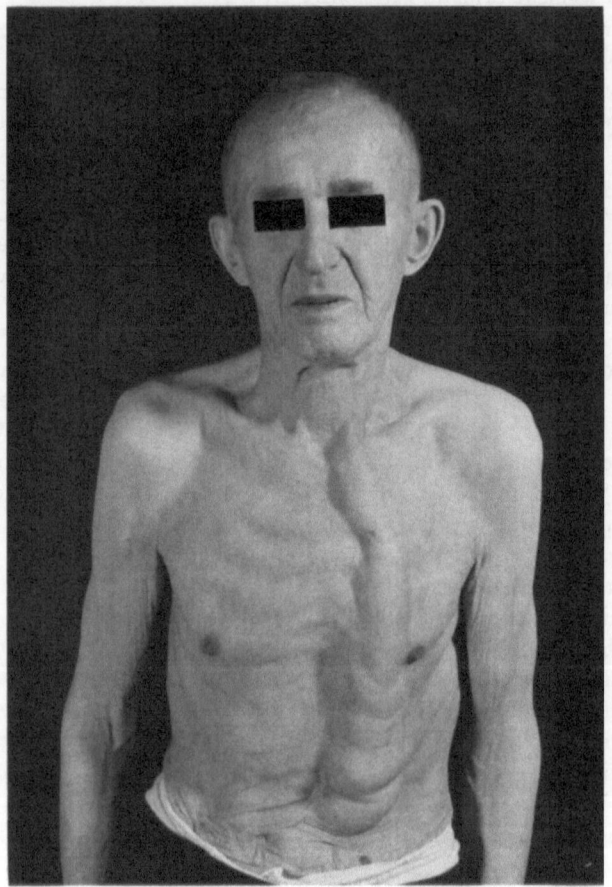

Fig. 1 a

Fig. 1. a) Total esophagectomy; 18-year cure. Early method of substitutive esophagus by subcutaneous jejunal transplant. (Courtesy Dr. THEODORE R. MILLER, Pack Medical Group.) b) Cancer of esophagogastric junction. Treatment: laparothoracotomy; esophagogastrectomy and intrathoracic anastomosis

evidently permits a quicker dissemination of the cancer to the mediastinal structures both by lymphatic spread and by direct invasion. Esophageal cancers involving the extreme lower segment of the esophagus are still attacked surgically through a left thoracoabdominal incision, with the anastomosis usually below the aortic arch. For cancers of the middle and superior thoracic esophagus, the right thoracic approach is preferable, for it facilitates mobilization of the esophagus with greater ease than when attempts are made to dissect the esophagus from beneath the arch of the aorta on the left side. The restoration of pharyngointestinal continuity has been accomplished by various ingenious methods such as complete mobilization of the stomach, preserving the integrity of the blood supply at its distal extremity and introducing the organ into the chest and neck for high anastomosis. The transverse colon or a well-vascularized limb of jejunum has also been introduced as a substitute for the esophagus. In some instances it has been routed through the anterior mediastinum in the retrosternal space, which is extrapleural. This route is the shortest distance

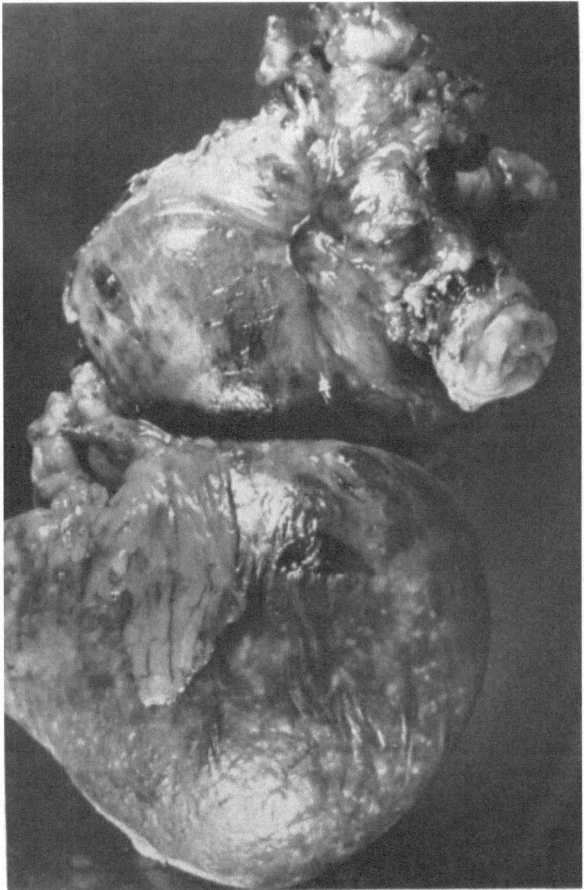

Fig. 1 b

between the abdomen and the neck, and the substitute organ may be carried upwards beneath the sternum through this avascular space.

Two additional measures of importance in lessening operative mortality, increasing curability, and diminishing the hazards of dissemination have been employed. Pre-operative irradiation, using megavoltage techniques either with 1 to 2 million volt X-ray machines or a cobalt beam, has been administered through two parasternal and two paravertebral ports subjecting the tumor to a cross fire, or circumferentially through rotation of the patient or of the cobalt source. These procedures are effective in delivering a considerable dose into the substance of the cancer. The treatment must not be given too quickly or the rapid dissolution of the cancer may lead to perforation and suppurative mediastinitis. The majority of esophageal cancers, if treated with small amounts of radiation over a relatively long time, can become disengaged with consequent resumption of swallowing, lessening of discomfort, prolongation of life, and avoidance of the serious and distressing complications that accompany cancer of the esophagus. In our experience, the prime importance of such irradiation is as a pre-operative measure lessening the hazards of dissemination and increasing the prospects of resectability. A second measure, a definite step forward, depends on the admission that the majority of esophageal cancers can be surgically removed but that an immediate anastomosis is a great hazard; therefore, the restoration of alimentary-tract continuity is postponed for a second operation until after the patient has completely convalesced from the first. After the esophagectomy, the patient is left with an anterior thoracic or cervical esophagostomy plus a gastrostomy for feeding purposes. The substitute esophagus is later introduced by the retrosternal route with an anastomosis performed at the base of the neck, thus avoiding the hazards of intrathoracic reconstruction performed at the time of surgical resection. The time elapsing between the first and second stages is usually three to six months, which allows the nutritive state of the patient to improve.

b) Cancer of the Stomach

Simple subtotal gastrectomy, such as has been commonly practiced for several decades, has not afforded a sufficiently high percentage of cures to satisfy any

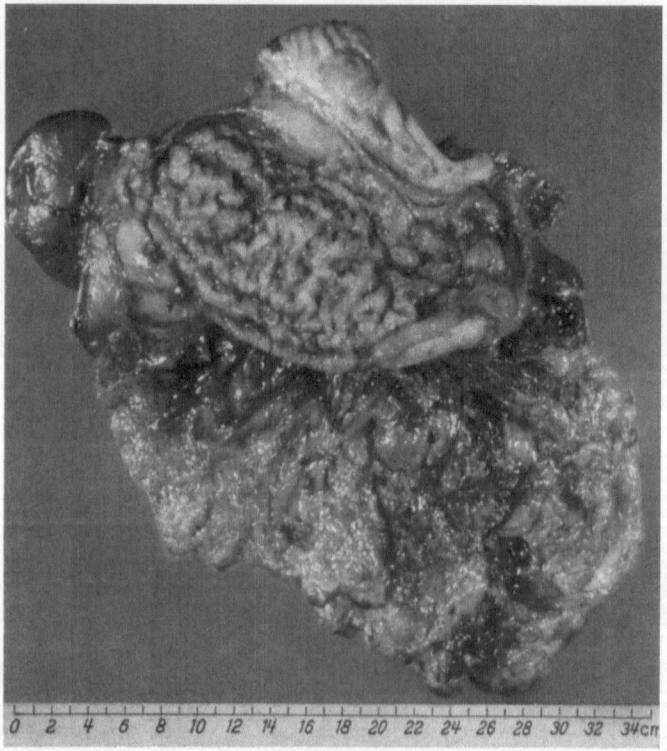

Fig. 2 a

Fig. 2. a) Anaplastic gastric cancer, Grade IV, diffuse, involving all layers. Laparothoracotomy; total gastrectomy, splenectomy, subtotal pancreatectomy. b) Leiomyosarcoma of stomach. Total gastrectomy, splenectomy, partial pancreatectomy. c) Diffuse lymphosarcoma of stomach requiring similar extended gastrectomy. Girl aged 21 years; living and well 12 years after operation. Three children. d) Recurrent lymphosarcoma of stomach. Partial gastrectomy in another country. Recurrent lesion treated by total gastrectomy, partial esophogectomy, intrathoracic esophagojejunostomy. Living and well 14 years

surgeon. Recurrence not only in the residual stomach but in the immediately adjacent lymph nodes has taken place so frequently that it has been obvious that the excision was not adequate enough to remove the cancer. The injection of a visible dye, such as Pontamin sky-blue, into the various segments of the living stomach shows the routes of lymph flow into specific regional groups of lymph nodes. The clearance of the surgical specimens by the Spalteholz technique following resection of the entire stomach, spleen, distal two-thirds of the pancreas, and perigastric tissues reveals unexpected metastases in lymph nodes quite far removed from the site of the primary cancer, and with such uniformity of occurrence as to indicate the need for the standardized procedure known as extended total gastrectomy. In short, for cancers of the middle and superior segments of the stomach, metastases occur so commonly along the entire lesser curvature and the greater curvature of the stomach, including the infrapyloric and retropyloric regions and the lymph nodes in the juxtacardiac groups (right and left) and in the hilum of the spleen and along

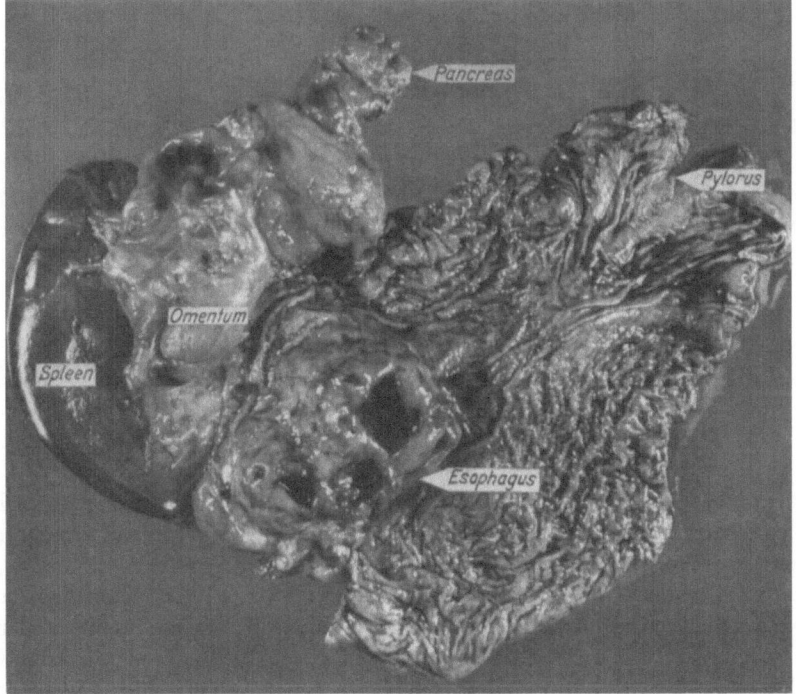

Fig. 2 b

the superior margin of the tail of the pancreas, as in all cases to necessitate total gastrectomy, splenectomy, and subtotal pancreatectomy of the distal pancreas, together with a liberal resection of cuffs of the esophagus and duodenum (PACK, 1965; PACK and ARIEL, 1965). Total gastrectomy such as this (Fig. 2 [a]—[d]) is also indicated for all malignant lymphomas involving the stomach, and for diffusely invading cancers regardless of their location. Cancers of the distal third of the stomach are now treated by a subtotal gastrectomy in which the entire lesser curvature of the stomach downward is included in the specimen and only the greater curvature side of the fundus is preserved for gastrojejunostomy. This operation is completed by a thorough dissection of the retropancreatic and para-aortic lymph

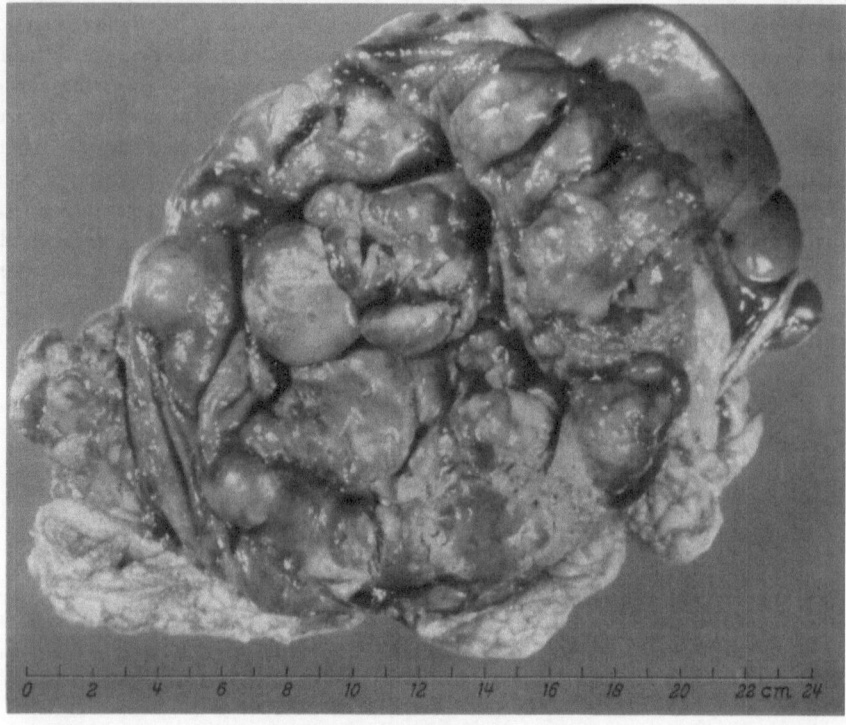

Fig. 2 c

nodes, together with those extending up to the hepatoduodenal ligament. We have some patients living and well for more than ten years after having their entire stomachs removed.

Substitute stomachs have been constructed by interposing segments of the jejunum, transverse colon, or right colon between the esophagus and duodenum or jejunum, in an attempt to afford a temporary reservoir and avoid some of the unpleasant sequelae of total gastrectomy, notably the dumping syndrome. In our hands, these substitute stomachs (with the exception of the Limo-Basto procedure) have seemed to delay rather than prevent the occurrence and the severity of the post-total-gastrectomy syndrome. The characteristic signs and symptoms of this complex are a feeling of weakness, collapse, pallor, perspiration, palpitation, and typical electro-cardiographic changes suggestive of transient coronary spasm. Rapid absorption of carbohydrates in the small intestine, with consequent alterations in potassium levels, hemoconcentration, hyperglycemia, etc., help to produce this symptom complex. The best treatment is to stop excessive sugar and starch intake and institute a high-protein diet with frequent small meals. There is apparently a lessened pancreatic external secretion in a majority of patients, with steatorrhea and slight creatorrhea. The operation as described offers a hope of cure to a greater number of patients.

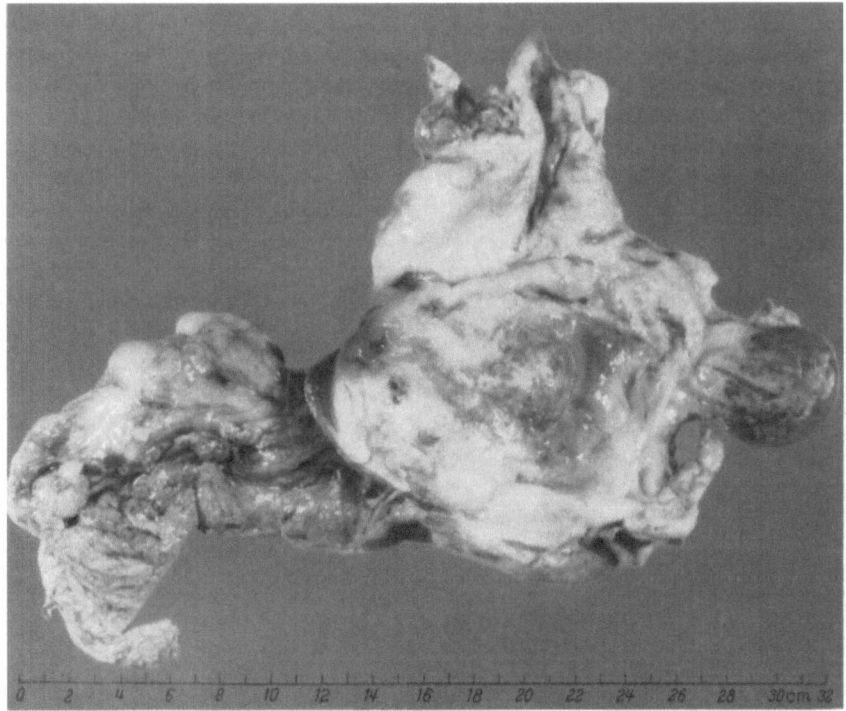

Fig. 2 d

c) Cancer of the Colon

Improvement in the management of cancers of the colon has resulted from the employment of antibiotics for the intestinal tract, the increasing use of a single-stage operation with a primary anastomosis rather than exteriorization, the exercise of proper precautions to prevent blood-borne metastases resulting from dislodgement of tumor emboli in veins during the operation, the adoption of prophylactic measures intended to lessen the hazard of implanting cancer in the line of the anastomosis, and the extension of the operation to ensure complete removal of the primary growth as well as of any metastasis that may be present. Investigators have with surprising frequency detected the presence of cancer cells within the mesenteric veins in the surgically resected segments of bowel. Furthermore, pathologists making many microscopic sections to study the intramural or invasive growth of cancers of the colon have found blood vessel invasion by the cancer in 20—30 % of patients. In the hope of lessening the frequency of hepatic metastases, the initial step in resection of the large bowel should be the immediate ligation of vessels of the mesentery before the cancer-bearing segment is manipulated. Ligation of the colon well above and well below the cancer is another precautionary step; the subsequent transection of the bowel is performed well above and well below the ligatures. The lumen of the bowel is antisepticized prior to the anastomosis. In theory, these measures prevent the breaking off of loose cancer tissue in the bowel and implantation in the line of the anastomosis.

Stimulated by the good results obtained through orthodox hemicolectomy for cancers of the right bowel, the magnitude of this operation being rendered necessary by the presence of one supporting artery, surgeons are now, in an effort to improve the cure rate, treating cancers of the descending and sigmoid colon by left hemicolectomy to an extent comparable with that for the right half of the colon. The rectum proper and the rectosigmoid are viable because of, and dependent solely on, the inferior and middle hemorrhoidal arteries. Knowing this, one may remove the splenic flexure, the descending colon, and the sigmoid colon, with anastomosis of the transverse colon to the rectosigmoid after proper mobilization. The marginal branch of the middle colic artery furnishes an adequate blood supply to the mobilized transverse colon employed for the anastomosis. The ligation of the inferior mesenteric artery at its origin from the aorta, with dissection of the para-aortic lymph nodes and a wide excision of the mesentery, enables the lymph nodes that may be implicated by metastases to be more completely removed. C. NAUNTON MORGAN, at St. Mark's Hospital, London, found that approximately 14% of 1000 surgically

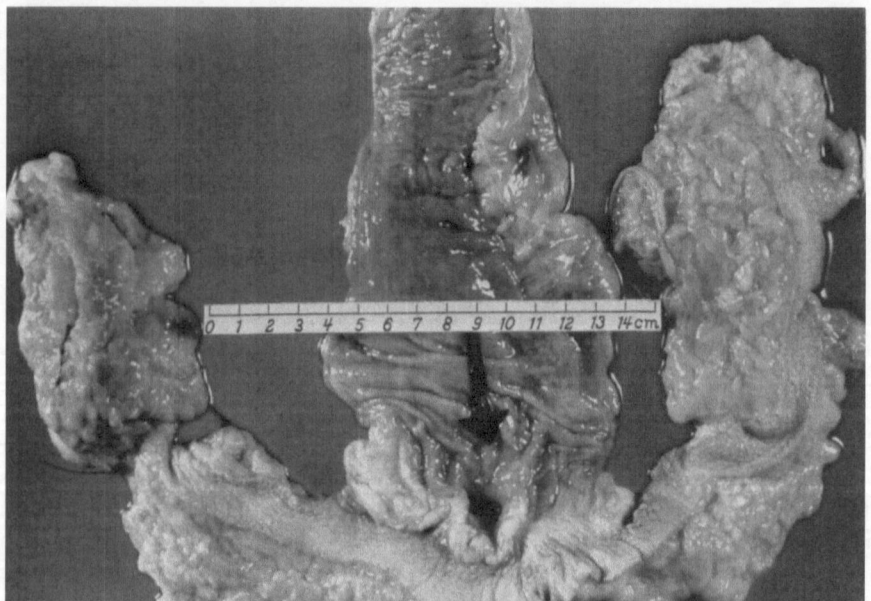

Fig. 3 a

Fig. 3. a) Rectal cancer involving anus. Abdominoperineal rectal resection in continuity with bilateral groin dissection. b) Postoperative view. Colostomy; wide sacrifice of perianal skin. Invasive cancers implicating anus and perianal lymphatics can metastasize to medial superficial inguinal lymph nodes. c) Multicentric cancers of colon and rectum associated with diffuse polyposis require total colectomy and rectal resection. d) Epidermoid carcinoma involving anus, rectum, and entire posterior vaginal wall neessitates panhysterectomy, abdominoperineal rectal resection, vaginectomy. e) This female patient had melanoma of anorectum, epidermoid carcinoma of anus, early polypoid adenocarcinoma of rectum, metastases in groin, and invasion of vagina. Living and well 9 years. Treated by abdominoperineal rectal resection, vaginectomy, bilateral groin dissection in continuity. Perineal view one year later. f) Same patient as in e). Healed groin dissections and colostomy
(arrow)

resected specimens had metastases in regional lymph nodes extending as far as the base of the inferior mesenteric artery. This proves that this more radical procedure would offer a better opportunity of cure. It is not employed in patients who are very obese or poor operative risks. Whenever colonic cancers are associated with diffuse intestinal polyposis, total colectomy is done with an attempt to preserve the rectum, and the operation is completed by ileoproctostomy. Any residual polyps in the rectum, if benign, are removed subsequently by endothermy excision and cauterization.

d) Cancer of the Rectum

The classic operation of abdominoperineal rectal resection has maintained its deserved reputation for the past two generations. As originally conceived and executed, it was a two-dimensional dissection, quite adequate upwards and also

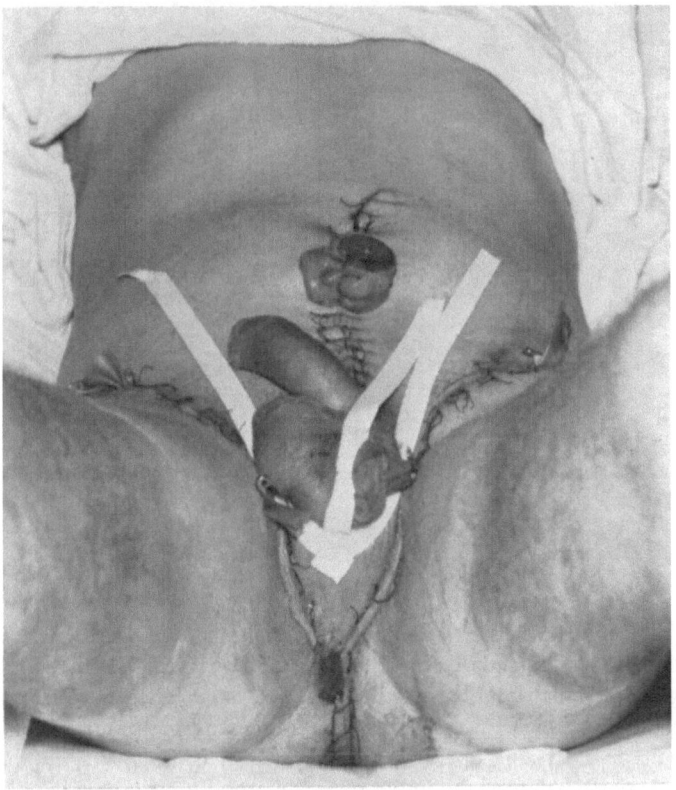

Fig. 3 b

below because it included the anus, but not sufficiently radical in removing the lateral spread of cancer or the uppermost group of vulnerable lymph nodes. The present three-dimensional rectal resection not only removes the rectum from the hollow of the sacrum and from the base of the bladder or the cervix and vagina but also the lymph nodes in the iliac and obturator groups. Fifteen to 20% of patients in whom the pelvic lymph nodes are excised are found to have metastatic cancer involving these nodes, even though the metastases were not clinically detectable at the time of the operation. The upper extent of the operation has also been increased to include the mesentery and lymph nodes as high as the origin of the superior hemorrhoidal

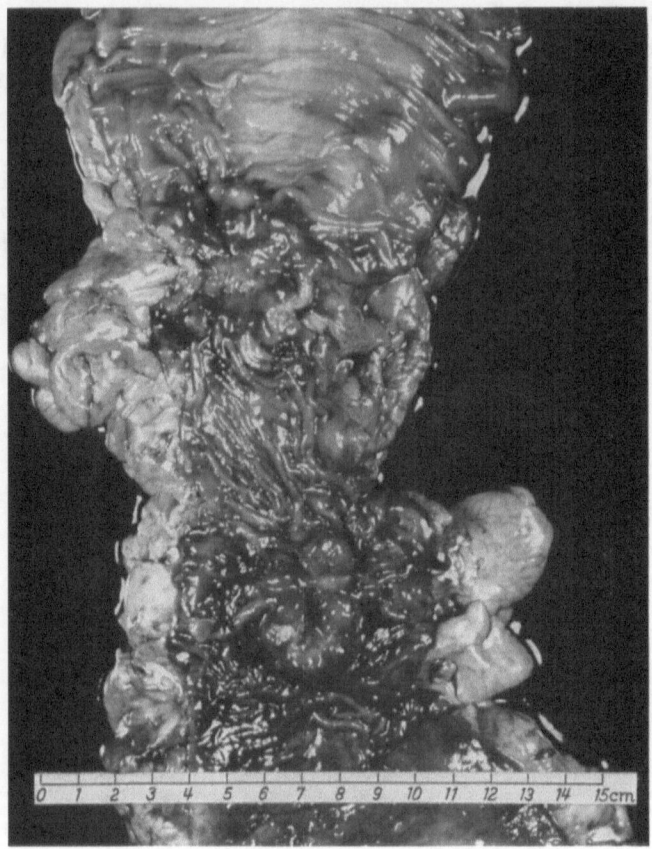

Fig. 3 c

vessels. If the cancer, whether it is adenocarcinoma or malignant melanoma (PACK and MARTINS, 1960), extends down into the anorectal canal, with dermal invasion implicating the perianal lymphatics, the operation is extended to include abdomino-perineal rectal resection, with dissection of the iliac and obturator lymph nodes and, in the female, at the same operative seance and in continuity with the anorectal specimen, a major portion of the vulva plus a bilateral groin dissection. The inguinal and femoral nodes are removed in continuity with the specimen, including the inter-vening lymphatics in the skin and subcutaneous tissues. If the patient is a male, the same operative technique applies, with bilateral groin dissection and a liberal sacrifice of perianal and scrotal skin in continuity.

There are four different operations from which may be chosen the one most suitable for the patient, depending upon the extent and location of the cancer (Fig. 3). They are: (1) total colectomy and rectal resection for rectal cancers asso-ciated with colonic polyposis; (2) abdominoperineal resection, supplemented by pelvic lymph node dissection; (3) pelvic evisceration for rectal cancers involving contiguous organs; and (4) conservative rectal resection with preservation of sphincter control. It may appear a strange paradox that one who advocates and practices

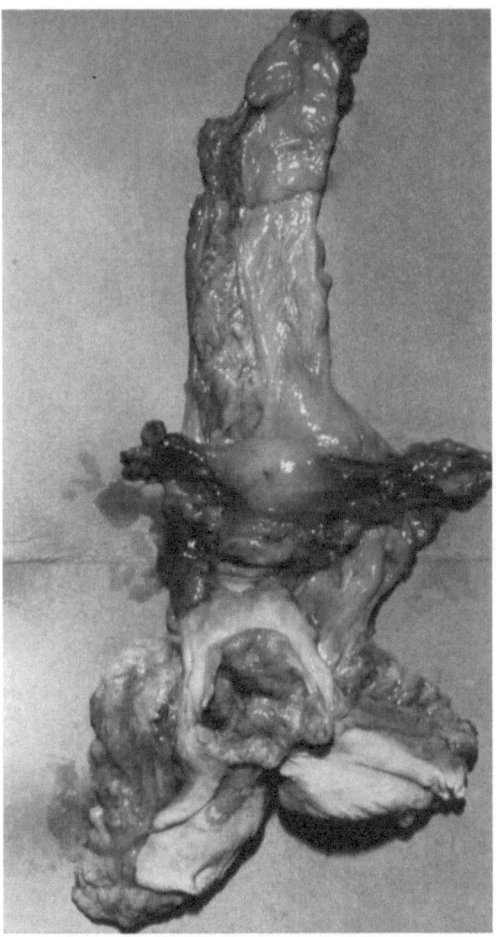

Fig. 3 d

radical surgical treatment for most cancers should at the same time advocate the conservative treatment of rectal cancers in *selected* cases. I am of the opinion that a definite place exists for preservation of the rectal sphincter. Some surgeons who have persistently advocated preservation of the rectal sphincter unfortunately have attempted to increase the indications for this operation until, ultimately, the recurrence rate becomes so high that the operation is abandoned altogether. A middle course is indicated. If a rectal cancer is polypoid, if it is freely movable, if it is sessile, if it does not encircle the bowel, if it is Grade II or Grade I, and if it is situated well above the anal sphincter, one of several measures may be adopted for removing it without sacrificing the rectal sphincter. If the cancer is at the level of the rectosigmoid or slightly above it - i. e., above the level of the peritoneal

reflection — and if it is a very early cancer, a superior segmental resection can be performed with primary anastomosis through an abdominal approach. Another procedure
we have sometimes employed is a modification of the ancient "pull through" operation

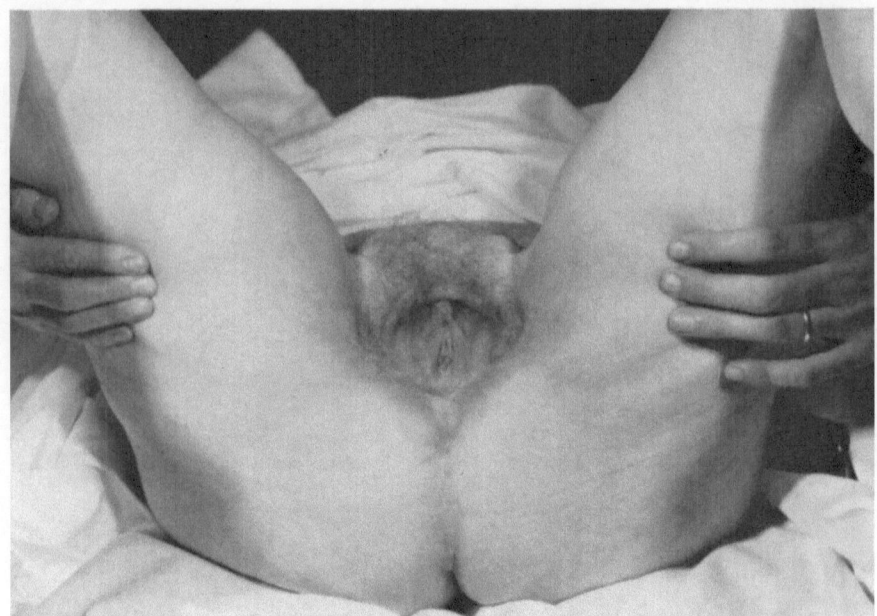

Fig. 3 e

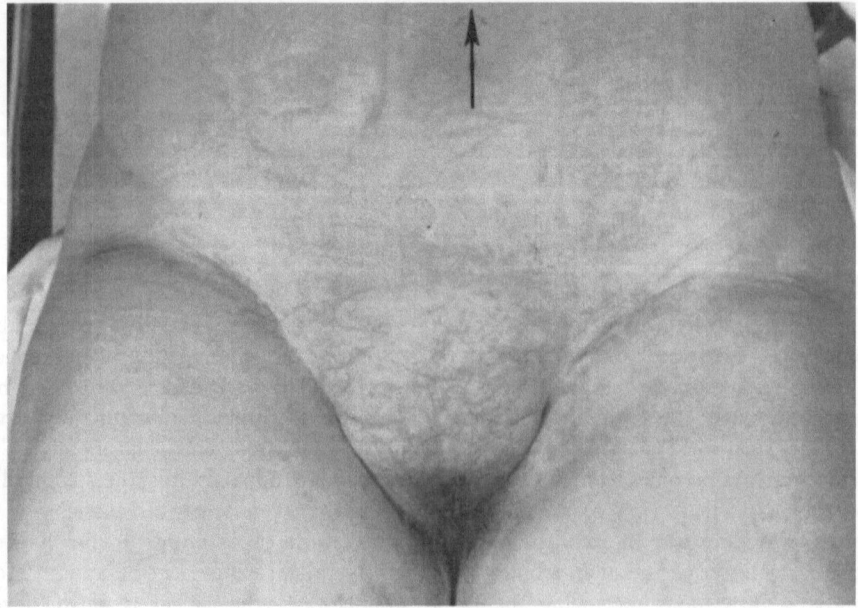

Fig. 3 f

of Hochenegg. The intussusception of the rectum or rectosigmoid cannot be prolapsed readily through the manually dilated but intact sphincter in patients who are fat or have much fat in the mesentery or round the rectum and the sigmoid colon. But in a thin subject with an early cancer of this type it is a very satisfactory and easy method of resection. Mobilization of the bowel in an abdominal approach must be more complete than in the ordinary abdominoperineal resection, and the bowel is dissected neatly and completely down to the pelvic floor. After abdominal mobilization of the rectosigmoid and rectum, the patient is placed in the lithotomy position and the rectum is intussuscepted by traction so that even the anal canal is turned inside out. The tumor is then readily visible on the outside surface. The resection and anastomosis are then done externally, and afterward the anastomosed bowel can easily be pushed upward through the temporarily relaxed sphincter. Although I advocate pelvic evisceration on the one hand and a conservative operation for selected early cancers of the rectum on the other, I should like to emphasize that meticulous surgical judgment must always be exercised in choosing cases for these procedures.

4. Surgical Treatment of Cancer of the Pancreas

The enthusiasm that followed the institution of the operation of subtotal pancreatectomy with duodenectomy for cancers of the head of the pancreas and of the ampulla of Vater has been tempered with the passage of time by the realization that

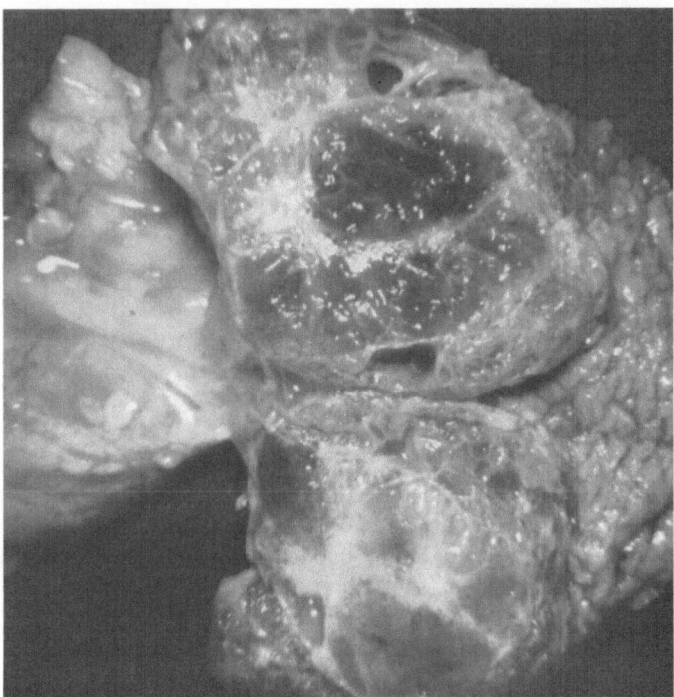

Fig. 4 a

Fig. 4. a) Successful pancreatoduodenectomy for huge cystadenoma of pancreas containing multicentric cancerous foci. b) Total pancreatoduodenectomy and splenectomy

this operation does not cure the majority of patients. Palliation is achieved, but few cancers of the pancreas proper are cured, though the salvage rate is much better for periampullary carcinomas. Surgical removal of the head of the pancreas together with the entire duodenum has not been sufficient to prevent even local extension of the disease, to say nothing of distant or visceral metastases. Examination of pancreatic juice obtained from the duct of Wirsung at the time of transection of the pancreas has shown viable cancer cells. Furthermore, the operation as originally conceived does not provide for an adequate dissection of peripancreatic lymph nodes. More recently, the operation (Fig. 4) has been extended to include total

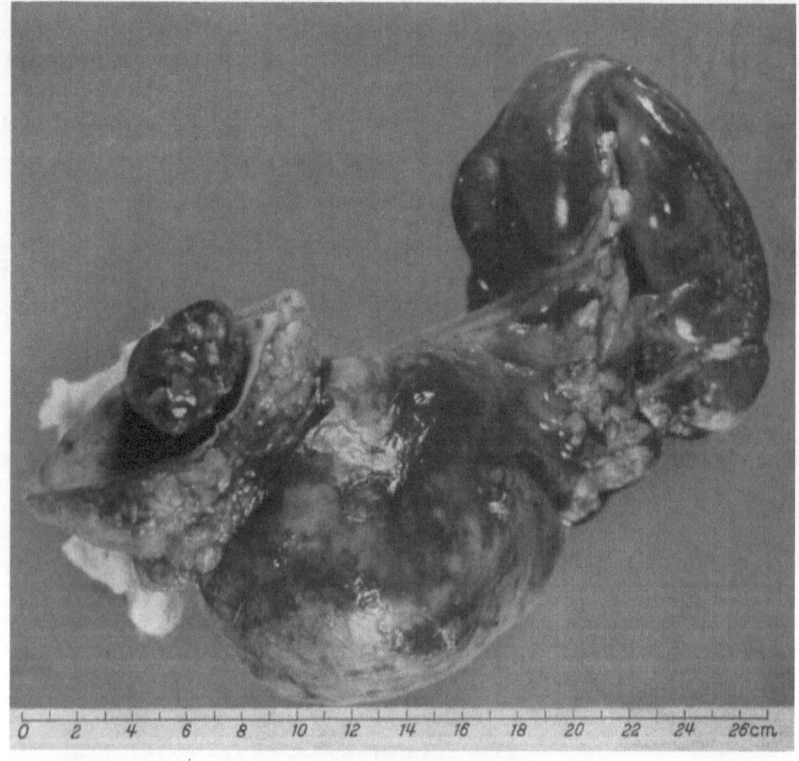

Fig. 4 b

pancreatectomy, splenectomy, and dissection of all the peripancreatic lymph nodes, particularly along the splenic pedicle and the superior margin of the pancreas and, after mobilization and resection of the duodenum and head of the pancreas from the superior mesenteric vein, of the retropancreatic and para-aortic lymph nodes as well as those extending up along the hepatoduodenal ligament.

The diabetes resulting from total pancreatectomy is more easily regulated with a standard dose of insulin and a dietary regimen than is the usual spontaneous diabetes occurring in a patient with a diseased pancreas. Thus it is not a great postoperative handicap. With the prolongation of life provided by this extirpative procedure, it has now become apparent that cancer of the pancreas is an extremely malignant neoplasm with a tendency for widespread visceral metastases that militate against the prospect of ultimate cure.

During the last three decades many variations and compromises have been suggested for postoperative reconstruction of the extrinsic biliary and upper gastro-intestinal tracts after pancreatoduodenectomy. The procedure we have routinely employed is the simplest possible. The transected jejunum below the ligament of Treitz is mobilized and brought up through the transverse mesocolon for a retrocolic type of direct or end-to-end choledochojejunostomy. A jejunal loop below the mesocolon is elevated and employed for a terminolateral type of gastrojejunostomy as an antecolic anastomosis. This reconstruction entails only two anastomotic procedures, one retrocolic and one antecolic, the latter to some extent ensuring that there will not be excessive regurgitation of gastric contents and food into the common bile duct, with the hazard of ascending cholangitis. The residual gallbladder is drained externally for the purpose of relieving undue pressure on the recent cholangiojejunostomy.

5. Hepatic Lobectomy for Tumors of the Liver

Surgeons have been reluctant to perform major hepatectomies, being intimidated by two possibilities: first, the danger of intractable and perhaps fatal hemorrhage

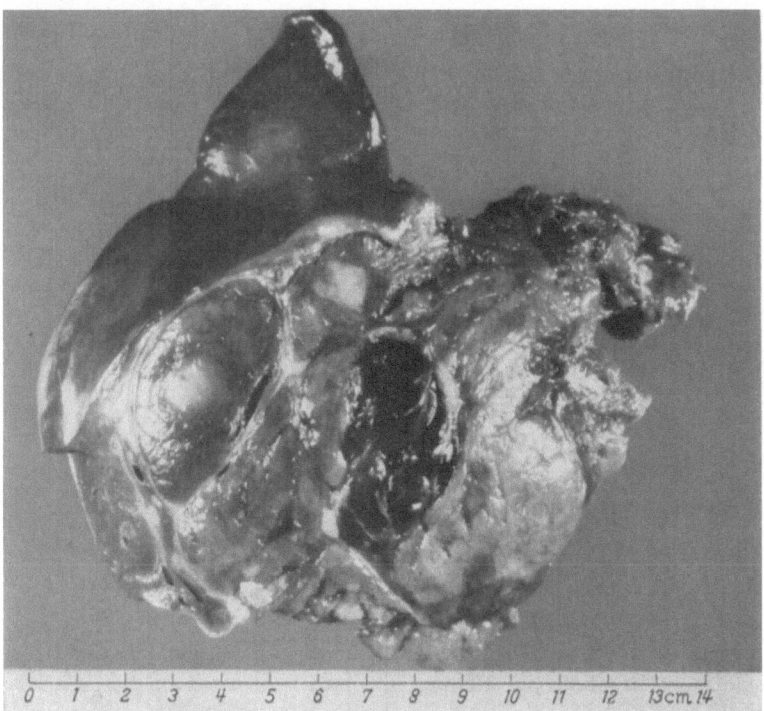

Fig. 5 a

Fig. 5. a) Hepatoma in infant requiring left hepatic lobectomy; 5½-year cure. b) Total right hepatic lobectomy for metastatic cancer of colon. c) Photograph of patient taken in operating room, to show residual left lateral segment after surgical removal of right lobe and medial segment of left lobe (extended right hepatic lobectomy). d) Photograph of patient 18 months after surgical removal of 80% of liver; to show globular regenerative hyperplasia of liver

because of the complexities of the triple circulation (i. e., the high-pressure arterial
flow through the hepatic artery, comprising 40% of the inflow, the low-pressure
venous flow through the portal vein, comprising 60% of the inflow, and the
intricate biliary circulation); and second, the danger of interfering with some of the
no fewer than 70 important functions attributed to the liver, many of which are
vital (PACK and ISLAMI, 1964).

As regards the surgical anatomy, the liver is a bipartite organ, because the
arterial supplies to the right and left lobes do not commingle across the interlobar
fissure (PACK and ISLAMI, 1962, 1964). However, the portal venous circulation does
traverse the main dividing septum, inasmuch as the left portal branch is comprised
of the union of several vessels such as the left umbilical vein carrying arterial blood
in the embryo, the ductus Arantii, and others; this composite left portal vein sends
recurrent intrahepatic branches across the septum to drain into the caudate and
quadrate lobes. If a surgeon wishes to remove the right lobe or do an extended right
hepatic lobectomy to include the medial segment of the left lobe or the left lobe
of the liver independently, he should exercise vascular control by preliminary
ligation of the corresponding hepatic artery, portal vein, and bile duct to that
particular segment. The only other vessels to be ligated in the operation are the

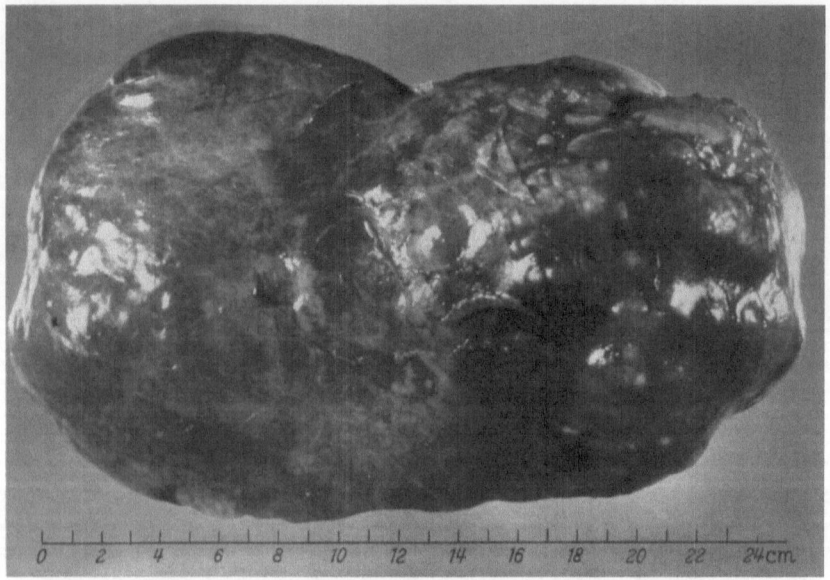

Fig. 5 b

several hepatic veins emptying into the vena cava on the right side and one important single large hepatic vein draining the lateral segment of the left lobe. The
operation is relatively bloodless and is safe if performed by this technique (Fig. 5)
(PACK and ISLAMI, 1965).

The indications for removal of the lobe of the liver include primary liver cancers,
either hepatocarcinomas or cholangiocarcinomas, when they are unilobar in origin
and distribution. Invasive carcinoma of the gallbladder with extension into the

liver substance calls for total right hepatic lobectomy, since invasion of the liver, which is a vascular sponge, inevitably results in intrahepatic metastasis or dissemination to the portal lobules (PACK and BRASFIELD, 1955 a). Nothing short of

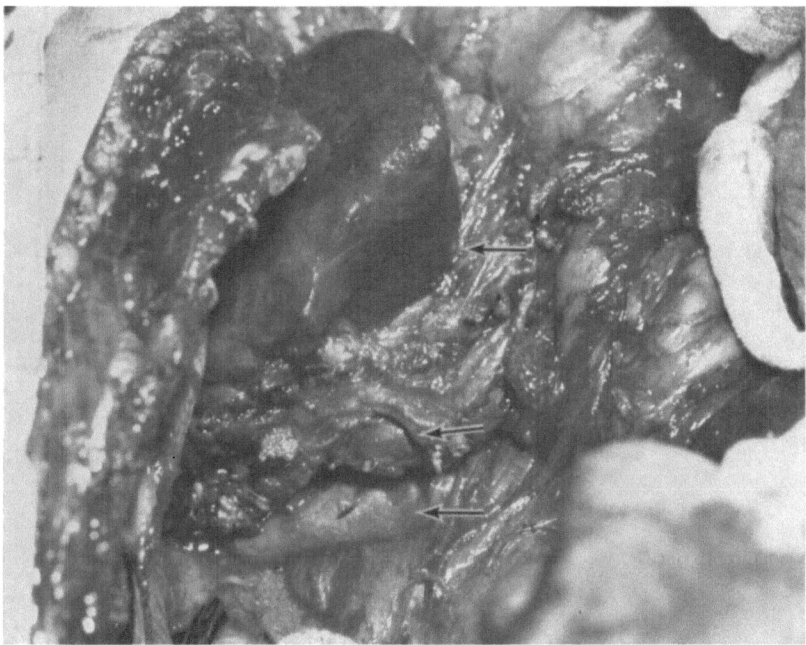

Fig. 5 c

removal of the entire lobe will give the patient a prospect of cure. I have removed the right lobe of the liver in several instances for malignant mesenchymal tumors such as fibrosarcoma and leiomyosarcoma.

Metastases to the liver may in some instances entail a total lobectomy, right or left. The decision to perform such a major operation for metastatic cancer, either sarcoma or carcinoma, requires critical judgement. Hepatic metastases, from the sequence of their appearance, may be termed precocious, synchronous, or metachronous (PACK and BRASFIELD, 1955 b). When a huge nodular liver is the first indication of a cancer of undiscovered origin, the primary cancer is usually so small as to be asymptomatic, but on the other hand it is often highly malignant, anaplastic, and very cellular, so that the prospect of affording palliative relief through removal of the primary cancer, wherever located, and hepatic lobectomy is not good. Still, we have had patients who have had a comfortable life of worthwhile duration following such double operations.

In the case of synchronous metastases in which the primary cancer in, for example the rectum or colon is discovered at the same time as the metastases, or at operation, the decision to proceed with hepatic lobectomy and, say, rectal or colon resection as a two-stage operation will depend on the judgement of the surgeon at the time. Metachronous metastases in which the patient has apparently been cured of the primary cancer with no evidence of local recurrence, only to have the metastasis in the liver appear at a much later date, would theoretically seem more favorable for such a major procedure as hepatic lobectomy. The procedure may be used for ocular melanomas metastatisizing to the liver of recent date.

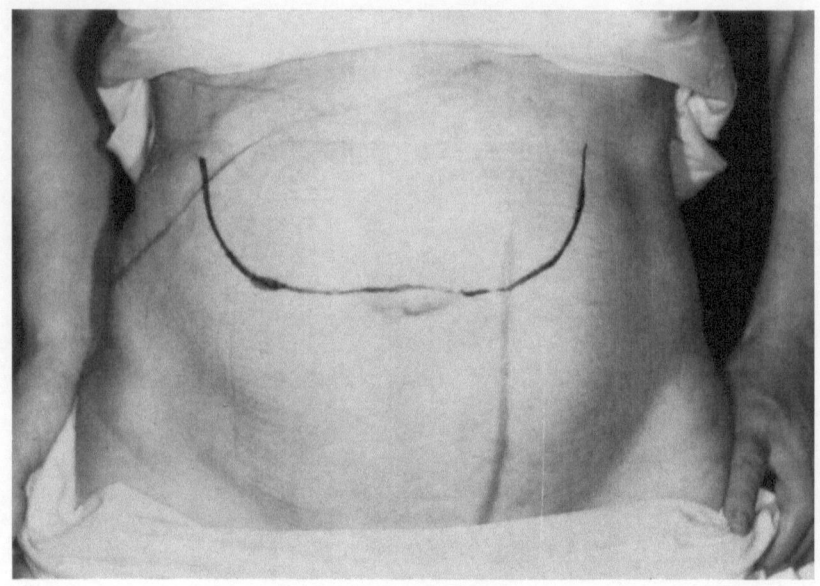

Fig. 5 d

The right lobe and the medial segment of the left lobe together comprise 80 % of the total weight of the organ. It is amazing that the lateral segment of the left lobe, comprising less than 20 % of the liver substance, is sufficient to maintain life and carry out all of the important functions of the liver. All of the portal blood, of course, is deflected to the lateral segment of the left lobe when an *extended* right hepatic lobectomy is done including the right lobe and the medial segment of the left lobe or all liver tissue to the right of the sagittal fissure. The remaining segment undergoes immediate regenerative hyperplasia (PACK, ISLAMI, HUBBARD and BRAS-FIELD, 1962). Even in the human, this segment of the liver may expand so as ultimately to have as large a volume as a previously intact normal liver. We have previously studied the factors that are influential in promoting regenerative hyper-plasia of the liver in laboratory animals.

6. Surgical Treatment of Cancer of the Breast

a) Extended Radical Mastectomy with Internal Mammary Lymph Node Dissection

The principle of *en bloc* excision and dissection in continuity for primary cancers metastasizing to adjacent regional lymph nodes has found general acceptance. The first standardized application of this principle followed the independent descriptions of so-called radical mastectomy by HALSTED and by WILLY MEYER in 1894. The operation embodies the sacrifice of the breast containing the primary cancer, together with complete dissection of the adjacent accessible regional lymph nodes in which metastases have occurred or might occur and, equally important, a wide swathe of intervening tissue with the communicating lymphatics. It has now been definitely established that the internal mammary lymph node chain and the corresponding axillary nodes constitute the two primary groups draining the lymphatics of the breast. Secondary extension from these two primary depots is to the supraclavicular nodes and ultimately into the jugulosubclavian venous junction. The extended radical mastectomy, therefore, aims essentially at resection in continuity of certain lymph channels and nodes which represent a primary echelon of metastatic spread (the internal mammary chain) or secondary or even tertiary echelons (PACK and BRAS-FIELD, 1963). Chest wall recurrences in the costochondral region, for example, are most likely to be manifestations of metastases to the internal mammary lymphatic

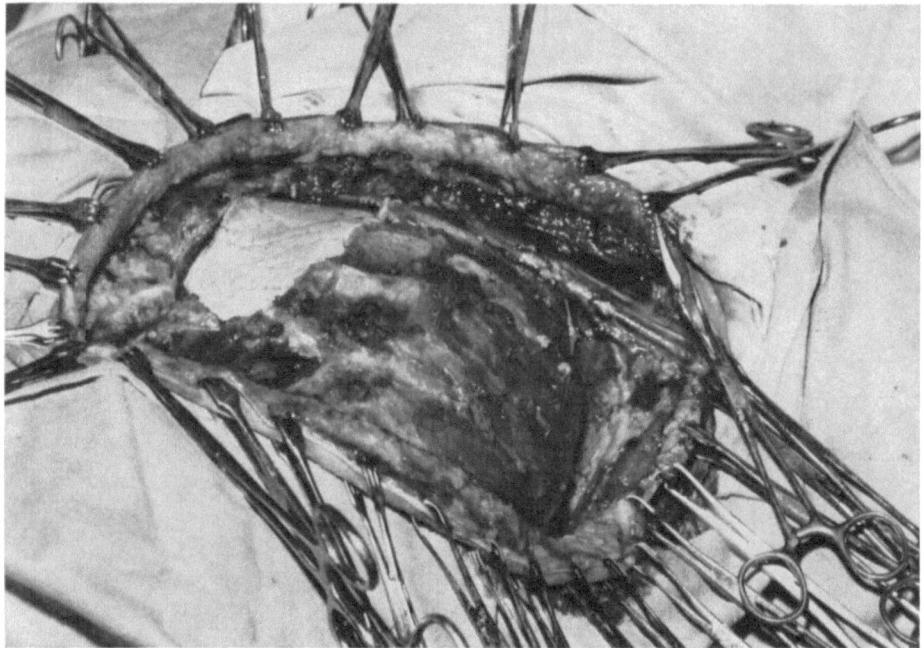

Fig. 6 a

Fig. 6. a) Extended radical mastectomy with internal mammary node dissection. Fascial graft to close the chest-wall defect. Metastasis in one internal mammary node. b) Same patient. Wound defect. [a) and b) from Pack & Brasfield (1963), courtesy. Archives of Surgery.] c) In 1937, at age 22 years, patient improperly received radiation therapy to both breasts for diffuse microcystic mastitis. Photograph 24 years later revealing bilateral diffuse ductal cancer. Treatment: simultaneous bilateral radical mastectomy

chain. The plastron no longer constitutes an insurmountable barrier to the attack upon breast cancer. One cannot ignore the high incidence of metastases to the internal mammary chain of lymph nodes which occurs in certain breast cancers and has been so thoroughly investigated by URBAN, HANDLEY, DAHL-IVERSEN, and others. It has been our routine practice, in all breast cancers situated in the medial segment of the breast and particularly those in the subareolar or central segment, to perform an extended radical mastectomy consisting of the orthodox procedure with axillary

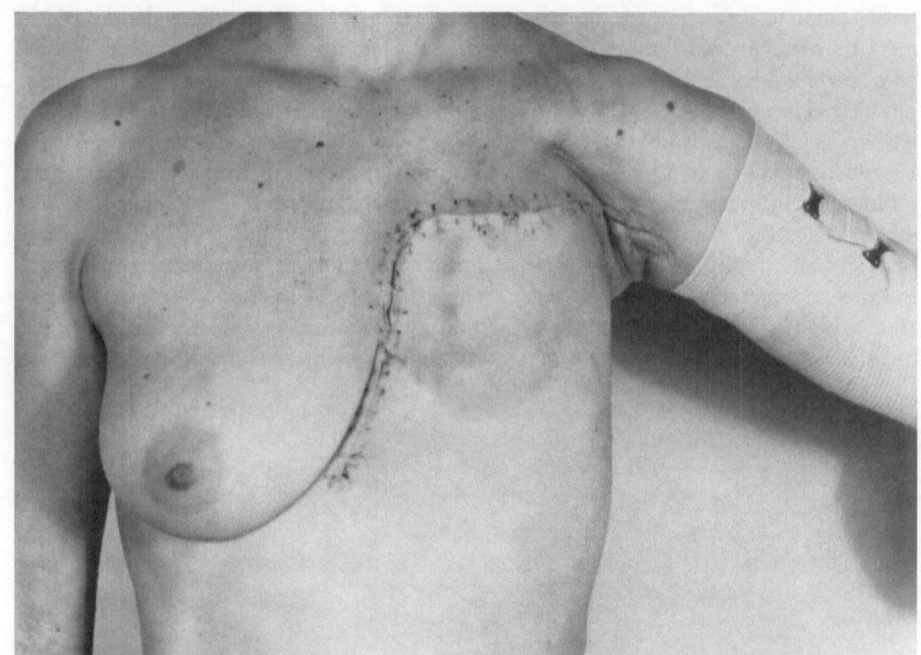

Fig. 6 b

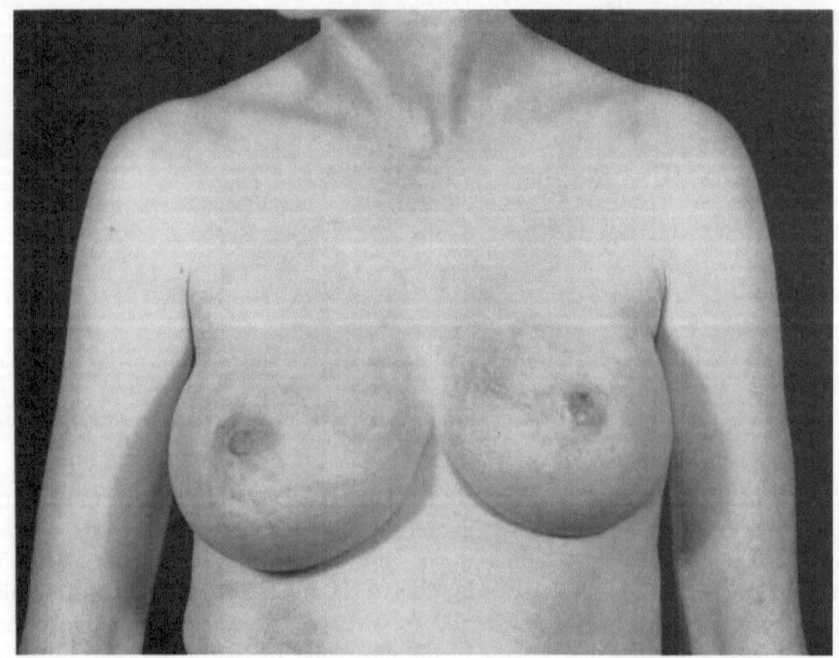

Fig. 6 c

lymph node dissection, plus the removal of a rectangular segment of the chest wall at the sternocostal junction incorporating the internal mammary chain of lymph nodes, which are involved by metastasis in approximately 40 % of patients (Fig. 6). The defect in the chest wall is closed by the insertion of a graft of fascia lata, either autogenous or ox fascia.

b) Argument for Bilateral Mastectomy

Thirty-five years ago, the proportion of women undergoing radical mastectomy for unilateral cancer who subsequently developed cancer in the remaining breast was approximately 3 %. With earlier diagnosis in succeeding years, the number increased to 8 %. The most common precancerous disease of the breast is that found in the remaining breast after mastectomy. It is an indisputable fact that both breasts are subject to the same carcinogenic, hormonal, and genetic influences (PACK, 1951). Meticulous studies of the breast other than the cancerous one, obtained either by surgical removal or at the necropsy table, have provided rewarding information about precancerous lesions, carcinomas in situ, that are not clinically identifiable. In a more recent survey described to me by G. F. ROBBINS, he and J. W. BERG found that among women under 45 years of age whose expectation of life under normal conditions would be good and whose cancers were confined to the breast alone or involved only the lowermost axillary lymph nodes, more than 20 % ultimately developed cancer in the remaining breast. This study indicates that these young women with early cancers live long enough for cancer in the opposite breast to develop, become detected, and treated. Once the objections of the lay public and a recalcitrant medical profession are overcome, the most important improvement in the therapy of breast cancers since the institution of internal mammary node dissection may well be immediate bilateral mastectomy with a transverse incision permitting simple mastectomy for the apparently inoffensive breast and conventional radical mastectomy for the cancerous member of the pair. It is my opinion that the opposite breast should *always* be removed, even if a secondary surgical procedure is involved, whenever the pathologist finds *multicentric* cancer in the first surgical specimen. X-ray mammography has so proved its worth that the therapist should *always* have the apparently normal breast subjected to this refined radiographic scrutiny before performing a unilateral mastectomy for known cancer. The number of unsuspected cancers detected by this means makes this procedure highly rewarding to the patient and surgeon alike.

7. Surgical Treatment of Pulmonary Cancer

The indications and technique for pneumonectomy for cancer are now well established and do not require recapitulation here. Simple pneumonectomy has been replaced by the more adequate operation of pneumonectomy plus meticulous dissection of the hilar and mediastinal lymph nodes, even in the absence of evidence of metastatic involvement. With the primary cancer well situated in the substance of the lobe, without hilar invasion, a lobectomy offers practically as good results as a total pneumonectomy, provided mediastinal nodal dissection is done. When there is extension of the cancer with deposits in the pleura, both visceral and parietal, some surgeons perform a pleuropneumonectomy as a palliative measure. Whenever a pneumonectomy is technically possible but the mediastinal lymph nodes are fixed and non-resectable, exposure permits interstitial infiltration of radioactive isotopes throughout the metastatic cancer in the mediastinum. A suspension of radioactive ceramic microspheres, each containing aliquot parts of radioactive yttrium-90, may be accurately distributed throughout the involved mediastinum and thus deliver a large and properly distributed dose of irradiation. This sometimes achieves worthwhile palliation.

8. The Principle of Excision and Dissection in Continuity (En Bloc Excision) for Cancers Metastasizing to Accessible Regional Lymph Nodes

Ever since the application of the principle of *en bloc* excision independently by HALSTED and WILLY MEYER for cancer of the breast and by Sir ERNEST MILES in the classic abdominoperineal resection, the principle has been employed, particularly

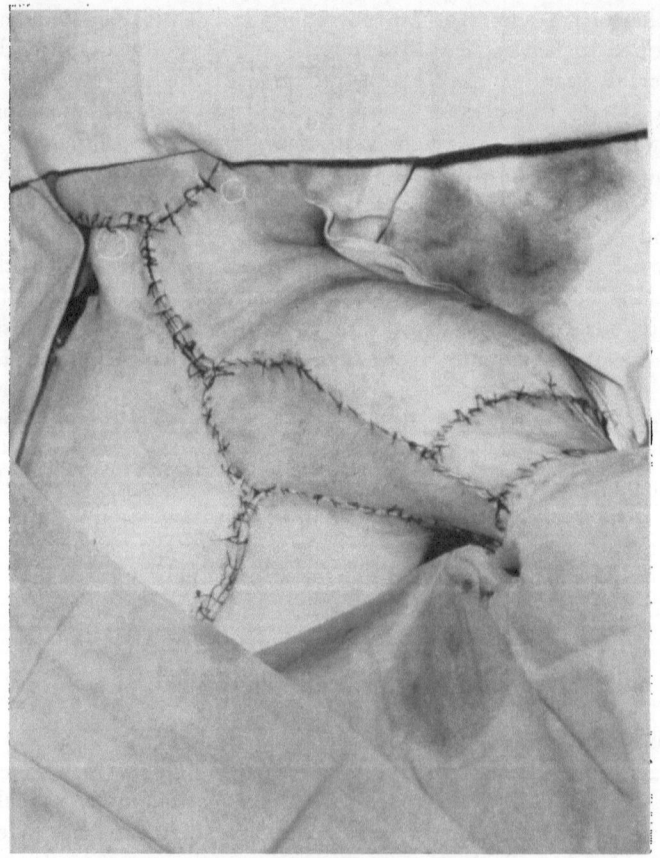

Fig. 7 a

Fig. 7. a) Melanoma of skin of left arm metastatic to axillary and lower cervical lymph nodes. Excision and dissection in continuity with axillary and neck dissection, claviculectomy, and skin grafting. b) Same patient; living and well 11 years later. [a) from PACK, G. T., CA — Cancer Journal for Clinicians 12, 11 (1962)], courtesy American Cancer Society.]

for cancers of the oral group (e. g., lip, tongue, floor of the mouth, inferior alveolus), thyroid cancer, certain cancers of the vulva and penis, cancers of the uterine cervix, and cancers of the rectum, for which pelvic lymph-node dissection is feasible. The operation embodies the sacrifice of the viscus or skin containing the primary cancer or an adequate removal of the tissue, e. g., skin, which contains it, together with complete dissection of the adjacent and accessible regional lymph nodes into which metastases have occurred or might occur and, equally important, a wide swathe of intervening tissue with the communicating lymphatics (PACK and ARIEL, 1958; PACK, SCHARNAGEL and MORFIT, 1945).

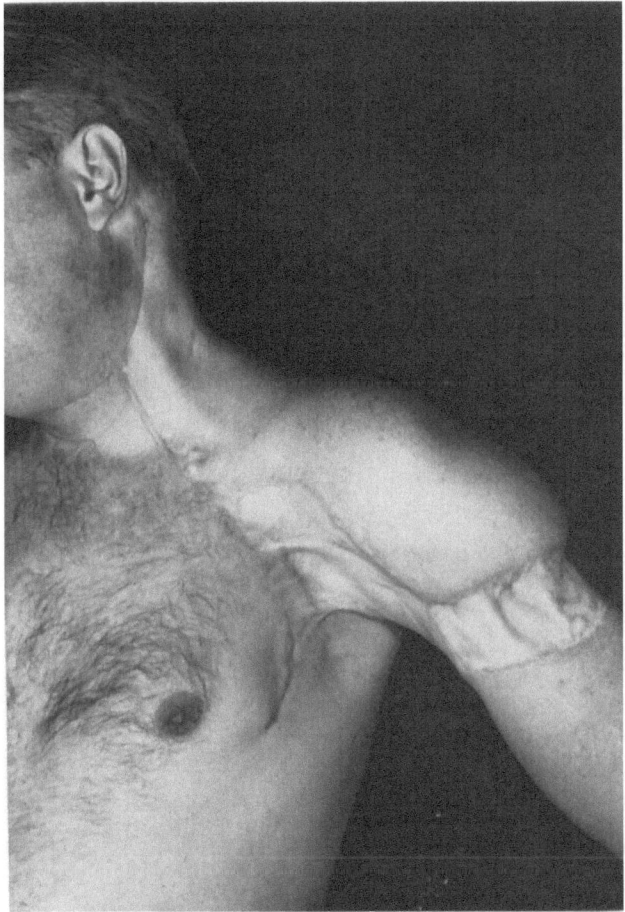

Fig. 7 b

a) Cancers of the Skin

Apart from superficial early epidermoid carcinomas, which can be treated satisfactorily by conservative excision or by irradiation, and basal cell cancers, there remains a group of anaplastic carcinomas and malignant melanomas capable of spreading, most commonly by the lymphatic route, to the regional lymph nodes,

which will be involved as a first relay in metastasis. The principle of *en bloc* excision
has found an application for many years in the treatment of melanomas of various
locations. Since melanomas may occur (although with different frequency) in the skin
of any region, it follows that many bizarre and planned incisions must be designed,

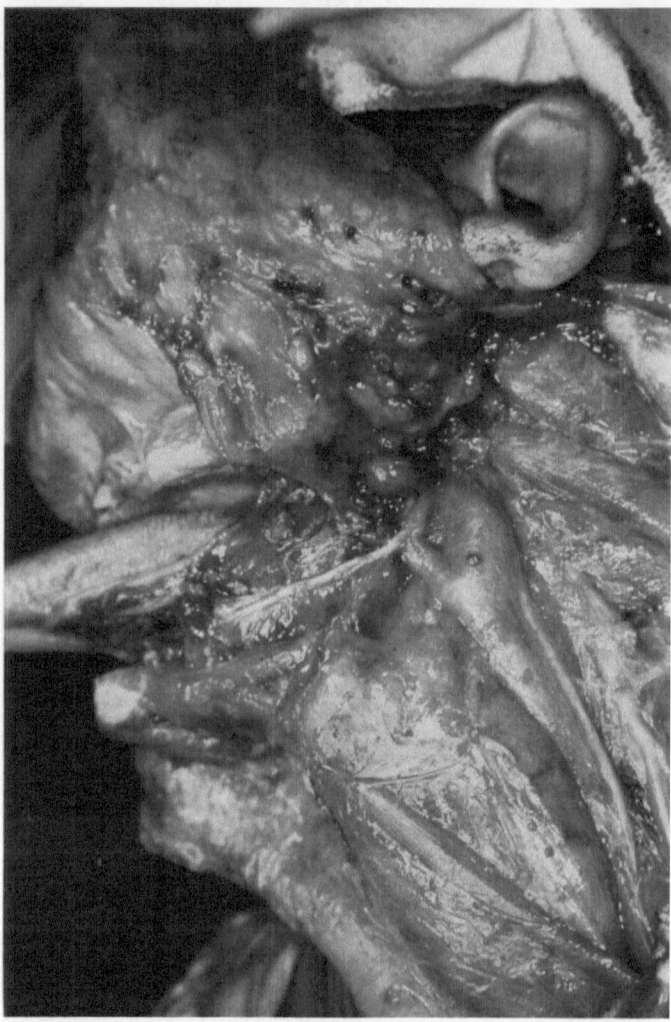

Fig. 8 a

Fig. 8. a) Cancer of the tongue and floor of the mouth with metastasis to cervical lymph nodes. Treatment by
composite resection and dissection in continuity with hemimandibulectomy. b) Another patient with a similar
distribution of primary oral cancer except that bilateral radical neck dissection was necessary. Postoperative
view. (Courtesy Dr. JOHN CONLEY, Pack Medical Group.)

each of sufficient scope to include the primary melanoma and the first relay of
lymphatic metastases. Some of these operations will also necessitate dissection of
cervical, axillary, inguinal, femoral, or iliac nodes and, in unusual circumstances,
of two such regional groups, e. g., (1) both axillae (midsternal or midvertebral

melanomas); (2) cervical and axillary (melanomas of the skin of the upper pectoral or scapular regions [Fig. 7]); (3) both groins (melanomas of the vulva, penis, and anal skin) (PACK and REKERS, 1964). For melanomas or anaplastic carcinomas remotely situated from the regional nodes involved or liable to future involvement, such as primary tumors on the hands and feet, excision and dissection in continuity manifestly cannot be performed. The lymph nodes are carefully dissected and removed, even if there is no clinical evidence of their enlargement or invasion. The

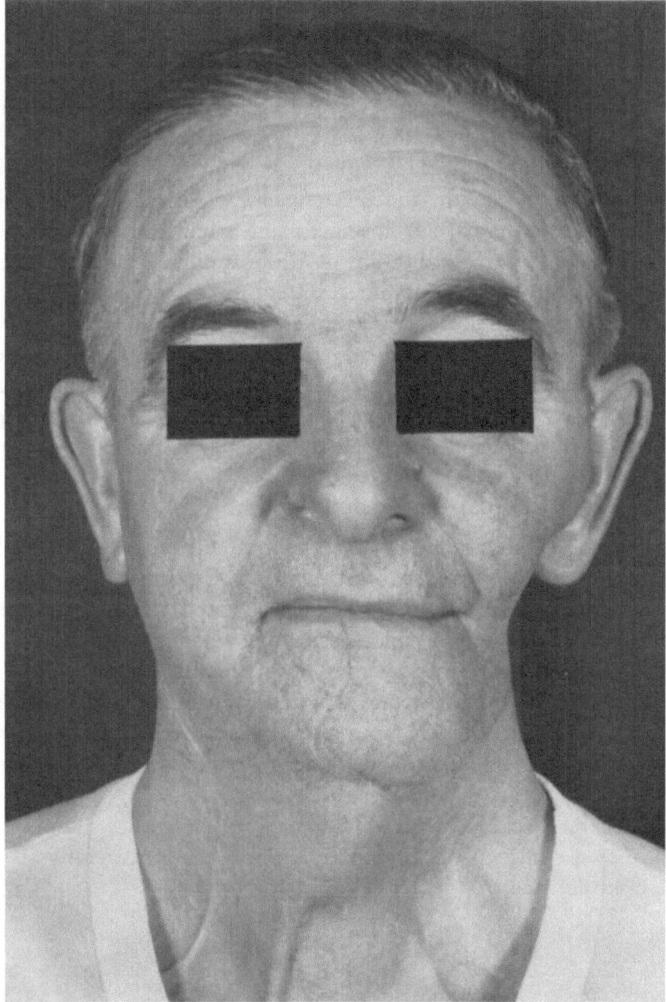

Fig. 8 b

percentage of metastases that occur in these nodes and remain undiscovered until revealed by microscopic examination is too great to run the risk of permitting them to remain if they can be removed by this elective procedure. Furthermore, in particular in the case of melanoma, if the regional and accessible lymph nodes are permitted to remain, the number that subsequently contain metastases is so great that an accusation of improper judgment can justly be made for leaving them.

b) Cancers of the Mouth and Related Structures

Superficial, non-invasive epitheliomas of the lip are still treated by relatively conservative measures — either surgical excision or irradiation using radium applicators or low-voltage short-distance contact X-rays. The deeply invasive cancers of the lip, as well as the epidermoid carcinomas of the cheek and of the anterior two-thirds of the tongue, the floor of the mouth, and the inferior alveolus, which are unilateral, metastasize with great frequency to the cervical lymph nodes. This being so, excision and dissection in continuity are readily accomplished, so that in addition to the radical cervical nodal dissection, which removes the jugular vein, the sterno-cleidomastoid muscle, and all of the lymphatic structures, a wide segment of the lip, the cheek, the floor of the mouth, and the tongue are removed in continuity during the dissection, even though in some instances this requires a hemimandibulectomy with either immediate or late restoration of the mandible by substitutive measures (Fig. 8). There are small lymph nodes intercalated, for example, along the lymphatic pathways in the tongue and floor of the mouth and along the course of the lymphatics draining into the neck, and they can be the source of metastatic deposits, resulting in diffuse recurrence of the cancer in many instances when a discontinuous operation is done, i. e., whenever primary cancers in the oral cavity or lip metastasizing to the cervical lymph nodes are removed as separate operative procedures.

c) Cancers of the Vulva

Many cancers of the vulva are non-invasive and multicentric, and develop on the basis of atrophic changes in the skin of the vulva. Experience and judgement are useful in determining when a simple vulvectomy may suffice in an aged subject. However, invasive epidermoid carcinomas of the vulva as well as all malignant melanomas, whether or not lymph nodes are palpable in the groin, should be treated by *en bloc* excision, with removal not only of the vulva in its entirety to include the introitus as far as the hymen but also of the intervening tissues to the groins, and with bilateral dissection of at least the femoral and inguinal lymph nodes. The medial superficial inguinal nodes are most commonly involved. Bilateral dissection is indicated because of the abundance of lymphatics draining the vulva and the well-known tendency of the cancer to spread contralaterally to the lymph nodes on the opposite side.

d) Cancers of the Penis

Excision and dissection in continuity for invasive cancers of the penis are the best accepted procedure and should be carried out in all except early lesions amenable to more conservative therapy. If a cancer is invasive, in many instances it requires total penectomy with bilateral groin dissection in continuity and the implantation of the urethra posterior to the scrotum (Fig. 9). Cancers, carcinomatous or melanomatous, that involve the urethra have a tendency to spread even to the prepubical nodes, which should be included in the dissection.

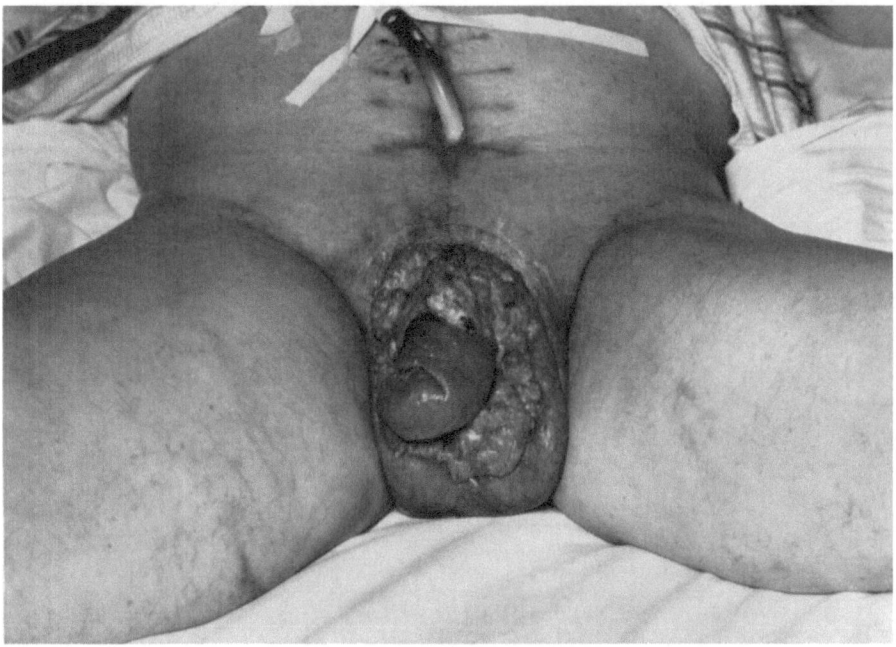

Fig. 9 a

Fig. 9. a) Advanced epidermoid carcinoma of penis and scrotum. Suprapubic cystostomy. b) Radical penectomy, excision of scrotum and testes, bilateral groin dissection in continuity. c) Closure of wound; perineal urethra. Ten-year definitive cure

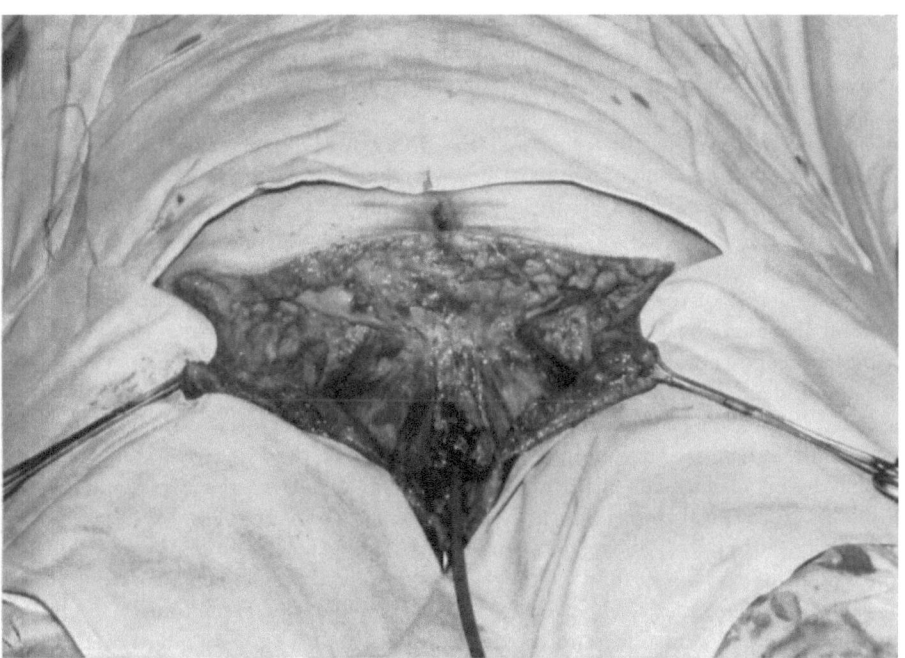

Fig. 9 b

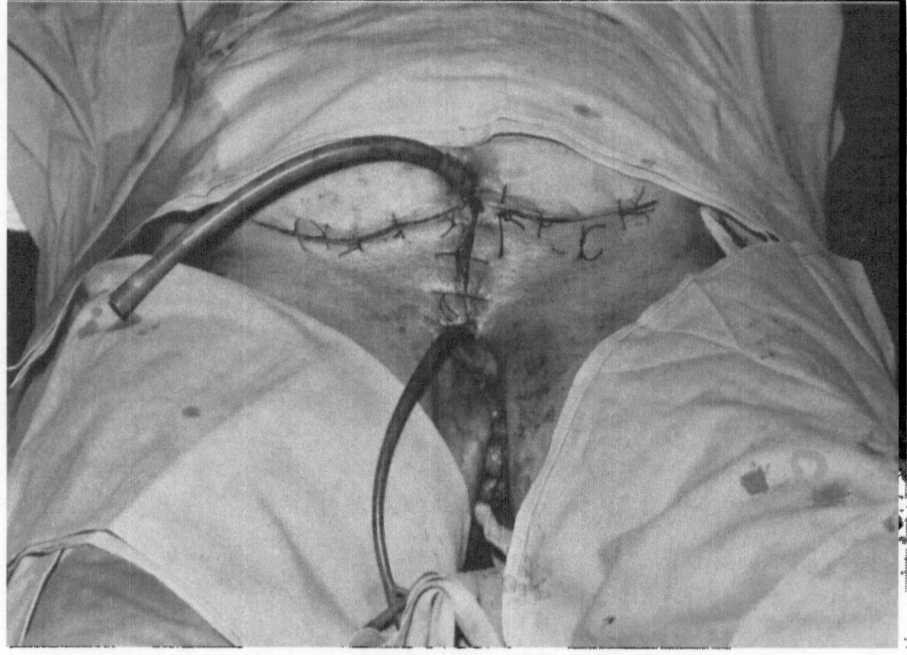

Fig. 9 c

9. Principles of Surgical Treatment for Soft-Tissue Sarcomas

For sarcomas of the soft tissues, the surgeon, in deciding whether to perform a radical surgical dissection or amputation, must take into consideration the histogenesis of the tumor, its degree of malignancy, its fixity or mobility, the original location, the question whether it is primary or recurrent, the incorporation or not of important nerves and arteries, and the presence of regional and distant metastases. He should be familiar with the behavior patterns of the sarcomas of different histogenetic types and plan his treatment accordingly. It is proper to secure consent for amputation prior to any operation on soft-part sarcomas of the extremities, because at the time of an attempt at local dissection it may be found that the extent and invasiveness of the tumor preclude the possibility of cure by local operation.

Soft-tissue sarcomas are usually not encapsulated, the covering of the tumor being a pseudo-capsule, composed of a condensation of fibrous components or the stroma of the neoplasm itself. This apparent encapsulation makes simple enucleation a great temptation because of the ease with which the tumor is dislodged from its bed. Such a temptation should be resisted, however, and the operation planned should be of an adequate character, with removal of all the tissue surrounding the sarcoma. If a radical dissection is performed for a sarcoma involving the extremities, a tourniquet is applied above the upper limits of the tumor and left in place during the taking of the biopsy and while the surgical dissection is being done, if at all feasible. If the superjacent artery can be exposed and temporarily occluded, hemostasis is well controlled and the dissection accomplished more quickly. If radical local removal of the sarcoma fails or it becomes increasingly evident as the operation proceeds that a conservative operation would be futile, amputation is immediately performed above the tourniquet.

If exploratory exposure of the sarcoma has been carried out without removal of the neoplasm; if a diagnosis has been previously established by a formal incisional biopsy; if a recurrence develops after incomplete excision of the tumor; or if the sarcoma fungates through the wound; and if successful radical dissection of the tumor is still considered feasible by the surgeon: it is an urgent necessity that the entire scar of the previous incision be completely removed with the specimen. The sarcoma is removed without the tumor being visible or encountered in the course of the dissection, i. e., the line of the dissection must extend well beyond the discernible boundaries of the neoplasm and it must be removed with the enveloping muscles, fat, and fascia (Fig. 10). The muscles which are involved or surround the

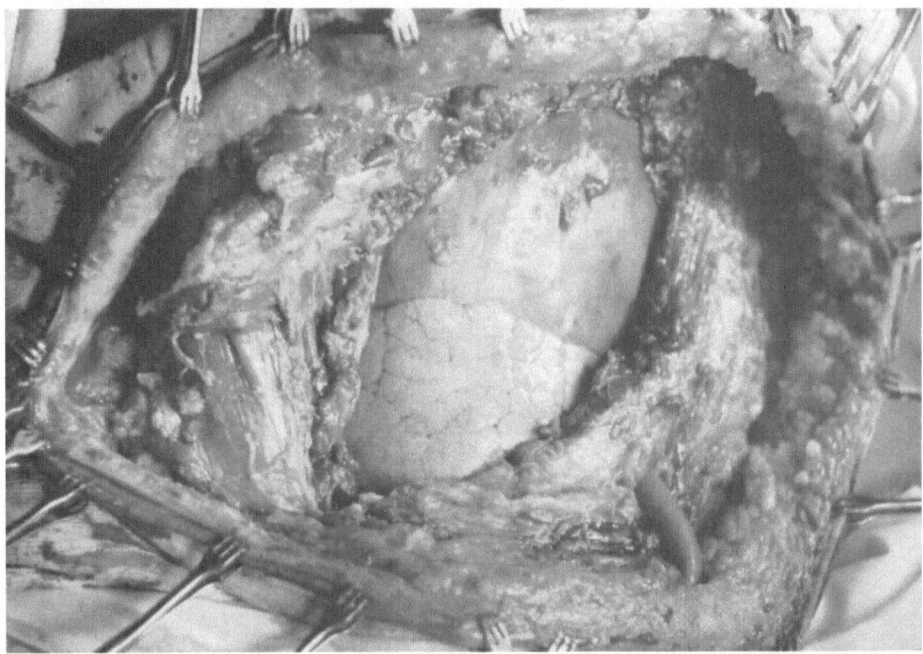

Fig. 10. Recurrent rhabdomyosarcoma of chest wall. Muscle group and rib resection. Closure of defect with fascial graft

sarcoma should be removed from their origin to their insertion. For sarcomas of the arms and legs, a radical surgical dissection is performed from above downwards.

Radiation, as an aid in the management of sarcomas of the soft tissues, must be given a proper place in the armamentarium. In our experience there have been many instances in which technically inoperable sarcomas have received preliminary irradiation which has permitted resection and ultimate cure. Pre-operative irradiation is considered mandatory for such vascular and anaplastic tumors as angiosarcomas and embryonal liposarcomas and, in fact, for any of the sarcomas of the soft tissues that show diffuse invasive tendencies. With a combination of irradiation and surgical excision, it has been possible to perform radical surgical dissection of certain sarcomas and to avoid amputation of the limb. This combination of treatment requires some knowledge of the radiosensitivity of sarcomas of varying histogenesis and some familiarity with the physical principles of irradiation.

10. Amputations for Malignant Tumors

a) Principles of Amputation for Sarcomas of the Extremities

Only experience can lead the surgeon to a decision as regards the choice of treatment for sarcomas involving the upper or lower extremity. Such factors as the location of the tumor, its histogenesis, its degree of malignancy, whether it is primary or recurrent, its encapsulation or its infiltrative method of growth may modify the ultimate choice of procedure. The decision on the superior limit of the amputation is important, as it may mean a difference between cure and local recurrence. We have constantly observed the principle that we should amputate above the origin of the muscle groups involved by the sarcoma. Some of the principles which have

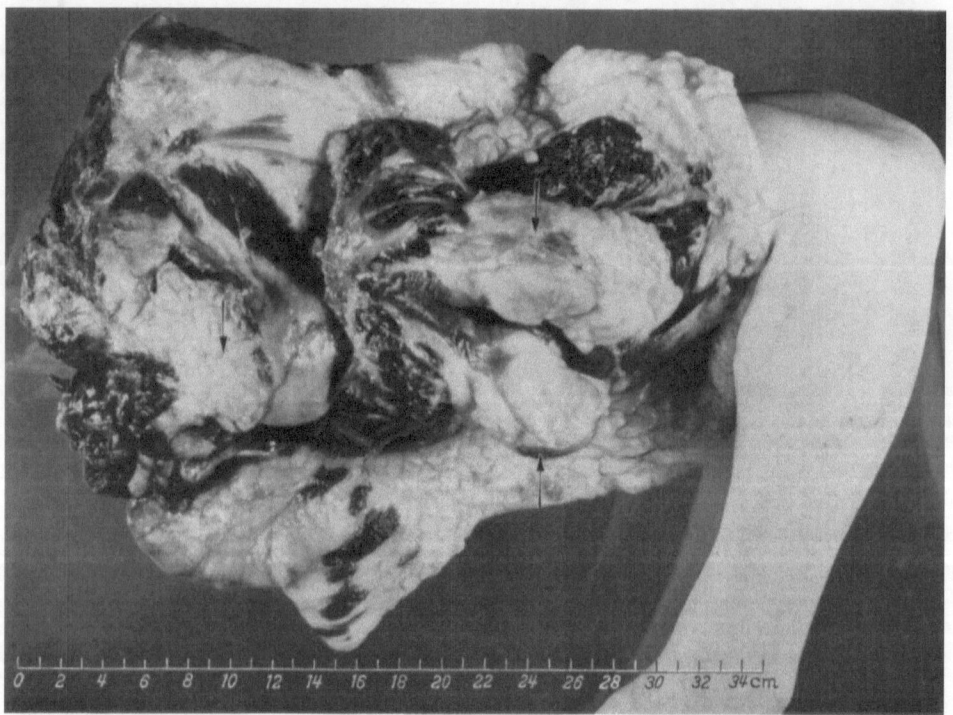

Fig. 11 a

Fig. 11. a) Interscapulothoracic amputation for malignant melanoma. b) Interscapulomammothoracic amputation for carcinoma of left breast, melanoma of left hand with satellitosis in skin of arm, liposarcoma of left fore-arm, left thyroid adenoma, metastases to left axillary nodes. Living and well 17 years later

been adopted over the years in the treatment of soft-tissue sarcomas of the extremity by amputation may be outlined as follows. (1) Rhabdomyosarcomas are sometimes of multicentric origin, so that it is imperative that all the muscle groups in which the tumor occurs should be removed in their entirety, else late recurrence may develop from the hidden foci, which are impalpable at the time of the dissection. (2) Sarcomas of the soft tissues tend to infiltrate along the fascial and muscular planes far above the palpable limits of the tumor. (3) Fascial fibrosarcomas are often so diffuse in their manner of growth and so prone to recur locally that the entire fascial sheath should be removed, even if this necessitates removal of the periosteal base of the superior attachment to bone. (4) In the amputation of an extremity for malignant neurilemmomas, the surgeon must exercise caution concerning the safe level of amputation, because of the tendency of these tumors to

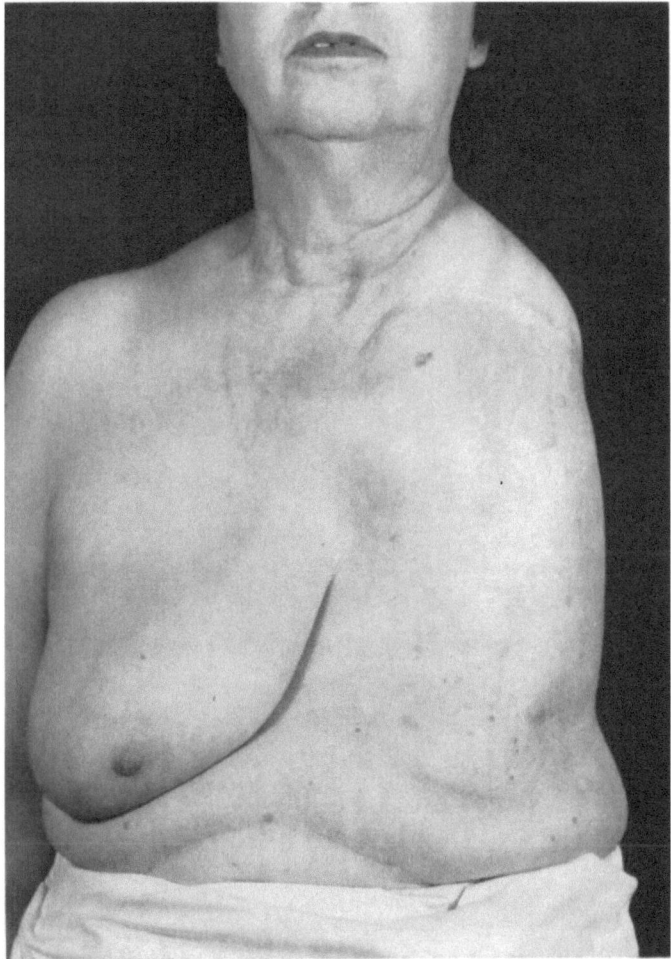

Fig. 11 b

extend centripetally upward along the nerve sheath and the coexistent moniliform beading of the nerve trunks by the neurofibromatous process characteristic of von Recklinghausen's disease. (5) The invasion of bone by these soft-tissue sarcomas permits a periosteal and intramedullary extension of the tumor along the shaft, in consequence of which amputation is performed either through or above the joint with which the diseased bone articulates. It is our opinion that there is no place among cancer operations for disarticulation of the humerus; in place of humeral disarticulation, we favor interscapulothoracic amputation (Fig. 11), on the ground that it is more radical, ultimately safer, and crippling to no greater degree. In the lower extremity, however, conservation of the upper portion of the thigh is of greater functional importance because the preservation of even a small stump is an advantage in adaptation to an artificial limb (PACK and ARIEL, 1958).

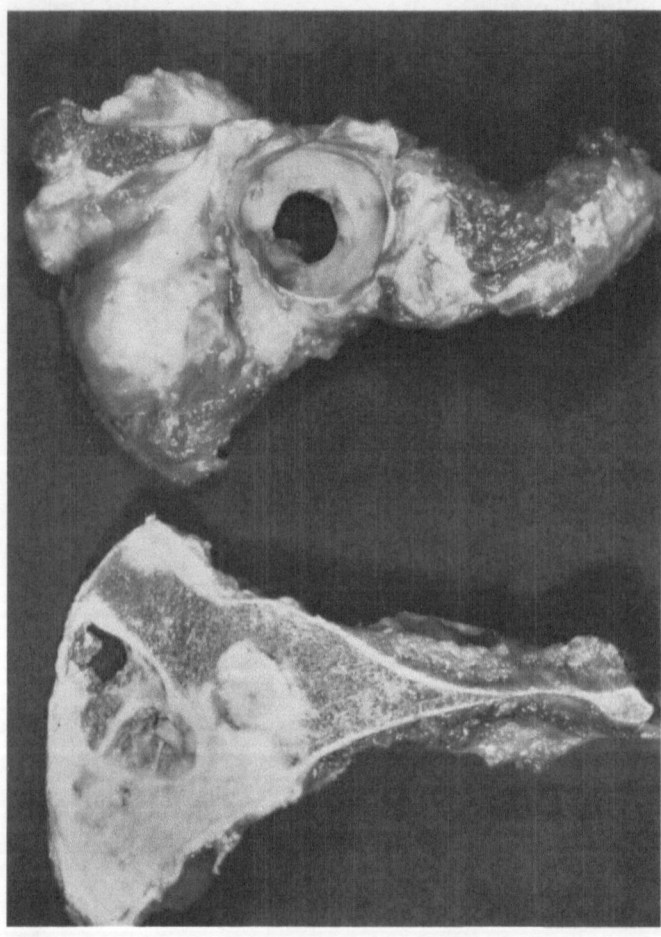

Fig. 12 a

Fig. 12. a) Interilioabdominal amputation (hemipelvectomy) for chondrosarcoma of os innominatum in January 1945. Later had successful hemicolectomy for adenocarcinoma and radiation therapy for tonsillar epithelioma. Died of heart attack in 1963 with no evidence of cancer. b) Hemipelvectomy for fibrosarcoma extending into iliac fossa; 21-year definitive cure. Wears satisfactory walking prosthesis. c) Recurrent malignant neurilemmoma of hip and buttock. Note cafe-au-lait stigmata and atrophy of leg. d) Same patient as in c). Hemipelvectomy. Note superior margin of malignant neurilemmoma. e) Hemipelvectomy for parosteal osteogenic sarcoma. f) Walking prosthesis after hemipelvectomy. Five years after the operation

b) Exarticulation of the Innominate Bone and Corresponding Lower Extremity (Hemipelvectomy) for Primary and Metastatic Cancer

The term hemipelvectomy is used to designate the complete removal of the lower extremity, the corresponding buttock, and the entire innominate bone in one stage. Various other names have been applied to this operation: interpelvioabdominal amputation, interiliosacropubic amputation, transiliac amputation, interinnomino-abdominal amputation, hindquarter resection, disarticulation of the innominate bone, and sacroiliac disarticulation. As surgical procedures of this radical extent become useful and are increasingly employed when the indications are clearly established, the operative mortality rate remains low and the end-results justify the deformity. The operation, which we have done for 205 patients, can now be performed with relative safety (Fig. 12). BILLROTH attempted it unsuccessfully for a soft-tissue sarcoma in 1891. It was first successfully accomplished by GIRARD in 1895. The first hemipelvectomy in the Memorial Cancer Center was performed by me in 1944.

Hemipelvectomy is indicated for those neoplasms which involve the hip joint, pelvic parietes, or soft tissues of the iliac region and which cannot be surgically

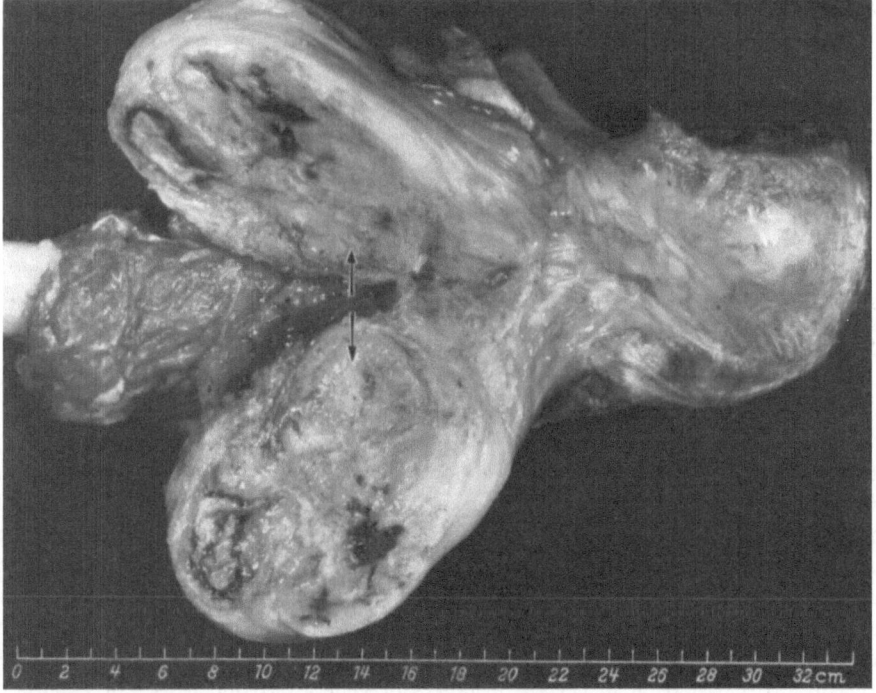

Fig. 12 b

extirpated by more conservative methods. The following are indications for its employment: (1) primary malignant neoplasms of the innominate bone such as osteogenic sarcoma and periosteal fibrosarcoma; (2) primary malignant neoplasms of the femur that have invaded the hip joint or innominate bone; (3) sarcomas of

the soft tissues of the upper part of the thigh, inguinal region, or buttock that have
invaded the hip joint or extended through the obturator foramen to invade the
pelvic parietes; (4) metastases to the iliac region which have infiltrated the hip joint

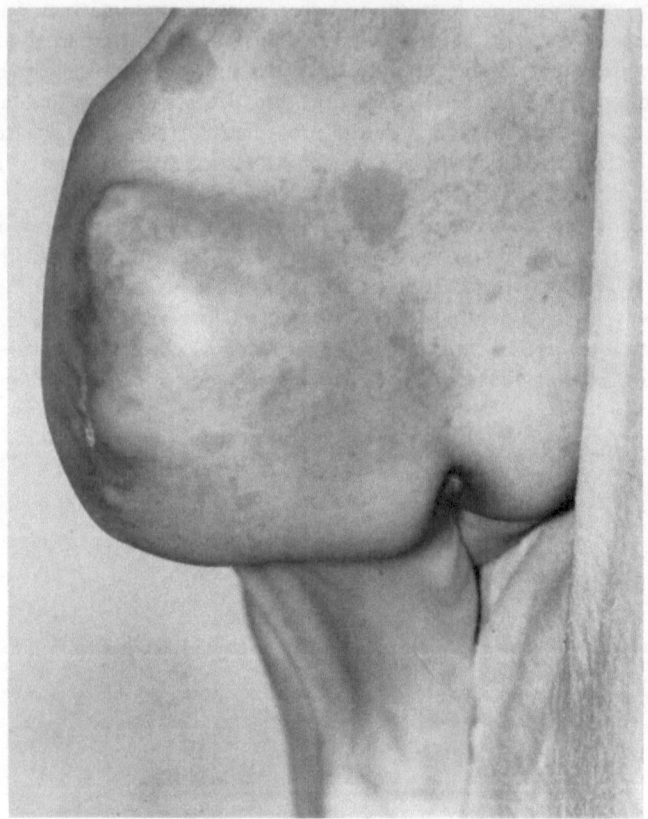

Fig. 12 c

or pelvic parietes or which, because of local extension, have precluded extirpation
of the cancer by less radical procedures such as radical groin dissection (in all
instances in which the operation is performed for the treatment of metastases the
primary neoplasm should be controlled or controllable); (5) certain massive benign
tumors of the innominate bone, such as chondroma and osteochondroma, or of the
soft tissues of the pelvic region, such as gross schwannomas, if they cannot be resected
adequately by less radical procedures and if the disability they entail warrants this
procedure; (6) palliation in certain instances of generalized metastases or extension
when involvement of the groin produces a bulky, infected, and painful mass that
cannot be controlled by any other means (this indication is seldom followed; in fact,
the opposite attitude is more commonly adopted, that is, the operation is seldom
performed if distant metastases are discovered); (7) certain infections and trauma
(none in our personal experience) (PACK, 1956; PACK and EHRLICH, 1946; PACK,
EHRLICH, and GENTIL, 1947; PACK and MILLER, 1964).

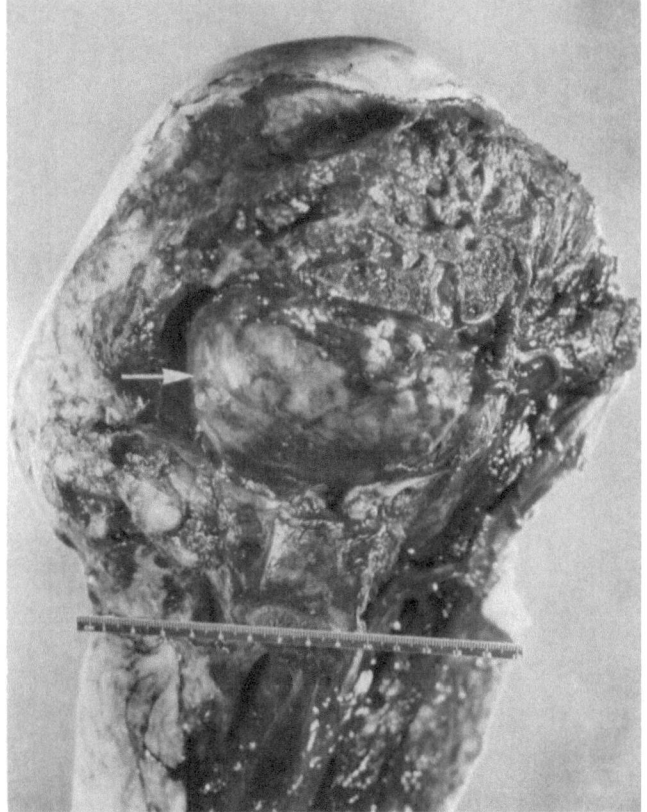

Fig. 12 d

c) The Tikhor-Linberg Resection of the Shoulder Girdle

The Tikhor-Linberg operation for resection of the shoulder girdle involves total scapulectomy, partial or complete excision of the clavicle, and resection of the head and neck of the humerus, with preservation of the arm, brachial plexus, subclavial artery, and vein (PACK and CRAMPTON, 1961). The operation was first planned by the Russian surgeon, Tikhor, and carried out afterwards by BAUMAN and LINBERG at the turn of the century. The purpose of the operation is threefold: (1) as the preferred method of treating certain tumors of the shoulder when the patient refuses amputation; (2) for certain cancers, or even unusually destructive inflammatory or traumatic lesions, when the neurovascular bundle remains intact; and (3) for the preservation of an upper extremity capable of limited but valuable function. The excision of these structures leaves the distal two-thirds of the upper arm, the elbow, forearm, and hand intact and attached to the body only by the untouched neuro-vascular bundle. The muscles of the arm are attached to the trunk by suture. The arm remains viable and functional, except that hyperextension cannot be carried out unless aided by the opposite arm. This operation (Fig. 13) can be performed only in carefully selected instances, but its feasibility and value should be borne in mind

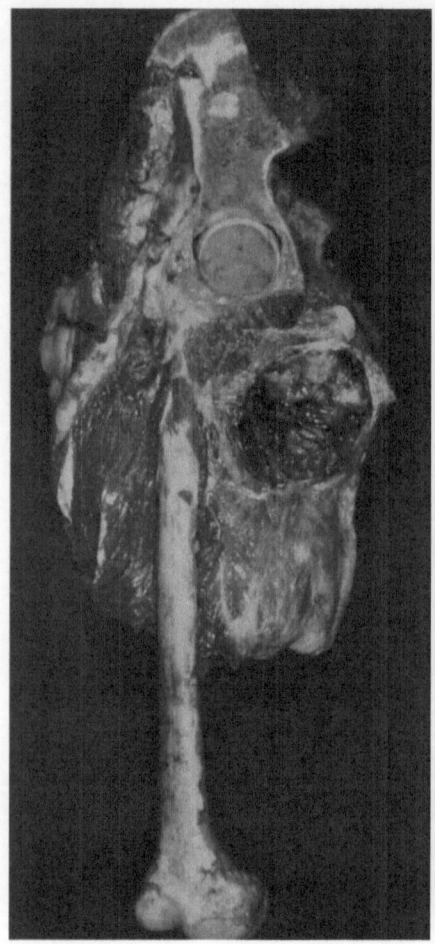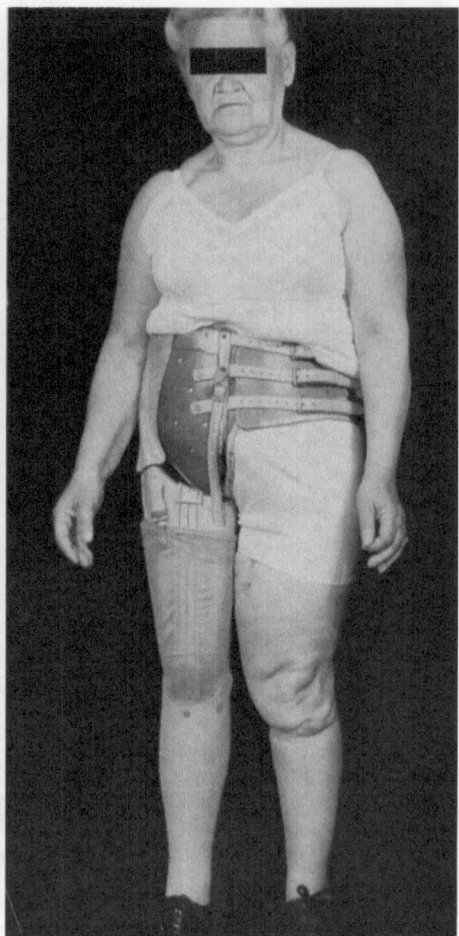

Fig. 12 e   Fig. 12 f

as it can be adequate and a more than satisfactory substitute for the disabling interscapulothoracic amputation.

Some of the lesions involving the shoulder girdle which have been considered for the Tikhor-Linberg shoulder girdle resection are:

1. *Inflammatory suppurative diseases* associated with massive bone necrosis, multiple fistulas, joint destruction, sepsis, etc. Since the introduction of antibiotics, this indication must have become infrequent; at least, we have never employed it.

2. *Metastasis to the shoulder girdle*. Crippling, destructive metastases to bone, constituting post-irradiation failures. If the patient could otherwise be considered to have a reasonable expectation of life, this operation might well be used more frequently as a palliative measure.

3. *Bone tumors*. Osteogenic sarcoma and chondrosarcoma of the scapula invading soft tissues and joints and unsuitable for scapulectomy. The radiosensitive endothelial myeloma does not qualify for an operation of this character.

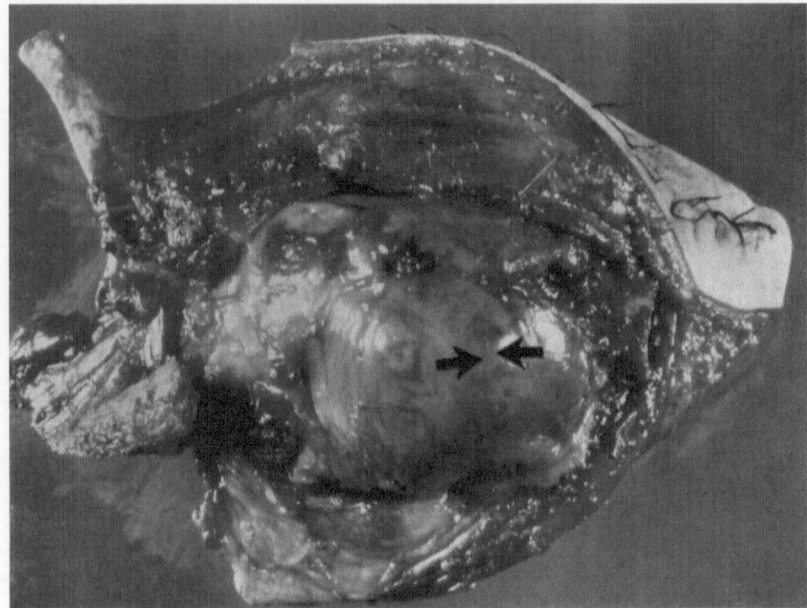

Fig. 13 a

Fig. 13. a) Tikhor-Linberg resection of shoulder girdle with preservation of neurovascular bundle and distal useful arm and hand. Gross specimen: chondrosarcoma. b) Another patient with chondrosarcoma. Roentgenogram of neoplasm. c) Another patient with massive chondrosarcoma of upper humerus. Resection of clavicle, scapula, and upper third of humerus *en bloc*. Note foreshortened and viable distal upper extremity. Six-year cure. (From Pack & Crampton, 1961, courtesy J. B. Lippincott Company.) d) Another patient. Resection of all components of shoulder girdle including soft tissues except for neurovascular bundle. Functional arm and hand. Six-year cure.

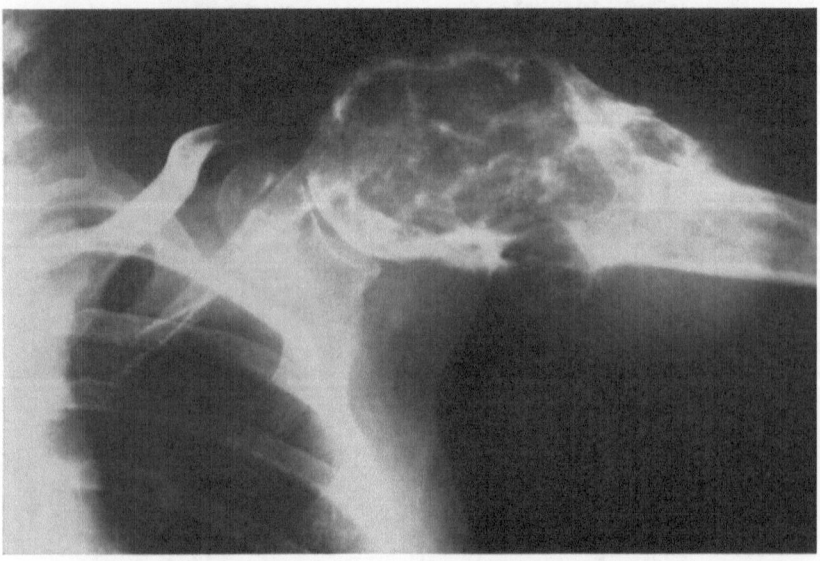

Fig. 13 b

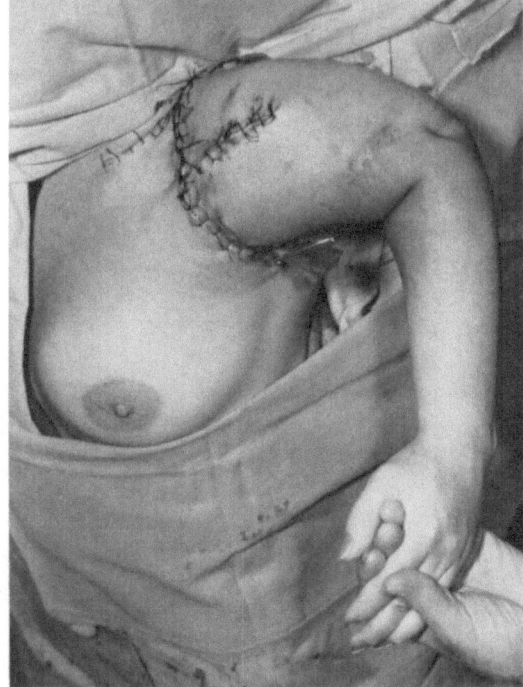

Fig. 13 c

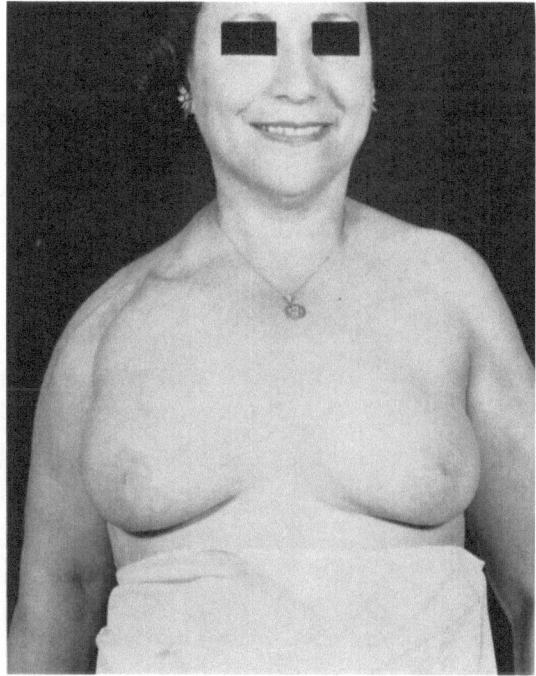

Fig. 13 d

4. *Synovial sarcoma* (malignant synovioma). Although this tumor is not of frequent occurrence around the shoulder joint, it would theoretically be the most suitable of all soft-tissue sarcomas for this specific operation.

5. *Liposarcoma.* The operation would generally be contraindicated for this tumor. Liposarcomas are most frequent in the shoulder and pelvic girdles but seldom involve the bone; they occasionally have an extraordinary degree of radiosensitivity and require extensive sacrifice of contiguous soft-tissue structures.

6. *Rhabdomyosarcoma.* This tumor would seldom be suitable for the Tikhor-Linberg operation because it usually does not involve the bone. It may be unicentric in origin. Experience has shown that it is fundamental in its surgical treatment to excise all of the muscle groups involved from their origin to their insertion, or to amputate proximally to their origin.

7. *Fibrosarcoma.* This tumor is commonly diffuse and invasive, and may produce a local condition in the shoulder girdle which will tempt the surgeon to perform shoulder girdle resection and preserve the arm. The pernicious tendency of this sarcoma to extend widely up and down the fascial planes beyond the range of the usual conservative operations should be borne in mind.

8. *Malignant neurilemmoma,* a tumor which may invade bone or erode it by continuity; it can be pseudo-encapsulated or invasive. Two hazards, namely, involvement of the brachial plexus and its predisposition to recur proximally along the nerve trunks, may render it unsuitable for this operation.

9. *Deeply invasive cancers of the skin.* Epidermoid carcinomas of the skin of the shoulder may involve the bones and shoulder joint. These cancers may have recurred after attempts at radiation therapy and are sometimes associated with radiation fibrosis and ulceration, necrosis, suppuration, fixation of the joint, intractable pain, and disability.

d) Hemicorporectomy (Lumbar Amputation) for Non-resectable Pelvic and Other Cancers

It has long been realized that a patient might possibly be cured of advanced cancers limited to the pelvis by a radical amputation between the lumbar vertebrae — a so-called hemicorporectomy. This would be feasible for advanced sacrococcygeal chordomas that have not metastasized, or for sarcomas of the bony pelvis or fixed sarcomas of the soft somatic tissues that are not unilateral at advanced stages of their development. More recently, THEODORE R. MILLER, an associate, has performed five such operations, chiefly for cancers of the urinary bladder previously treated by total cystectomy, colostomy, pelvic evisceration, and the construction of ileobladders, and with the advanced recurrent cancers strictly limited to the pelvis (Fig. 14). Amputations of the lower half of the body through the intervertebral lumbar spaces, with removal of both innominate bones, both lower extremities, and all the pelvic contents, have been successfully performed in five patients. Rehabilitation measures have been instituted with amazing results aided by the stoicism of these patients, their will to live, and their determination to adjust themselves to a continued existence without the lower half of their body. When lumbar amputation is considered, all its consequences should be carefully explained not only to the patient but also to those persons charged with his later physical and economic care, who should fully understand what is involved.

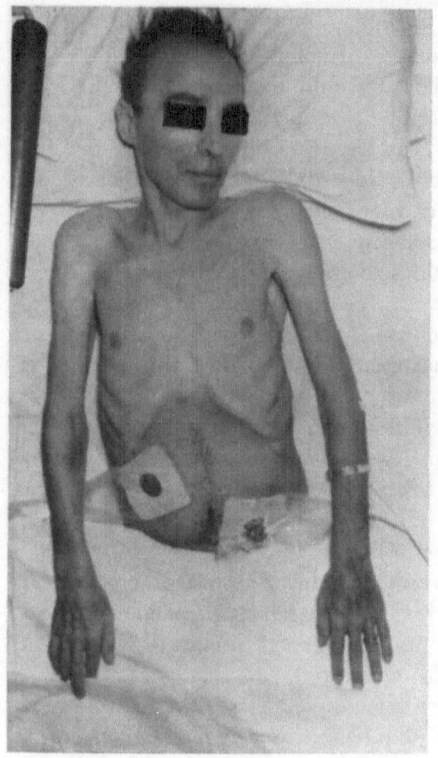

Fig. 14 a

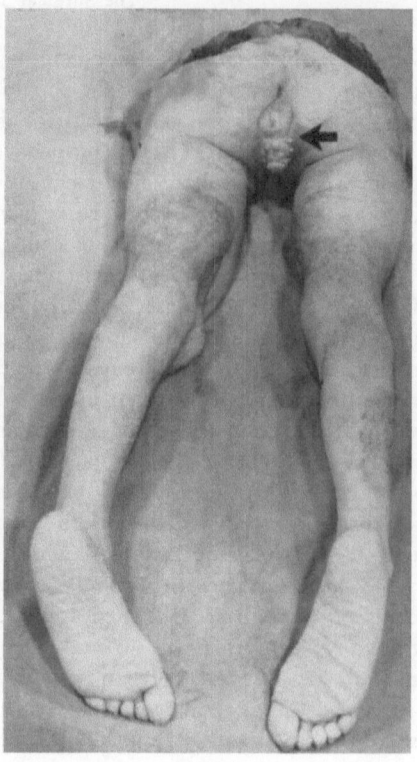

Fig. 14 b

Fig. 14. a) Hemicorporectomy; postoperative view. Transection of human body through 4th lumbar interspace. Ileal bladder; colostomy. b) Gross surgical specimen. Recurrent cancer of urinary bladder fungating through perineum. Loss of both lower extremities, bony pelvis, pelvic viscera, genitals. Upper abdomen intact. c) Convalescing patient. Rehabilitation; will wear prosthesis. (Courtesy Dr. THEODORE MILLER, Pack Medical Group.)

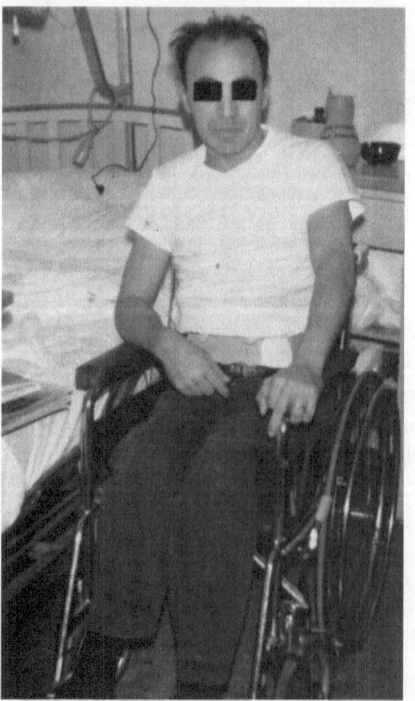

Fig. 14 c

11. Surgical Treatment of Ovarian Cancer

In young unmarried or childless women with an apparently unilateral ovarian cancer of low-grade malignancy, there are grounds for performing a unilateral oophorectomy, with preservation of the opposite ovary and the uterus to enable them to bear children. The majority of ovarian cancers, however, are rather advanced when detected and the cure rate is regrettably low. A more successful operation is panhysterectomy, with removal of both ovaries, the Fallopian tubes, and the uterus in its entirety even when it appears normal; in approximately 15 % of cases there is microscopic evidence of involvement of the uterus. At such operations it has been our practice to remove the great omentum, in the belief that omentectomy is a useful measure in lessening the hazard of subsequent peritoneal carcinosis with ascites, since the omentum has a tendency to pick up the loose cancer cells so frequently detected in the peritoneal cavity of patients who have ovarian cancer. As a prophylactic measure, a small polyethylene tube is often left in the peritoneal cavity, even in the absence of evidence of peritoneal carcinosis, and radioactive isotopes, such as radioactive chromic phosphate (a colloidal preparation) or a suspension of ceramic microspheres in which each particle contains radioactive yttrium-90, are administered. At all costs, the primary cancer should be removed, as well as the opposite ovary; but if the latter is not technically resectable at the initial exploration, a biopsy is followed by intensive external irradiation and, at the time of maximal regression (possibly six weeks later), a second operation can justifiedly be carried out in order to remove it. Cancer of the ovary is one neoplasm for which removal of the primary lesion is most essential if a good result is to be achieved, even though secondary and even tertiary laparotomies need be done subsequent to irradiation.

12. Surgical Treatment of Cancer of the Uterus

a) Endometrial Cancer

The five-year survival rates for the average carcinoma of the endometrium or body of the uterus have been improved by the pre-operative insertion of a tandem of radium or radioisotope capsules into the uterine cavity for, usually, 3600 milligram or millicurie hours. Within four to six weeks, a radical panhysterectomy is performed, with removal of the uterus, tubes, ovaries, cervix, and a liberal cuff of the vagina. When wound healing is complete, we have given supplementary intravaginal radiation therapy, using either a specially devised cobalt vaginal bomb or a Curie colpostat. The purpose is to lessen or prevent, if possible, the retrograde lymphatic dissemination of endometrial cancer down to the introitus, a complication which has occurred too frequently in the past.

b) Cancers of the Uterine Cervix

Well-planned and carefully executed irradiation is an excellent method of treating cancers of the uterine cervix in Stage I. The decision is not one implying the possible superiority of one form of therapy over the other, i. e., of radiation over surgery but, more particularly, one on the best method of treatment for the particular individual with cancer of the cervix. When confronted with a patient with this type of cancer, the clinician must decide when to advise surgical treatment; he must be aware of the limitations of surgical excision for cancer of this site; he must have the experience and ability to determine, if possible *a priori,* how extensive an operation is necessary to afford the patient a reasonable prospect of cure. It is generally admitted that 10—15% of patients with cancers of the uterine cervix in clinical Stage I have hidden metastases in the pelvic lymph nodes; in this group surgical excision would be preferable to radiation therapy.

The surgical procedures for early cervical cancers include the Wertheim abdominal hysterectomy with pelvic lymph-node dissection and the Schauta-Amreich radical vaginal hysterectomy, in two stages as the second stage is a bilateral retroperitoneal pelvic lymph-node dissection. These operations have proved their effectiveness for cancers limited to the cervix or to the tissues in the immediate proximity of the cervix. When the Wertheim operation is performed for a cancer of the cervix preoperatively classified as clinical Stage I and the pelvic lymph nodes contain microscopic metastases, the cure rate, 50%, is still commendable and cannot be rivalled by radiation therapy; whereas if the nodes removed at the time of the operation have no metastases the five-year survival rate is as high as 80% (LANGDON PARSONS, 1965). In performing this operation, it is more important to do an adequate dissection of the para-uterine tissues than to remove the distant nodes with meticulous care, because there is no great value in dissecting distant lymph nodes unless the primary cancer is so adequately removed as to afford a reasonable prospect of cure. Disturbing complications follow both radical radiation therapy and radical surgical treatment. The dissection round the base of the bladder may result in vesicovaginal and ureterovaginal fistulae and there may be an embarrassing atony of the bladder. Radiation therapy, too, may injure the bladder and intestines in a way that is difficult to rectify.

13. Pelvic Evisceration (Exenteration of the Pelvis for Cancer)

The operation of pelvic evisceration has been justified, and has sometimes been curative, in the treatment of locally recurrent cancers of the rectum, ovary, uterus, and urinary bladder, often after radiation therapy has failed and even when multiple fistulous communications exist between the bladder, vagina, and rectum. Pelvic cancers that were formerly considered inoperable because of invasion of neighboring organs are now being resected. For example, at least 30% of women dying of cancers of the uterine cervix have the cancer still confined within the true pelvis at the time of death.

The most radical operation for pelvic cancer is pelvic evisceration, all the structures of the pelvis being removed (Fig. 15). The operation in many cases is admittedly no more than a palliative procedure. The surgical procedure differs in the sexes only because of the different organs implicated. In the male, the urinary bladder and prostate are removed with the rectum, and all the pelvic lymph nodes are dissected away. In the female, the operation involves removal of the rectum, vagina, internal genitals, urinary bladder, urethra, and sometimes the vulva.

In pelvic evisceration the terminations of the ureters are removed with the cancer. In earlier years there was considerable difference of opinion as to how this should be done. Whenever the urinary bladder was removed for pelvic cancer other than of the rectum, and when the rectum could be preserved, bilateral ureteral implantation within the colon was performed, because the rectum and colon served as an excellent reservoir for urine; but if a permanent abdominal colostomy is to be

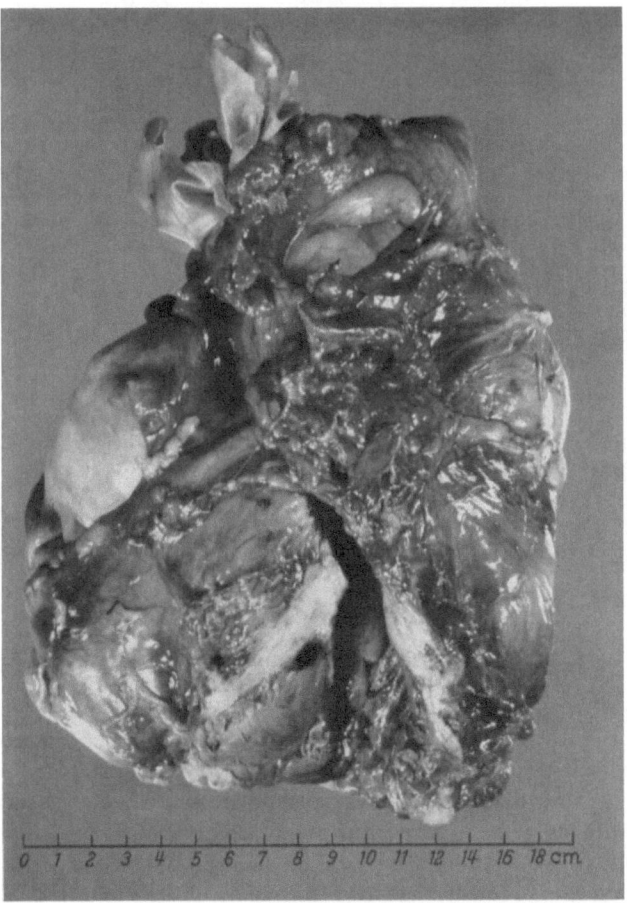

Fig. 15 a

Fig. 15. a) Pelvic evisceration in female patient. Gross specimen. Carcinoma of cervix uteri involving vagina, corpus of uterus, urinary bladder, and both parametria. b) Pelvic evisceration. Extensive vaginal cancer involving uterus, bladder, urethra, rectovaginal septum. Gross specimen after exenteration; 16-year cure

done, a decision must be taken on whether the ureters should be implanted in the colon, giving the patient a wet colostomy, or whether an ileal bladder — an isolated segment of ileum into which both ureters empty — should be constructed. The latter procedure has found almost universal favor within recent years, and there is less risk of ascending infections and pyelitis or pyelonephritis.

Reluctant as a surgeon may be to inflict this major disability upon his patients, he has no right to make the decision himself for the individual patient, whose attachment to life may lead him or her willingly to accept the disability in return

for a period of relief or a chance of cure. The operation is not technically difficult — in fact, it is less so than radical panhysterectomy with pelvic lymph-node
dissection.

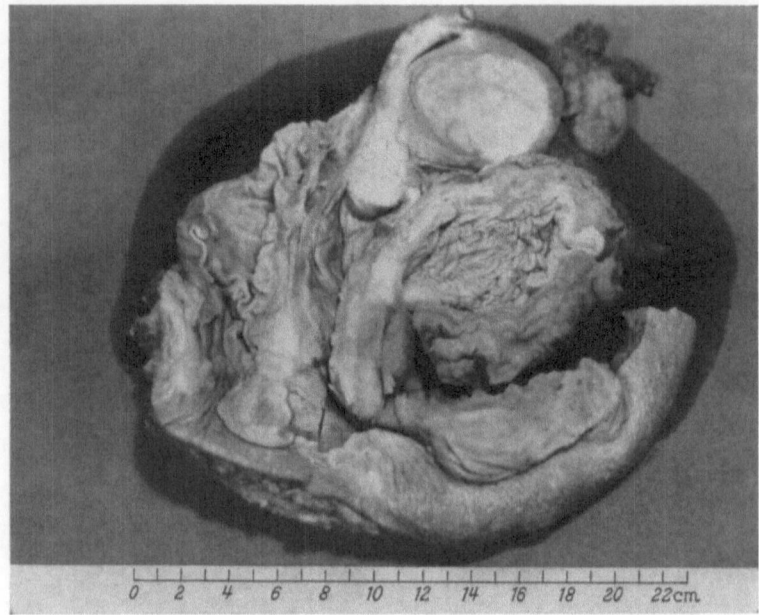

Fig. 15 b

14. The Synchronous Combined Abdominoperineal Surgical Approach for Certain Pelvic Tumors

For the surgical extirpation of certain presacral teratomas, benign or malignant;
for many rectal cancers in which difficulty in removal is anticipated; for early rectal
cancers when it is intended to conserve the rectal sphincter and construct an anocolic
anastomosis without a colostomy; for pelvic evisceration for cancers of uterine,
rectal, ovarian, prostatic, or vesicular origin implicating the adjacent viscera; and
for sacrococcygeal chordomas, we have for many years employed a synchronous
combined abdominoperineal surgical approach employing two teams of surgeons
(PACK and MILLER, 1965).

Using the two-team, synchronous abdominoperineal technique, we have removed
massive presacral teratomas and teratocarcinomas previously declared non-resectable
by competent surgeons. This method increases the operability of such tumors and
simplifies the technical problems, as well as reducing the time taken for the operation
by half or even more. There is infinitely less blood loss because of better hemostasis,
less shock, less difficulty with anesthesia, and less risk of contamination. The same
advantages are found in the application of this technique to abdominoperineal rectal
resection, especially when the cancers are large, infected, and adherent and implicate
adjacent viscera. In our view, an absolute indication for the two-team abdominal
approach is the sacrococcygeal chordoma. Here, the surgeon working through the
abdomen can achieve good hemostasis by bilateral ligation of the internal iliac

arteries and the middle sacral artery, and mobilize and dissect the superior third or half of the chordoma, while his colleague, working below, is not impeded by constant hemorrhage and the inaccessibility of the upper limits of the tumor.

15. Surgical Excision of Unicentric Visceral Metastases

Segmental excision or hepatic lobectomy for metastatic cancer in the liver has been described. The removal of a metastasis to the brain, if unifocal as suggested by arteriography and radioisotopic localization, has been successful in affording some long-term operative survivals. A solitary metastasis of thyroid cancer was removed from the brain of one of my patients, an 11-year-old girl, and she is still in good health now, 25 years after the craniotomy.

The majority of patients who die as a result of sarcomas of the soft tissues as well as of osteogenic sarcoma do so because of pulmonary metastases rather than of locally recurrent sarcomas or continued growth of the original neoplasm. It is a common occurrence with these tumors that the local radical surgical treatment or amputation is often successful but visceral metastases, usually to the lung, become apparent in succeeding years. Some patients, even at post-mortem examination, reveal no evidence of local recurrence. The pulmonary metastases are usually fairly well demarcated as spherical bodies rather than as diffuse infiltration of the lung parenchyma. If a metastasis in the lung from a sarcoma of the soft tissues or a bone sarcoma appears to be a single focus, or if two or three metastases are confined within the lobule, the surgeon may properly attempt a lobectomy or a segmental resection. Before performing a thoracotomy with this intent, it is wise to have anteroposterior and lateral tomographic studies made in order to reveal any metastatic foci that might not be seen with the orthodox chest roentgenograms. In our series of patients, lobectomy and segmental excision have proved to be of definite palliative benefit when the procedure has been employed with such specific indications.

16. Homotransplantation of Entire Organs in Humans

Experimental removal of the entire liver or lung or both kidneys (for bilateral malignant tumors) has been done with replacement by homologous organ grafts in humans. These transplantations may ultimately succeed with increasing knowledge of factors responsible for host rejection by the recipient. Most of the technical, physiological, and immunological problems had been studied in dogs prior to attempting the operation in the human. It must be accepted that for the present, and for some time to come, these heroic procedures must be done under academic auspices because of the complexities of the problems involved, the number of highly competent specialists in the various fields of medicine required to work simultaneously for the single patient, and the expense of the procedure.

The removal of a nephritic kidney and its replacement by a homologous kidney graft from a monozygotic twin was a successful procedure that heralded a series of organ graft operations. Bilateral renal cancers, however, might require some other procedure. WILLET WHITMORE, at the Memorial Cancer Center in New York, had a child patient who had bilateral Wilm's embryomas of the kidneys. He replaced the kidneys by a homologous renal graft from an unrelated child dying in the hospital, using the presently accepted technique of placing the transplanted kidney in the pelvis with arterial and venous anastomoses between the internal iliac and renal vessels.

If one lung is removed for any purpose, of course, it does not require replacement, as it is a paired organ. HARDY *et al.* (1963) transplanted a homologous lung to a human patient, proving that the operation is technically feasible. Perhaps in the future bilateral discrete spherical metastases in the lungs, appearing long after a primary sarcoma or carcinoma has apparently been cured locally, may be treated surgically by staged operations in which one lung is replaced by a homologous transplantation from another patient. Unhappily, the transplantation of lungs in dogs, although technically successful, has not provided lungs sufficiently capable of proper aeration and oxygen absorption; it is hoped that this difficulty will subsequently be overcome.

Total hepatectomy for cancer and other diseases, with orthotopic replacement, has been performed by STARZL and his colleagues at the University of Colorado School of Medicine (1961, 1963) and by MOORE and colleagues at Harvard Medical School (1960). On the basis of previous experiments with dogs (WELCH, 1956), following the initial work by GOODRICH and his associates (1956), they have mastered the intricate problems of surgical technique and are equipped with the means of overcoming the immunological rejection of the graft. They have stated that the homograft liver removed immediately from the dead donor should be cooled and perfused quickly and be ready for putting into place with vascular anastomosis in order to prevent severe and irreparable hepatocellular damage, the diseased organ having in the meantime just been removed by another team. STARZL comments that the greatest technical hazard is the vena cava anastomosis at the diaphragm, and one postoperative complication that is dangerous is intravascular clotting.

Methods of preventing rejection of these various homografts and of paralysing or inhibiting the natural immune response include splenectomy (not always) and preoperative and postoperative administration of azathioprine (Imuran), azaserine, and actinomycin C.

17. Surgical Aid in Hormonal Therapy

Among the many ways in which the surgeon can be of help in the care of the individual patient should be mentioned that of assisting the endocrinologist treating cancers responsive to hormonal therapy. Here the surgeon can remove certain organs which elaborate hormones that may be necessary for the continued growth of the cancer, removal upsetting the hormonal balance so as to bring about regression or reduced growth of the cancer. He may be called on to castrate either the male or female patient, especially for cancers of the breast, ovary, and prostate, or to perform bilateral adrenalectomy or hypophysectomy. These are forms of palliative surgery in the management of cancer.

References

ARIEL, I. M., and G. T. PACK: Treatment of tumors of the soft somatic tissues. Rev. Surg. **21**, 157 (1964).

ENGELL, H. C.: Cancer cells in the blood. A five to nine-year follow-up study. Ann. Surg. **149**, 457 (1959).

GOODRICH, E. O., H. F. WELCH, J. A. NELSON, T. S. BEECHER, and C. W. WELCH: Homo-transplantation of the canine liver. Surgery 39, 244 (1956).

HARDY, J. D., W. R. WEBB, M. L. DALTON, jr., and G. R. WALKER: Lung homotransplantation in man. Report of the initial case. J. Amer. med. Ass. 186, 1065 (1963).

MOORE, F. D., H. B. WHEELER, H. V. DEMISSIANOS, L. L. SMITH, O. BALANKURA, K. ABEL, J. B. GREENBERG, and J. J. DAMMIN: Experimental whole-organ transplantation of the liver and of the spleen. Ann. Surg. 152, 274 (1960).

PACK, G. T.: Definition of inoperability of cancer. Ann. Surg. 127, 1105 (1948).

— Argument for bilateral mastectomy. Surgery 29, 929 (1951).

— Major exarticulations for malignant neoplasms of the extremities: interscapulothoracic amputation, hip joint disarticulation and interilioabdominal amputation. J. Bone Jt Surg. 38-A, 249 (1956).

— The extension of radical surgery in the treatment of cancer. J. Iowa med. Soc. 47, 291 (1957).

— The surgeon's role in the mangement of cancer. New York J. Med. 64, 375 (1964).

— Cancer of the stomach. Amer. J. Gastroenterol. 44, 18 (1965).

— Cancer therapy: a perspective and prospective view. In ARIEL, I. M. (ed.): Progress in clinical cancer, Vol. I. New York: Grune and Stratton 1965, pp. 1—14.

—, and I. M. ARIEL: Tumors of the soft somatic tissues. New York: Hoeber 1958. Section II: General principles of treatment of tumors of the soft somatic tissues (including techniques of local excision, excision and dissection in continuity, hip joint disarticulation, hemi-pelvectomy, interscapulothotacic amputation), Chaps. 7—13.

— — Treatment of gastric cancer. Minnesota Med. 48, 747 (1965).

—, and R. D. BRASFIELD: Total right hepatic lobectomy for cancer of the gallbladder. Ann. Surg. 142, 6 (1955).

— — Metastatic cancer of the liver. The clinical problem and its management. Amer. J. Surg. 90, 704 (1955).

— — Radical mastectomy. Arch. Surg. 86, 214 (1963).

—, and R. S. CRAMPTON: The Tikhor-Linberg resection of the shoulder girdle. In DEPALMA, A. F. (ed.): Clinical orthopaedics. Philadelphia: Lippincott 1961; Chap. 12, pp. 148—161.

—, and H. E. EHRLICH: Exarticulation of the lower extremities for malignant tumors: hip joint disarticulation (with and without deep iliac dissection) and sacroiliac disarticulation (hemipelvectomy). Ann. Surg. 123, 965 (1946).

— —, and F. de C. GENTIL: Radical amputations of the extremities in the treatment of cancer. Surg. Gynec. Obst. 84, 1105 (1947).

—, and A. H. ISLAMI: Surgical treatment of tumors of the liver. In PACK, G. T., and I. M. ARIEL (ed.): Treatment of cancer and allied diseases, 2d ed. New York: Hoeber 1962; Vol. 5, Chap. 20.

— — Operative treatment of hepatic tumors. Ciba Clinical Symposia 16, 35 (1964).

— — Surgical treatment of hepatic tumors. In POPPER, H., and F. SCHAFFNER (eds.): Progress in liver diseases. New York: Grune and Stratton 1965; Vol. 2, Chap. 29.

— —, J. C. HUBBARD, and R. D. BRASFIELD: Regeneration of human liver after major hepatectomy. Surgery 52, 617 (1962).

—, and F. G. MARTINS: Treatment of anorectal malignant melanoma. Dis. Colon Rect. 3, 15 (1960).

—, and T. A. McGRAW: Interscapulomammothoracic amputation for malignant melanoma. Arch. Surg. 83, 694 (1966).

—, and T. R. MILLER: Middle hepatic lobectomy for cancer. Cancer 14, 1295 (1961).

— — Exarticulation of the innominate bone and corresponding lower extremity (hemi-pelvectomy) for primary and metastatic cancer. J. Bone Jt Surg. 46-A, 91 (1964).

— — A plea for the synchronous combined abdominoperineal surgical approach for certain pelvic tumors. Surgery 57, 613 (1965).

—, and P. E. REKERS: Radical groin dissection. In Cooper, Philip (ed.): The craft of surgery. Boston: Little, Brown & Co. 1964.

—, I. SCHARNAGEL, and M. MORFIT: The principle of excision and dissection in continuity for primary and metastatic melanoma of the skin. Surgery 17, 849 (1945).

Parsons, Langdon: Surgical treatment of cancer of the cervix. J. Amer. med. Ass. **193**, 598 (1965).

Starzl, T. E., H. A. Kaupp, jr., D. R. Brock, J. V. Linman, and W. T. Moss: Studies on a rejection of the transplanted homologous dog liver. Surg. Gynec. Obst. **112**, 135 (1961).

—, T. L. Marchioro, K. N. Von Kaulla, G. Herman, R. S. Brittain, and W. R. Waddell: Homotransplantation of the liver in humans. Surg. Gynec. Obst. **117**, 659 (1963).

Welch, C. S.: Homo-transplantation of the canine liver. Surgery **39**, 244 (1956).

Wood, Sumner, jr., E. D. Holyoke, and J. H. Yardley: Mechanisms of metastasis production by blood-borne cancer cells. Canadian Cancer Conference, Vol. 4, pp. 167—223 (1961).

Problems in the Treatment of Disseminated Cancer of the Breast: Selection of Patients for Hormone Treatment [1]

H. J. Tagnon, A. Coune, J. C. Heuson, and M. van Rymenant

The treatment of disseminated breast cancer consists first of modification of the hormonal environment of the patient. This can be done either by hormonal deprivation — oophorectomy, adrenalectomy, or hypophysectomy — or by the administration of hormones, usually steroids, androgens, estrogens, and corticosteroids. Only when these therapeutic measures have failed is it advisable to have recourse to non-hormonal cytotoxic agents, such as the alkylating drugs and 5-fluorouracil. One exception to this rule may be the group of patients less than one year postmenopausal. These are notoriously resistant to hormonal manipulation, whether surgical (hormonal deprivation) or medical (hormonal administration). This is why a clinical investigation is now being conducted with the aim of discovering whether the use of 5-fluorouracil or of some alkylating agent should precede hormone treatment in this particular group of patients, as the only exception to the general rule.

The great limitations to hormonal treatment of disseminated breast cancer should not be minimized. Less than 45 % of patients respond, and in those responding the favorable effects are temporary. No five-year cure has been observed. The remission usually lasts a few months, rarely a few years. *Even so, the hormonal treatment of advanced breast cancer represents the most remarkable success achieved so far in the care and control of advanced cancer.* It is possible that the same is true for cancer of the prostate, but the data on this disease are fewer and the effects of treatment have not been fully evaluated.

The non-hormonal chemotherapeutic agents available at present are much more toxic and much less specific than hormones for cancer of the breast.

The hormonal treatment of disseminated breast cancer is based on the concept of hormone dependence. Huggins (1965), who made the original observations on cancer of the prostate in dog and in man, expresses this concept as follows. When

[1] This work was supported by Grant Ca 4896-03 of the National Institutes of Health, Bethesda, Md., United States of America, for a co-operative study organized in Europe, and by Contract Euratom-ULB-Pise no. 026-63-4 BIAC. The European Breast Cancer Group is now part of the *Groupe Européen de Chimiothérapie anti-cancéreuse.*

the cells of origin of a cancer are dependent on hormones for their metabolic activity, in a certain proportion of cases the cancer itself may similarly be dependent and will undergo atrophy associated with clinical regression when hormonal support is withdrawn. Clinical regression is not the only manifestation of hormone dependence. In the case of the prostate, measurements of enzymes produced by the tumor have shown a striking and immediate alteration of enzyme activity following modification of the hormonal environment (TAGNON et al., 1953; TAGNON and STEENS-LIEVENS, 1963).

The term "hormone dependence" has been criticized because it tends to over-simplify an otherwise very complicated situation. It is true that in disseminated breast cancer the main argument for hormone dependence is derived from the observation of the often favorable effects of oophorectomy in premenopausal women. However, confirmation that this effect is due to deprivation of estrogens alone is not available (TAGNON, 1964 b). The ovaries are producers not simply of estrogens but also of other steroid hormones; oophorectomy should not be equated with estrogen deprivation. It is well established that in certain patients small amounts of estrogens may activate the disease, while larger amounts have an inhibitory effect (KENNEDY, 1962). This and other data show that the concept of hormone dependence is not simple. Perhaps, as has been suggested, the term "hormone-dependent tumors" should be changed to that of "hormone-sensitive tumors". The concept nevertheless remains a useful one, has tended to unify our concepts, and has had a stimulating effect on research. As the area of exploration broadens, the concept will need fresh adjustments. This does not impair its essential validity.

Advanced breast cancer is an important problem of medicine. At least 75 % of all patients die of their disease; this is due to the fact that mammary cancer differs from others in its development. Certain forms have an acute course and kill the patient in a few months. In contrast, many have a very slow course, which explains why more than 15 % of patients may survive five or more years without any treatment (BLOOM, 1964). This slow development also explains the persistence of recurrences after radical treatment when the patient seems cured according to the usual criteria. Five-year survival rates have not the same significance in cancer of the breast as in other forms of cancer. In spite of five symptomless years following radical treatment, metastases keep occurring and affect 2 % of patients every year, and the threat of recurrence is always present for as long as the patient lives. The free interval, i. e., the time between radical treatment for the localized primary tumor and the first appearance of metastases, is more variable in this type of cancer than in any other, and may extend from a few months to several decades.

From these considerations some principles emerge that should provide guidance in treatment (SEGALOFF, 1960).

1. Hormonal treatment is palliative: it should therefore be employed for the patient with advanced disease that is beyond the resources of surgery and radio-therapy. Localized tumors should not be treated with hormones for either diagnostic or therapeutic purposes.

2. Isolated metastases, bone metastases in the weight-bearing areas of the body, or imminent pathological fractures should be treated by local deep X-ray therapy. This is usually very effective and does not prevent the institution of hormonal treatment if disseminated metastases are present.

3. Before hormonal treatment is given it is essential to obtain proof that the disease is progressing. This is done by measuring the metastatic lesions after a given interval, say from 2 to 4 weeks, and noting their growth. Metastases that are quiescent should not be treated. Visible metastases may remain quiescent for months or even years and non-interference is indicated, in the interest of the patient. This quiescence of breast cancer metastases, falsely interpreted as the result of treatment by physicians unfamiliar with the natural history of the disease, is the most important cause of serious errors in the evaluation of old and new hormonal agents (Segaloff, 1960; Van Rymenant et al., 1963).

4. Evaluation of the results of treatment should be by objective measurement of all measurable lesions in centimetres and millimetres. The methods have been published elsewhere (Segaloff, 1960; Van Rymenant et al., 1963). An objective method of evaluation is necessary for scientific reasons, but it is just as necessary in the best interests of the patient, because continuation or change of the therapeutic method rests on evaluation of the observed effects and it is just as important to pursue effective treatment as it is to discontinue ineffective treatment — regardless of the misleading indications given by subjective improvements that are not con-firmed objectively by the course of the lesions.

The selection of patients for the different types of hormonal treatment is best discussed on the basis of the general scheme of therapeutic planning shown in Table 1. Premenopausal and postmenopausal women differ in their response, and within each of these two groups subgroups can be delimited that respond differently and have a different prognosis. The plan proposed here is subject to revision and parts of it represent a choice between alternatives that may, on the basis of present-day knowledge, be equally acceptable. *In premenopausal women* oophorectomy produces a remission in from 35% to 45% of cases. Oophorectomy is preferred to sterilization by X-rays because castration is more rapid and the operation is better tolerated than is X-irradiation.

Table 1. *Treatment of Advanced Breast Cancer*

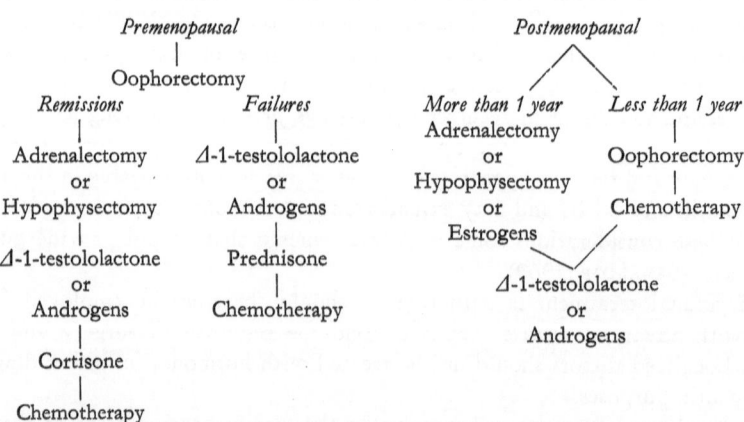

There is general agreement that oophorectomy is the obligatory first step in this group of patients, because probably no other treatment gives as high a rate of remission. Patients resistant to oophorectomy very rarely experience a remission with adrenalectomy or hypophysectomy, and we therefore believe that they should not undergo these operations. They may be given 100 mg of testosterone propionate intramuscularly three times a week. However, the group of premenopausal patients resistant to oophorectomy has a bad prognosis and is usually also resistant to administered hormones. The same holds true for patients with disseminated cancer who are less than one year past the natural menopause. This composite group of patients less than one year postmenopausal behaves quite differently from those more advanced in the postmenopausal period. It is in this group that the use of non-hormonal chemotherapy may be justified as the first treatment.

Premenopausal women who respond to oophorectomy and relapse have an approximately even chance of a second remission if adrenalectomy or hypophysectomy is carried out (MacDonald, 1962); while the chances of achieving a second remission by the administration of androgens are probably approximately 15 % to 20 % (Segaloff, 1960; Groupe Européen du Cancer du Sein, 1962, 1964). Dao and co-workers have shown the superiority of adrenalectomy over fluoxymesterone, an orally active androgen, in these patients (Dao and Tan, 1962). There are many remissions and they last longer. Androgens are indicated in patients who refuse the operation, or in geographical areas where the operation is not available. Severe virilization, distressing to the patient, and, occasionally, aggravation of the tumor growth with an acute course are the price to be paid for the remission they make possible. Hypophysectomy is carried out surgically or, with less certainty, by intrasellar injection of yttrium.

In postmenopausal women oophorectomy is rarely beneficial. Yet the major ablative procedures appear to be equally effective in postmenopausal and premenopausal women (MacDonald, 1962). Adrenalectomy can be performed without concomitant oophorectomy in patients more than one year postmenopausal because they rarely have significant ovarian activity left.

Hormones can also be administered to these patients as the first step in treatment, but the rate of remissions is reduced as compared with that for ablative procedures. Estrogens were thought to give a higher rate of remissions than androgens, at least in the first few postmenopausal years (MacDonald, 1962). Recent observations on randomized patients seem to show the essential similarity of results obtained by either estrogens or androgens in postmenopausal women. The rate of remission with either is approximately 20 %—25 %, and improves with advancing age to reach a maximum of 30 %—35 % in patients over eight years past the menopause. Estrogens do not have the disadvantage of virilization and we prefer them to androgens. The latter may be tried if estrogens fail, but there is little hope of success with them.

The general experience is that hormone administration is rarely successful in patients relapsing after a major ablative procedure, and that if one type of hormone is ineffective the other type will be equally ineffective (European Breast Cancer Group, to be published).

Estrogens are given in the form of an oral dose of 3 mg daily of ethinylestradiol. Certain authors have suggested that β estradiol may be a more effective estrogenic agent than others and have described spectacular regressions following its use in association with high doses of progesterone (Huggins, 1965).

The studies of the co-operative groups on breast cancer on patients treated with androgens show a significantly longer survival for responders than for non-responders

(SEGALOFF, 1961). This could be just as well attributed to the nature of their cancer as to the effect of treatment, since there is the possibility that hormone-sensitive cancers may, as a class, develop more slowly than hormone-resistant cancers, irrespective of the treatment given. This is suggested by the longer free interval seen in responders.

While estrogens in postmenopausal women rarely produce toxic effects, they may have a stimulating effect on the growth of the tumor, with dangerous results in as many as 50 % of premenopausal patients (PEARSON, 1957). This is considered a manifestation of hormone dependence. However, the results of oophorectomy in patients showing this estrogen sensitivity are not uniformly good. This again confirms the importance, at present, of not equating oophorectomy with estrogen deprivation. These toxic effects are usually observed with small therapeutic doses of estrogens. Very large doses of estrogens appear less toxic than smaller doses in premenopausal women.

Toxic manifestations associated with stimulated tumor growth are also seen with androgens, but less commonly. From a small number of personal observations, we believe that if androgens stimulate the growth of the tumor in a given patient estrogens will do the same, but the reverse is not true. Therefore, if a patient shows toxic manifestations due to accelerated tumor growth after administration of androgens, she should not be given estrogens instead (KARHAUSEN et al., 1955).

In recent years, the compound Δ-1-testololactone has gained increasing recognition as a valuable agent with the same indications as testosterone propionate (SEGALOFF, 1961). Actually the remission rate with both compounds appears to be identical. Δ-1-testololactone has the great advantage of complete lack of toxicity, and no hormonal effects are observed in patients (Groupe Européen du Cancer du Sein, 1962, 1964). Suggestive evidence exists that patients responding to testosterone propionate also respond to Δ-1-testololactone (Groupe Européen du Cancer du Sein, 1964). The evidence is enough to justify its substitution for testosterone and so produce elimination of the latter's undesirable hormone effects in the routine treatment of advanced cancer of the breast. The dose is 100 mg of Δ-1-testololactone three times a week intramuscularly. The oral dose is 2 mg daily. The equivalence of parenteral and oral administration is not completely established (SEGALOFF, personal communication).

No inhibition of gonadotrophin production is observed in patients receiving Δ-1-testololactone, whether they have remissions or not. There are other effective sex hormones that produce remissions without affecting the gonadotrophins, for instance fluoxymesterone and 2-methyldehydrotestosterone. This shows that inhibition of gonadotrophins is not essential for antitumoral action (TAGNON, 1961). Patients in whom testosterone propionate has produced a temporary regression may experience a fresh regression on withdrawal of the hormone. Several such cases have been observed. It is important to take this into account when treatment is changed from testosterone to another drug. An intermediate period of observation between the two treatments should be allowed in order to enable this "withdrawal regression" to take place. It is beneficial to the patient and may last several months (SEGALOFF, 1958).

The place of corticosteroids (mainly prednisone) in this treatment is under discussion. In our opinion, prednisone and other corticosteroids are not indicated for long-term treatment because: (1) they do not produce a real remission as defined by the co-operative groups on breast cancer, prerequisites of which are non-progression of any lesion and regression of at least 50 % of all measurable lesions, and (2) their effect is of short duration (VAN GILSE, 1962). NISSEN MAYER is of another opinion and thinks that small doses of prednisone may be equivalent to an adrenalectomy. His criteria of evaluation are different from ours (NISSEN MAYER and VOGT, 1959).

There are, however, important indications for the use of prednisone. It is of value in the following dangerous and acute developmental phases of breast cancer: (a) extensive lung metastases reducing the vital capacity to below $1^1/_2$ litres; (b) hypercalcemia; and (c) brain metastases. In these three groups major ablative procedures carry a big operative risk, and administration of hormones may, as pointed out above, occasionally stimulate growth and, in patients with a small reserve, produce a rapidly irreversible condition. These patients should receive prednisone in large doses, from 1 to 3 mg per kg; not infrequently this treatment will produce a sufficient temporary improvement to allow specific hormone treatment to be carried out, surgical or medical. Hypercalcemia is a dangerous complication associated with the development of bone metastases, although other factors are important in its appearance. We have observed it in ambulatory patients and others. This condition needs urgent treatment; fluids must be pressed and prednisone administered (TAGNON, 1961).

The hormone treatment of disseminated breast cancer is still a subject in which clinical investigation and careful observation of the patients are predominant. The choice of treatment in any given case is based on an estimation of the probable response, an objective evaluation of the response, and a step-by-step scale of treatment, as shown in Table 1. One of the most important advances in treatment would be the development of a laboratory test enabling prediction of the type of treatment to be given to a patient. Tests of this kind, based mainly on hormone measurements in the blood and urine, are the subject of much research at present and may become available soon (BULBROOK, 1965).

That is why the adoption of acceptable objective criteria for the evaluation of lesions and remissions is very important. We have for many years used the criteria adopted by the co-operative groups of the National Institutes of Health, United States of America, and have found by experience how invaluable strict adherence to objective, uniform criteria is, not only from the point of view of scientific progress but also from that of the good of the individual patient. This is so because the selection of patients for hormone treatment is based on the recognition of the objective success or failure of the successive therapeutic steps. Co-operative studies that speed up the evaluation of new compounds are based on a plan of treatment that can be adopted by several institutions in one or different countries, working and publishing their results together. In Europe the European Group of Cancer Chemotherapy (G. E. C. A.) [1] is the clearing-house for such co-operative studies and the distribution of experimental plans.

When hormone treatment has either been unsuccessful or has ceased to be effective, the last resort is conventional non-hormonal chemotherapy, which is based

---

[1] Headquarters: Institut J. Bordet, 1, rue Héger-Bordet, Brussels, Belgium. Secretary: P. Straüli, Schmelzbergstraße, Zurich, Switzerland.

mainly on the use of 5-fluorouracil or alkylating agents. The chemotherapy of disseminated cancer of the breast produces a certain number of remissions (20 % with 5-fluorouracil), with perhaps a higher proportion in the groups less than one year postmenopausal than in the others. These remissions are of short duration and attended by the usual hematological and general toxic side effects of cytotoxic agents. In interpreting the action of these agents in disseminated cancer of the breast, their complex action on the organism should be taken into account. Part or all of the observed results could conceivably be due to an effect on other structures than the tumor itself. For instance, it is well known that the gonads and other endocrine glands are sensitive to the action of alkylating agents (KENIS et al., 1956).

In conclusion, it may be said that there are no laboratory methods at present available capable of predicting the response of patients with disseminated mammary cancer to the different forms of hormone treatment. The selection of patients for treatment must be based on clinical experience derived from careful observation correctly interpreted. Objective evaluation of the results of treatment is necessary to guarantee the best possible treatment to the patient. Close observation of the patient by someone familiar with the natural history of the disease and the pharmacology of the therapeutic agents is indispensable to ensure the maximal therapeutic effect without prohibitively toxic side effects.

References

BLOOM, H. J. G.: Natural history of untreated breast cancer. Ann. N. Y. Acad. Sci. 114, 747 (1964).

BULBROOK, R. D.: Hormone assays in human breast cancer. Vit. and Horm. 23, 329 (1965).

DAO, T. L., and E. TAN: A comparative evaluation of adrenalectomy and androgens in advanced mammary cancer. Cancer Chemother. Rep. 16, 309 (1962).

European Breast Cancer Group: Testosterone propionate therapy of breast cancer: a progress report. Cancer Chemother. Rep. 16, 273 (1962).

European Breast Cancer Group: Study No. 3 (to be published).

Groupe Européen du Cancer du Sein (Coordinateur: H. J. TAGNON): Le traitement hormonal du cancer du sein en phase avancée. Comparaison des résultats obtenus au moyen de la delta-1-testololactone et du propionate de testostérone. Rev. franç. Etud. clin. biol. 7, 1067 (1962).

Groupe Européen du Cancer du Sein (Coordinateur: H. J. TAGNON): Le traitement hormonal du cancer du sein en phase avancée. Comparaison entre le propionate de testostérone et la combinaison propionate de testostérone — delta-1-testololactone. Rev. franç. Etud. clin. biol. 9, 88 (1964).

HUGGINS, C. B.: Propositions in hormonal treatment of advanced cancers. J. Amer. med. Ass. 192, 1141 (1965).

KARHAUSEN, L., Y. KENIS, J. SMULDERS, et R. PARMENTIER: Hypercalcémie et néphro-calcinose: étude de 4 cas de cancer du sein avec métastases osseuses. Acta clin. belg. 10, 296 (1955).

KENIS, Y., P. DUSTIN, J. A. HENRY, et H. J. TAGNON: Action du Myleran dans 22 cas de leucémie myéloïde chronique. Rev. franç. Etud. clin. biol. 1, 435 (1956).

KENNEDY, B. J.: Massive estrogen administration in premenopausal women with advanced breast cancer. Cancer Chemother. Rep. 16, 283 (1962).

MACDONALD, I.: Endocrine ablation in disseminated mammary carcinoma. Surg. Gynec. Obstet. 115, 215 (1962).

NISSEN MEYER, R., and J. H. VOGT: Cortisone treatment of metastatic breast cancer. Acta Un. int. Cancr. 15, 2240 (1959).

PEARSON, O. H.: Observations on the role of androgens and estrogens in body balance. Arch. intern. Med. 100, 724 (1957).

SEGALOFF, A.: Testosterone propionate therapy of breast cancer. A report for the cooperative breast cancer group. In PINCUS, G., and E. P. VOLLMER (ed.): Biological activities of steroids in relation to cancer. New York and London: Academic Press 1960.
— et al.: Study No. 2 of the Cooperative Breast Cancer Group. Cancer Chemother. Rep. 11, 109 (1961).
— Breast cancer. St. Louis: C. V. Mosby: 1958, pages 193—195.
TAGNON, H. J., P. SHULMAN, W. F. WHITMORE, and L. A. LEONE: Prostatic fibrinolysin. Role in hemorrhagic diathesis of cancer of the prostate. Amer. J. Med. 15, 875—884 (1953).
— Traitement hormonal du cancer du sein en phase avancée. Brux. méd. 41, 817 (1961).
—, and A. STEENS-LIEVENS: Studies of fibrinolysis and acid phosphatase in cancer of the prostate. Biology of the prostate and related tissues. Washington: National Cancer Institute 1963 (Monograph No. 12).
— La dépendance hormonale dans les cancers mammaires. Méd. et Hyg. (Genève) 22, 1001 (1964 a).
— Clinical results with hormones in disseminated mammary cancer. In PLATTNER, P. A. (ed.): Chemotherapy of cancer. Amsterdam and New York: Elsevier 1964 b.
VAN GILSE, H. A.: Long term treatment with corticosteroids of patients with metastatic breast cancer. Cancer Chemother. Rep. 16, 293 (1962).
VAN RYMENANT, M., A. COUNE, H. J. TAGNON, et S. SIMON: Le traitement hormonal du cancer du sein en phase avancée. Méthodes d'étude: comparaison de la delta-1-testololactone avec le propionate de testostérone. Acta clin. belg. 18, 469 (1963).

Hormone Treatment of Cancer of the Prostate

CLARENCE V. HODGES and DIETER KIRCHHEIM

The hormone treatment of prostatic cancer is based on the dependence of prostatic cells on the stimulus of androgens for their development and maintenance. The prostate gland remains small in eunuchoid individuals throughout puberty and shrinks after castration or the suppression of androgens, direct or indirect, by administration of estrogens (HUGGINS and CLARKE, 1940). The extension of this study to the treatment of prostatic cancer as described by HUGGINS and HODGES (1941) showed that castration or estrogen therapy produced a dramatic response in about 80 % of patients with disseminated prostatic cancer. If prostatic cancer is not amenable to cure by radical prostatectomy (stage A or B in WHITMORE's classification, 1963), hormone therapy should be instituted. BARNES (1959) has shown that delay in instituting anti-androgen therapy after prostatic cancer has been diagnosed results in a shorter average survival than if it had been begun immediately.

The initial choice in anti-androgen therapy is bilateral orchiectomy, estrogen administration, or a combination of the two. Each choice has its advantages and disadvantages. Castration is definitive and irreversible; its application is not dependent upon the patient's memory or willingness to continue therapy. However, it involves a surprising amount of psychic trauma for many men in the prostatic cancer age group. Impotence is usually (but not always) a sequel of the procedure.

Estrogens have the advantage of being non-mutilating and relatively inexpensive. They often cause hypertrophy and tenderness of the breast, along with water retention. Some patients develop striking psychic depression on estrogens. Chronic estrogen administration results in atrophy of the testis and penis and, usually, impotence.

Many centers prefer to use a combination of estrogens and castration as soon as the diagnosis of prostatic cancer has been made. This type of therapy is based on Nesbit and Baum's collective review (1950) in which a better five-year survival rate (44 %) was found for combined therapy than for orchiectomy alone (31 %) or estrogens alone (29 %).

At our institution, the regimen for treating freshly diagnosed inoperable prostatic cancer consists of estrogens first. The rationale for this treatment is derived from the observation that occasional patients who become refractory to estrogens obtain a further regression of their cancerous lesions when orchiectomy is performed. For the same reason, we do not combine estrogens and orchiectomy as initial therapy. About 80 % of patients will show objective improvement from hormone therapy. Unfortunately, no prostatic cancers appear to have been destroyed by hormone therapy and about 80 % of those initially improved will show exacerbations of their disease within one year.

Histological proof of prostatic cancer is required before treatment is instituted since other lesions, particularly tuberculous and non-specific granulomatous prostatitis, may be impossible to differentiate by other means. A false diagnosis of malignancy imposes a tragic sentence on the unfortunate patient.

Castration

Bilateral epididymo-orchiectomy under general anesthesia is the method of choice. Current anesthesiologic skills make the usual minor discomfort and occasional major pain of orchiectomy under local anesthesia unnecessary. The operation is done rapidly but with meticulous attention to hemostasis. Orchiectomy alone has been advocated, leaving the epididymis in the scrotum for cosmetic purposes, but this seems unnecessary in the usual patient. Intracapsular parenchymectomy (scooping out the testicular substance from the incised capsule and fulgurating the rete testis) is hardly necessary for cosmetic reasons and may leave androgen-forming cells behind (O'Conor, Chiang and Grayhack, 1963). Closure without drainage and firm compression with elastic adhesive dressings complete the operation.

The chain of events relating to steroid hormone metabolite excretion before and after castration has been studied by Gallagher and associates (1963). These authors examined individual metabolites of steroid hormones in a group of patients with untreated prostatic cancer before and after orchiectomy and continued these studies at intervals following orchiectomy until death. All the patients had too extensive a neoplasm for radical excision. Each of 13 patients exhibited a decrease in the combined output of androsterone and etiocholanolone after orchiectomy. However, the authors state, "in this series of patients there was no evident correlation between the level of urinary androgen metabolites before orchiectomy and recurrence or lack of remission." And "there was, further, no evident correlation between the fall in androgen excretion after orchiectomy and remission or failure to improve." Patients who were followed with serial examinations of the urine for androgen metabolites for most of their lifetime after castration failed to show changes in output of androgen metabolites which might be correlated with an exacerbation of malignant disease.

Estrogens

In 1941 HUGGINS and HODGES demonstrated the effectiveness of natural estrogens (estradiol benzoate, 1.66 to 3.32 mg daily) and synthetic compounds with estrogen-like biological activities (stilbestrol, 1 mg daily) in lowering elevated serum acid phosphatases in patients with metastatic carcinoma of the prostate. The theoretical concept which had led to the endocrine therapy of prostatic carcinoma has been discussed in the introduction. The "biologic titration" studies by HUGGINS and CLARKE (1940) suggested a quantitative reciprocal relationship between stilbestrol and testosterone as measured by the secretory output of the prostate in castrated dogs. On the basis of these experiments, HUGGINS spoke of the "neutralization" of androgens by exogenous estrogen administration. While the endocrine treatment of inoperable (stage C or D) prostatic cancer has changed little since its introduction, the mechanism of action of estrogens or stilbenes remains controversial. Several investigators (CHRISTENSEN [1944], O'CONOR et al., [1953], SCOTT [1956], KIRCHHEIM and SCOTT [1965], ROTHAUGE et al., [1963]) studying gonadotrophin excretion in patients or histological and histochemical changes in the rat prostate following various hormonal manipulations arrived at the conclusion that natural and synthetic estrogens act by pituitary inhibition of ICSH. GOODWIN (1961) supported HUGGINS' original findings in dogs. In this species estrogens can inhibit the androgen-maintained prostatic secretion in the hypophysectomized dog. ROTHAUGE et al. (1963) investigated the effect of three estrogenic substances (diethyl-dioxystilbene-diphosphate, diethyldioxystilbenedipropionate, and estradiol-unde-cylate) upon testicular histology, Leydig cells, and urinary gonadotrophins. They concluded that these estrogens inhibit the secretion of ICSH by the pituitary. The typical histological changes in the prostate of man following castration for prostatic carcinoma cannot be distinguished from those following prolonged estrogen administration.

In summary, one may say that accumulated evidence indicates in indirect action of estrogens on prostatic cancer in man by way of the inhibition of pituitary gonadotrophins, resulting in testicular atrophy and loss of androgen production. A direct effect of estrogens upon prostatic cancer cells has never been proven, but has been considered as a result of tissue culture and in vitro metabolic studies (LASNITZKI [1954], FRANKS [1959], MACDONALD and LATTA [1956], KNOBIL [1952]).

Higher survival rates of patients with stage C or D prostatic cancers have been reported (NESBIT and BAUM [1950], SCHIRMER et al. [1965]) following castration plus estrogen treatment than following either castration or estrogen alone. This suggested to some urologists that estrogens must, in addition to the above-mentioned indirect effect, have a direct effect on the cancer cells or, according to GRAYHACK et al. (1955), another inhibitory effect on the production of LTH (prolactin) or adrenal androgens. The latter appears unlikely, since estrogens cause adrenal hyperplasia in laboratory animals (BIRKE, 1955). Estrogens have also been tried to "shrink" stage C tumors and make them amenable to radical prostatectomy (COLSTON and BRENDLER, 1946). Histological examination of specimens after such prostatectomy showed a variable and random response of the cancer cells; the treatment did not result in destruction of all the cancer cells which had invaded the tissues beyond the confines of the prostate.

A co-operative study reported by Brendler (1965) showed that conventional or high doses of estrogens had no effect on patients in relapse after temporary remission following orchiectomy.

Two compounds with estrogenic activity merit special mention. One is diethyl-dioxystilbenediphosphate, a water-insoluble phosphorylated stilbene first employed clinically by Druckrey and Raabe (1952), and credited with specific effects on the prostatic cancer cells. They and other clinicians assumed that it would penetrate into the normal and neoplastic prostatic epithelial cell and become dephosphorylated by their acid phosphatases. This would then result in a precipitation of the "active" stilbene compound in the prostatic cell. For this reason high intravenous dosages were administered. Most urologists have not noticed superior clinical results with high dosages of intravenous diethyldioxystilbenediphosphate than with the conventional 5 mg of stilbestrol daily. The investigations previously mentioned by Rothauge et al. (1963) gave support to the view that the action of this stilbene compound was indirect, by way of the hypophysis. Fergusson (1961) injected C-14-labeled stilbestrol diphosphate intravenously and found that the concentration of free stilbestrol in prostatic tissue was five times higher than in other tissues during the first half hour after intravenous administration and then fell rapidly within three hours. Behnam et al. (1962) demonstrated the localization of radioactive phosphorus when diethylstilbestrol-diphosphate-P 32 was injected into the isolated prostatic circulation by radioautographic techniques.

The second compound is polyestradiol phosphate. Jöhnson et al. (1963) reported the unusually high five-year survival rate of 52 % following injection of 80—200 mg of polyestradiol phosphate (Estradurin) intramuscularly once monthly. On the basis of extensive urinary steroid excretion studies (fractionated) they concluded that "estradurin exerts its favorable therapeutic action mainly through direct effects on cancer cells and *not* via reduced testicular androgen production." No histological studies of the testes were reported. The authors emphasized the value of intramuscular injections in unreliable patients. Since this compound is a polymerization product of phosphorylated estradiol, their findings are in disagreement with those of Rothauge et al. (1963) on estradiol.

Several other natural and synthetic estrogens are available, which are similar in their mode of action to those discussed above.

Adrenalectomy

After failure of estrogens, castration, or a combination of the two to control prostatic cancer, the next step is naturally to attempt removal of extragonadal sources of androgen. Since about two-thirds of the 17-ketosteroids excreted in the urine are of adrenal origin, extirpation of the adrenals is a measure that follows logically. Bilateral adrenalectomy was described by Huggins and Scott (1945) but since they could not use cortisone for support their patients could be maintained for only a limited period of time. The availability of corticoids allowed Huggins and Bergenstal (1951) to describe a successful maintenance regimen after bilateral adrenalectomy. About 50% of patients with disseminated prostatic cancer will show subjective benefit from this treatment, and about 15 % may show objective improvement (Dao, 1957). However, the improvement is short-lived, lasting on the average about 30 days. Since most of these benefits can be obtained by "medical adrenal-ectomy" — the administration of corticoids and the induction of adrenal atrophy —, this operation has relatively little application at the present time.

Administration of Corticoids

As indicated above, the administration of cortisone or similar steroids will occasionally produce subjective and objective evidence of remission in disseminated prostatic cancer. Prednisone and prednisolone are currently used in dosages of 25—50 mg per day. Diabetes, hypertension, psychosis, and the presence or history of a peptic ulcer are contraindications to this therapy. An ulcer-preventing regimen must be followed while the patient is on corticoids. It is difficult to separate the euphoria induced by corticoids from the therapeutic results when subjective impro-vement is being assessed. Evidence for objective improvement is usually lacking.

Hypophysectomy

In comparison with carcinoma of the breast, only a few studies have been done on the beneficial effects of hypophysectomy on carcinoma of the prostate — in most instances when reactivation of a tumor growth has occurred after castration and estrogen treatment. The rationale of pituitary ablation lies in the elimination of the following hormones:

1. ACTH
2. Gonadotrophins
3. Prolactin
4. Growth hormone

This will result in abolition of androgen production by the adrenals and gonads.

The absence of the latter two hormones is probably responsible for the occasional remissions reported. Experimentally, GRAYHACK et al. (1955) and PEARSON et al. (1956) have demonstrated the synergistic effect of these hormones on prostatic growth. The limited number of cases treated by hypophysectomy precludes a critical evaluation of the benefit of this procedure in relapsed or castration-estrogen refrac-tory cases. SCOTT and SCHIRMER (1962) have reported their experiences at Johns Hopkins Hospital with 17 patients who had disseminated prostatic cancer. The two longest survivors were alive 22 and 23 months after hypophysectomy. Seven patients showed objective and subjective improvement. The authors felt that a previous good response to castration-estrogen therapy and evidence of continued androgen pro-duction indicated that the response to hypophysectomy would be favorable. PEAR-SON et al. (1956) performed hypophysectomy on 79 patients with advanced neoplastic disease, four of whom suffered from carcinoma of the prostate. One patient in relapse after castration-estrogen therapy, with tumor invasion of the spinal canal and complete paraplegia, obtained objective remission as manifested by restoration of bladder and rectal control and partial motor power. They found "the surgical removal of the pituitary by way of a transfrontal craniotomy a satisfactory means of accomplishing total hypophysectomy with minimal morbidity and mortality." SMITH et al. (1959) did a left frontal hypophysectomy on five patients with advanced metastatic carcinoma. They stated that "all four who survived the operation have shown worthwhile subjective and objective improvement." A simpler approach using yttrium-90 with nearly complete destruction of the pituitary has been reported by Forrest et al. (1958), but others (Young, 1957) found the extent of pituitary destruction by radioisotopes variable and unpredictable. However, reactivation of growth usually occurs without biochemical indications of a return of pituitary function (Smith, Gurling and Baron, 1959).

Replacement treatment consists of cortisone and thyroid hormone. If the stalk is not, or is only minimally, traumatized polydipsia and polyuria occur only transiently in about 50% of cases. Replacement therapy with posterior pituitary powder by nasal insufflation may be necessary. Insulin tolerance is reduced, but hypoglycemic responsiveness is normal. In diabetic patients insulin requirements are markedly reduced.

Further work is necessary in this field.

Androgens

Testosterone was reported by Huggins and Hodges (1941) to cause exacerbation of prostatic cancer both clinically and as indicated by the acid and alkaline phosphatase levels. There have been occasional reports since (Munger, 1947; Brendler, Chase and Scott, 1950), describing both subjective and objective remissions. This aspect will be reviewed more thoroughly in the light of the findings of the co-operative study cited below.

Anabolic agents with less androgenic action, such as norethandrolone, have been reported by Brendler and Winkler (1953) to bring about symptomatic improvement but little evidence of objective remission. These authors and we have observed that the urinary 17-ketosteroid excretion is decreased in all patients on this compound, but there is little change in the objective indices of disseminated cancer.

The Co-operative Study of Reactivated Prostatic Cancer

In 1956, twelve medical institutions[1] under the sponsorship of the Cancer Chemotherapy National Service Center undertook a co-operative study. Since the main problem in prostatic cancer relates to the ultimate lack of response to hormonal management, it was decided to study the effects of various hormone regimens in patients who had either regressed after previous improvement or had never benefited from hormone therapy. The basic qualifications for inclusion of a patient in the study were that he should have undergone orchiectomy at least six weeks prior to entry into the study and have failed to benefit from castration or hormone therapy, as evidenced by the increasing size or consistency of his primary tumor, the increasing size or number of bone or soft tissue metastases, or the continued elevation of the serum acid phosphatase. The plan of study was prepared and approved by all the investigators prior to each phase of the study. Biometrical supervision was provided by a staff of statisticians who worked with the group from

---

[1] 1) New York University, 2) State University of Iowa, 3) University of California at Los Angeles, 4) Northwestern University, 5) Vanderbilt University, 6) University of Oregon, 7) Columbia University, 8) University of Rochester, 9) University of Miami, 10) Johns Hopkins University, 11) University of Kansas, 12) Memorial Center (New York).

the outset in preparing each plan, retrieving information, and assessing the results. Pathologists selected to participate in the study reviewed each pathological specimen submitted on entry of the patient into the study.

Trial one: stilbestrol versus placebo

The first trial compared 100 patients who received 5 mg of stilbestrol daily with 100 patients who received the same amount of lactose. The study was carried out in a double blind fashion in which the compounds were not known to the investigator and the patient was randomly allocated to the drug or the placebo by the statistical center. The drug and placebo were administered for four weeks and various physical and laboratory parameters were compared before and after the study. The essence of the statistical findings was that there was no significant difference between stilbestrol in small doses and lactose in the patient with reactivated cancer.

Trial two: small versus large doses of stilbestrol

The patients were again those who had relapsed or had not been benefited by previous hormone therapy. One hundred patients received 5 mg of stilbestrol daily, as compared with 500 mg of stilbestrol daily. No difference was found between the two groups and, in fact, it was impossible to tell by clinical observation whether the patient was in one group or the other.

Trial three: testosterone

As mentioned above, occasional patients have been reported to be benefited by the administration of testosterone. In this study, an open sequential design was employed in an attempt to demonstrate differences in the effect of 300 grams weekly of testosterone propionate as opposed to 30 mg of stilbestrol weekly, both given by intramuscular injection. No benefit was found with either agent and in only a few of the patients was there an exacerbation requiring discontinuance of the testosterone.

Trial four: prednisone

An open sequential design was again employed in comparing the efficacy of 30 mg of prednisone daily with 5 mg daily of stilbestrol, both by mouth. No benefit was obtained with either compound. A few cases appeared to be exacerbated by prednisone.

Trial five: medroxy progesterone acetate

Pilot studies with this progestational agent at dosages of 200 mg and 1000 mg daily were tried. No significant effects were observed in periods of up to three months.

Pilot trials

Each group in the co-operative study conducted separate small studies using various synthetic steroids. These were chiefly compounds known to have estrogenic activity and testosterone analogues without significant androgenic activity. No significant benefits were observed.

Androgens and ^{32}P

Testosterone has been used to stimulate malignant prostatic cells prior to intravenous administration of radioactive sodium phosphate. Early reports were encouraging (WILDERMUTH et al. [1960]; MAXFIELD et al. [1958]). Subjective relief of pain is occasionally observed, but there has been little objective effect.

Androgens and Regional Perfusion with ^{32}P

At this institution we have been interested in the stimulation of stage C prostatic cancers with testosterone, followed by regional perfusion of the isolated pelvic circulation with a radioactive phosphate (HODGES et al., 1964). Previous studies (BEHNAM and OCKER, 1960; BEHNAM, HODGES and THYE, 1962) had shown that perfusion of the isolated prostatic circulation in the dog resulted in a high concentration of phosphorus within the prostate and that the radioactivity was actually within prostatic epithelial cells.

Testosterone propionate (50 mg) is administered intramuscularly every day during the five days prior to perfusion. At surgery, the pelvic circulation is isolated and oxygenated blood containing the radioactive phosphate is perfused through the pelvic circulation for 30 to 50 minutes. The end point of perfusion is determined when the peripheral radioactivity reaches one-third of the pelvic radioactivity.

Fifteen patients with stage C or stage D lesions have been subjected to regional perfusion in the manner described above. While it is too early to assess the long-term survival, five out of 15 patients are still living and symptom-free three to five years following perfusion. All patients had undergone orchiectomy and the majority had received estrogens prior to perfusion. Interestingly, marked shrinkage of the primary tumor did not occur following perfusion in two patients until estrogens were administered again; prior to perfusion, estrogens had become ineffective in these patients.

Conclusions

Laboratory investigations have increased our understanding of the relationship between hormones and the normal and neoplastic prostate cell, and clinical application of the findings has conferred considerable palliative benefit on and prolonged the life of many patients suffering from prostatic cancer. New problems and questions have arisen, such as androgen independency and reactivation of the cancer after initial response to endocrine treatment. Progress has recently been, and is being, made in the study of steroids (e. g., the measurements of testosterone in plasma) and enzymes.

The application of such basic research will no doubt help us in making further progress in the treatment of prostatic cancer.

References

BARNES, R. W., and W. C. EMERGY: Management of early prostatic cancer. Calif. Medicine (Baltimore) 91, 57 (1959).

BEHNAM, A. M., C. V. HODGES, and J. THYE: Microradioautography in internal irradiation of the prostate. J. Urol. (Baltimore) 88, 805 (1962).

—, and J. M. OCKER, jr.: Perfusion of the isolated prostatic circulation with radioactive phosphorus (P32). J. Urol. (Baltimore) 84, 753 (1960).

BIRKE, G., C. FRANKSSON, and L. O. PLANTIN: Estrogen therapy in carcinoma of the prostate. Acta chir. scand. 109, 1 (1955).

BRENDLER, H.: Steroids in reactivated prostatic cancer. In Methods in hormone research, Vol. 4. New York: Academic Press 1965, pages 105—122.

—, W. E. CHASE, and W. W. SCOTT: Prostatic cancer. Further investigations of hormonal relationship. Arch. Surg. 61, 433 (1950).

BRENDLER, H., and B. S. WINKLER: Effect of norethandrolone on 17-ketosteroid excretion in prostatic cancer patients. J. clin. Endocrin. **19**, 183 (1953).

CHRISTENSEN, B. G.: Hypofysectomi og Oestrinbehandlung, Copenhagen: Munksgaard 1944.

COLSTON, J. A. C., and H. BRENDLER: Endocrine therapy in carcinoma of the prostate: preparation of patients for radical perineal prostatectomy. Trans. Amer. Ass. gen.-urin. Surg. **38**, 241 (1946).

DAO, T. L.-Y.: Present status of adrenalectomy in the palliation of the metastatic carcinoma of the prostate. In Proceedings of the 3rd National Cancer Conference. Philadelphia: Lippencott 1957, page 282.

DRUCKREY, H., and S. RAABE: Organ spezifische Chemotherapie des Krebses (Prostata-carcinom). Klin. Wschr. **30**, 882 (1952).

FERGUSSON, J. D.: Tracer experiments showing the distribution and fate of injected phosphorylated oestrogens in cancer of the prostate. Brit. J. Urol. **33**, 442 (1961).

FORREST, A. P., D. W. BLAIR, and J. N. VALENTINE: Screw-implantation of the pituitary with yttrium-90. Lancet **2**, 192 (1958).

FRANKS, L. M.: The effects of age on the structure and response to oestrogens and testosterone of the mouse prostate in organ cultures. Brit. J. Cancer **13**, 59 (1959).

GALLAGHER, T. F., W. F. WHITMORE, jr., B. ZUMOFF, and F. HELLMAN: Studies in prostatic cancer before and after orchidectomy. Nat. Cancer Inst. Monogr. **12**, 131 (1963).

GOODWIN, D. A., D. S. RASMUSSEN-TAXDAL, A. A. FERREIRA, and W. W. SCOTT: Estrogen inhibition of androgen maintained prostatic secretion in the hypophysectomized dog. J. Urol. (Baltimore) **86**, 134 (1961).

GRAYHACK, J. T., P. L. BUNCE, S. W. KEARNS, and W. W. SCOTT: Influence of the pituitary on prostatic response to androgen in the rat. Bull. Johns Hopk. Hosp. **96**, 154 (1955).

HODGES, C. V., R. J. MOORE, A. M. BEHNAM, and T. H. LEHMAN: Regional perfusion of inoperable prostatic cancer with radioactive phosphorus. J. Urol. (Baltimore) **92**, 540 (1964).

HUGGINS, C., and D. M. BERGENSTAL: Surgery of the adrenals. J. Amer. med. Ass. **147**, 101 (1951).

—, and P. J. CLARKE: Quantitative studies of prostatic secretion. II. The effect of castration and estrogen injection on normal and hyperplastic prostate glands of dogs. J. exp. Med. **72**, 747 (1940).

—, and C. V. HODGES: I. The effect of castration and of estrogen and of androgen injection on serum phosphatases in metastatic carcinoma of the prostate. Cancer. Res. **1**, 293 (1941).

—, and W. W. SCOTT: Bilateral adrenalectomy in prostatic cancer: clinical features and urinary excretion of 17-ketosteroids and estrogens. Ann. Surg. **122**, 1031 (1945).

JÖHNSON, G., E. DICZFALUSY, L. O. PLANTIN, L. RÖHL, and G. BIRKE: Estradurin ® (poly-estradiol phosphate) in the treatment of prostatic carcinoma. A. Clinical and steroid metabolic study. Acta endocr. (Kbh.) Suppl. **83**, 3 (1963).

KIRCHHEIM, D., and W. W. SCOTT: The effects of castration and sex hormones upon aminopeptidases and phosphatases of the rat prostate. Invest. Urol. **2**, 393 (1965).

KNOBIL, E.: The relation of some steroid hormones to beta-glucuronidase activity. Endo-crinology **50**, 16 (1952).

LASNITZKI, I.: The effect of estrone alone and combined with 20-methylcholanthrene on mouse prostate glands grown in vitro. Cancer Res. **14**, 632 (1954).

MACDONALD, D. F., and M. J. LOTTA: Aerobic glycolysis of human prostatic adenoma: in vitro inhibition by estrogen and by androgen and estrogen. Endocrinology **59**, 153 (1956).

MAXFIELD, J. R., jr., G. S. MAXFIELD, and W. S. MAXFIELD: The use of radioactive phosphorus and testosterone in metastatic bone lesions from breast and prostate. Sth. med. J. (Bgham, Ala.) **51**, 320 (1958).

MUNGER, H. V.: Are some prostatic carcinomas estrogen dependent? Trans. S. cent. Sect. Amer. urol. Ass. **100**, 100 (1947).

NESBIT, R. M., and W. C. BAUM: Endocrine control of prostatic carcinoma. J. Amer. med. Ass. **143**, 1317 (1950).

O'Conor, V. J., jr., S. P. Chiang, and J. T. Grayhack: Is subcapsular orchiectomy
   a definitive procedure: Studies of hormone excretion before and after orchiectomy.
   J. Urol. (Baltimore) 89, 236 (1963).
—, R. E. Desantels, J. W. Pryor, P. L. Munson, and J. H. Harrison: Studies of hormonal
   changes in relation to cancer of the prostate: a progress report. J. Urol. (Baltimore) 81,
   468 (1953).
Pearson, O. H., S. R. Bronson, C. C. Harrold, C. D. West, M. C. Li, G. P. MacLean,
   and M. B. Lipsett: Hypophysectomy in treatment of advanced cancer. J. Amer. med.
   Ass. 161, 17 (1956).
Rothauge, C. F., O. Weller, and E. Schuchardt: Die Wirkung von Diäthyldioxystilben-
   diphosphat (Honvan®) auf die Keimdrüse und die Gonadotropinausscheidung beim
   Manne. Klin. Wschr. 41, 90 (1963).
Schirmer, H. K. A., G. P. Murphy, and W. W. Scott: Hormonal therapy of prostatic
   cancer. A correlation between histologic differentiation of prostatic cancer and the
   clinical course of the disease. Urol. Digest, 15, September 1965.
Scott, W. W.: Regulators of prostatic growth. Trans. Amer. Ass. gen.-urin. Surg. 47, 168
   (1956).
—, and H. K. A. Schirmer: Hypophysectomy for disseminated prostatic cancer. In Essays
   in experimental biology. Chicago: University of Chicago Press 1962, page 175.
Smith, E. J. R., K. J. Gurling, and D. N. Baron: The effect of hypophysectomy in advanced
   carcinoma of the prostate. Brit. J. Urol. 31, 181 (1959).
Whitmore, W. F., jr.: The rationale and results of ablative surgery for prostatic cancer.
   Cancer (Philad.) 16, 1119 (1963).
Wildermuth, O., D. Parker, J. O. Archambeau, and C. Chahbazian: Management of
   diffuse metastasis from carcinoma of the prostate. J. Amer. med. Ass. 172, 1607 (1960).
Young, S.: Pituitary necrosis due to implants of radioactive gold and yttrium. Lancet 1,
   548 (1957).

Recent Advances in the Treatment of Malignant Hemopathies

Jean Bernard

With 1 Figure

The treatment of malignant hemopathies can be considered under two main
headings. One class of therapy aims at the destruction of the malignant cells;
examples are radiotherapy and chemotherapy. The other has the vaguer and perhaps
loftier aim of cell regulation and attempts to make use of the defense mechanisms
of the host organism against the cancer. In the following discussion the examples
will be drawn especially from Hodgkin's disease and leukemia, and the destructive
forms of treatment will be dealt with first.

I. Destructive Forms of Treatment

1. Radiotherapy of Hodgkin's Disease

For a long time the radiological treatment of Hodgkin's disease was carried out
with moderate doses. This imposed no strain on the radiologist or on the patient,
but it meant that there was no hope of the patient having periods of more than
temporary improvement. The justification for this attitude, which could today be
termed "defeatist", appears to have been the view, then very fashionable, that the

blood diseases were systemic — that suddenly, as if by a stroke of a magic wand, all the bodily constituents were affected by the malignant blood condition. Since, then, the patient was doomed, why treat him too actively and tire him by over-zealous radiotherapy?

Around the year 1929 GILBERT (1938, 1939) in Switzerland and CHEVALLIER (1932) in France questioned this view, but met with the opposition of the radiologists. Indeed, it has been only quite recently that studies in America have shown that they were right. These studies have been carried out by two groups of investigators in particular: that of VERA PETERS (1966) at Toronto and that of HENRY KAPLAN at Palo Alto (KAPLAN, 1962, 1966 a, b; KAPLAN and ROSENBERG, 1966). The former especially has reported a number of remarkable examples of survival of patients in good condition 15 years after treatment. As in the time of GILBERT, these results were at first received with scepticism, but the large number of confirmatory observations finally brought conviction. In this respect, the Hematological and Radiological Societies of France a short time ago held a joint meeting in which most of the hematologists and radiologists concerned with these questions in the world — from the USA, Canada, England, France etc. — participated (LUKES et al., 1966; MATHÉ, 1966 a, b; SCHWARTZ, 1966). The meeting was preceded by an investigation in which three eminent pathologists (an American, a Belgian, and a Frenchman) met and, with no information given to them previously, examined the original microscope sections from the tissues of patients who had survived for more than 15 years after the diagnosis of Hodgkin's disease. The results of this study were remarkable in two respects: (1) the three pathologists, working separately, agreed on every case; and (2) practically every case was indeed Hodgkin's disease.

As far as radiotherapy is concerned, therefore, the new contributions to treatment are the following:

(1) A *high* dose of radiation is absolutely essential. It should be of the order of 3000—4000 rad per field (ENNUYER et al., 1966; FAYOS et al., 1965; GARY-BOBO, 1966; GLINSKA, 1966; LAUGIER et al., 1966; PAPILLON et al., 1966; PAPILLON, CROIZAT et al., 1966; PIEMONTE, 1966; TUBIANA et al., 1966).

(2) It is extremely important to irradiate not only the area affected but also the *adjacent* zones. It has long been the subject of speculation whether Hodgkin's disease should be considered as a systemic disease or as a localized disease starting, like any other cancer, at some exact point. The truth seems to lie between these two extremes: Hodgkin's disease very quickly spreads to the regions adjacent to the first affected. It follows that radiotherapy must be preventive and that if, for example, the left cervical lymph nodes are affected not only must they be irradiated but so too must all the other suspect areas.

(3) *Lymphography* has shown how frequent and how extremely serious are subdiaphragmatic retroperitoneal localizations of the disease. The prognosis in cases of subdiaphragmatic gland involvement and of combined subdiaphragmatic and supradiaphragmatic node involvement is poor. It is difficult to expect any lengthy survival for patients so affected.

While the need for high doses of radiation and for systematic preventive irradiation of neighbouring regions and the seriousness of the prognosis in cases with subdiaphragmatic involvement are now well established, there are other characteristics of Hodgkin's disease about which less information is available. Thus we are still ignorant of the real significance of the so-called systemic signs of the disease — fever, biochemical changes, increased sedimentation rate, and alterations in the serum proteins (BERNARD, 1966). On the other hand, we know that visceral involvement is very ominous and weighs heavily against the patient; it is difficult to expect a long period of survival for him if his disease involves the liver or the lung (GRACE and MITTELMAN, 1966; JELLIFFE, 1966; JOHNSON and BRACE, 1966; KARNOFSKY, 1966; LACHER and DURANT, 1965).

When the hope of long remissions for Hodgkin's disease became a reality, it became necessary, as in other fields of cancer, to establish an international classification of the stages of disease. This has now been more or less achieved. Four major stages are distinguished: stage I, localized; stage II, regional; stage III, generalized; and stage IV, with visceral involvement. Two categories are differentiated at the regional stage, according to whether the zones affected are contiguous (II-I) or not (II-II). But a clear distinction is made between stage II, in which the involved lymph nodes are demonstrable on only one side of the diaphragm, and stage III, a generalized form in which lymph nodes on both sides of the diaphragm are involved. The spleen is accepted as being a lymphatic organ and its involvement leads a patient to be considered in stage III, not IV. Finally, in all cases the letter A or B is added according to whether there are general signs or not. In stage I and II we apply at present a therapeutic protocol designed to reinforce cobalt therapy by sandwiching it between two courses of treatment with drugs. We begin with intravenous injections of 0.5 mg/kg body weight of nitrogen mustard, given for five days, then follow with a heavy and extensive dose of cobalt, as stated above, and then attempt to consolidate the result obtained by a dose of 10 mg vincaleucoblastine once a month for the succeeding twenty months. It would be premature to express an opinion on the results of this method of treatment, but the point worth stressing is that it marks a necessary change in our attitude towards Hodgkin's disease. A casual and defeatist attitude is no longer permissible towards patients with Hodgkin's disease in stages I and II; this is a condition that is not invariably fatal, in which it is possible to hope that 20% of patients will survive for 15 years (EASSON, 1966 a, b, c; EASSON and RUSSELL, 1963).

2. Treatment of Acute Leukemia

Three periods in the history of the treatment of acute leukemia can be distinguished. The first dates from 1947, when the first exchange transfusion was performed, to 1959. It was a period of high hope, for nearly every year brought a new therapeutic approach and there were reasonable expectations that a definitive solution was not too remote. Unfortunately, in the second period, between 1954 and 1962, progress ceased. No new drug, no new method appeared, and treatment was reduced to combinations of the drugs known previously. Happily, however, in the past four years, which form the third period, fresh advances have been made. They are of two kinds. On the one hand new drugs are now available; on the other, new ideas have been propounded on the association and combination of these drugs.

The three new drugs that have recently come into use in the treatment of acute leukemia are vincristine, methyl-bis-guanyl- hydrazone (a synthetic compound), and cytosine arabinoside, an antimetabolite and antagonist of cytidine. Vincristine (also known as Leurocristine or Oncovin) is an alkaloid from the periwinkle very nearly allied to the vincaleucoblastine employed in the last few years in the treatment of Hodgkin's disease. Whereas vincaleucoblastine is of moderate toxicity and effective almost exclusively against Hodgkin's disease and reticulosarcoma, vincristine is more toxic but possesses a much wider spectrum of activity, embracing the acute leukemias and a large number of lymphoblastic sarcomas. Vincristine is administered once weekly in the form of a slow intravenous perfusion in isotonic glucose or physiological saline solution. The average dose is of the order of 1—2 mg per m^2 body surface per week.

When vincristine alone is employed in treating an attack, complete remission lasting for about two months is obtained in 65—70% of cases. At the first relapse 50—60% of cases again undergo remission. Vincristine may on the one hand, like all the drugs used in the treatment of leukemia, cause aplasia (which may be very grave) and, on the other, it has side effects on other systems of the body than the hematopoietic system, particularly the nervous system. Since it is neurotoxic, it is necessary regularly to test the patient's tendon reflexes, which often disappear, and to observe him for ptosis. Absent tendon reflexes and ptosis are the first signs of the development of polyneuritis, which often takes the form of a pseudo-myopathy and which fortunately in the great majority of cases regresses. Much more rarely (in ten out of 120 cases), we have seen convulsions, in the form of generalized epileptic attacks; in addition, the patient may present with abdominal syndromes, which at the beginning led to unjustified surgical intervention; and he generally suffers from transient alopecia. On the whole, however, in spite of these drawbacks, it is not too difficult to employ vincristine in treatment; most of the children under our care at present suffer from only a moderate number and degree of side effects of this kind.

At present we feel that to obtain a first remission it is preferable not to use vincristine alone, but to associate it with prednisone. The combination consists of the usual dose of prednisone, i. e., 3 mg/kg body weight, with the dose of vincristine shown above, which varies from 1 to 3 mg/m^2. In a recent series complete remission was achieved in 40 children out of 41 and 7 out of 9 adults (Table 1). The very high percentage of complete remissions is noteworthy. Comparative study of the various advances made in the past few years in the treatment of malignant blood diseases shows that, while prednisone alone gave 74% of remissions in 62 cases, prednisone and vin-

Table 1. *Acute Lymphoblastic Leukemia Treated Initially with Prednisone and Vincristine in Combination*

	Children	Adults
Number of patients	41	9
Failure	1	—
Deaths during induction	—	2
Complete remissions	40	7
Deaths during consolidation	2	0
Maintenance treatment	38	7
Lost sight of	1	1
Deaths during remission without relapse (chickenpox after reinduction)	1	0
Relapses	13	1
In remission	23	5

cristine together gave 94% in a recent series of 83 cases. The association of these two drugs thus achieves the remarkable result of producing complete remission in almost all cases of acute lymphoblastic leukemia in children and adults.

The second new drug is a synthetic one belonging to the group of triguanidines: methyl-glyoxal-bis-guanyl hydrazone, commonly known as methyl-GAG. This drug was shown to be effective in the treatment of the very grave disease acute myeloblastic leukemia, which without treatment is generally fatal in one or two months. The treatment available before — 6-mercaptopurine, methotrexate — produced remission in only 10—12% of cases at the most. Methyl-GAG is given as an intravenous perfusion or if need be intramuscularly, the dose varying between 100 and 350 mg/m² body surface weekly. It is by far the most toxic of all the drugs we have had to use in this field: it causes considerable digestive upsets, nausea, vomiting, and abdominal pain. It may give rise to very serious and refractory aplasia of the bone marrow. Finally, it may cause mucosal and skin disturbances, erythema or necrosis, the lesions vaguely resembling some forms of acrodynia with swelling, edema, rubor, and excruciating pain in the extremities. But weighing against these severe side effects is the fact that it gives distinctly better results than any treatment previously used. Thus, in a first series of cases where we used methyl-GAG alone, we obtained 22% of complete remissions in acute myeloblastic leukemia in children and adults. We later combined methyl-GAG with 6-mercaptopurine, giving high doses of the former (350 mg/m² intravenously three times a week) and the usual doses of 6-mercaptopurine. Out of 42 cases we obtained remission in 14. While this result is not exactly brilliant, it is not negligible; a 33% remission rate in acute myeloblastic leukemia is well above any previously obtained. Several of the patients are still alive, 15 to 18 months after the treatment.

The last of the new drugs is cytosine arabinoside (BERNARD et al., 1966). As stated above, it is an antimetabolite and an antagonist of cytidine that has recently been discovered. As a drug, its interest is twofold: it is very active in the treatment of several experimental cancers; and it has as well powerful antiviral activity, particularly against herpes and related viruses.

Cytosine arabinoside is given intravenously, the average dose being 30 mg/m² per diem; the perfusion is given over the whole of the day, the patient receiving perfusions for 12 out of each 24 hours during 18—20 days. Unlike methyl-GAG, cytosine is fairly well tolerated. It may indeed cause blood and marrow aplasia of considerable extent and alopecia, but practically no digestive, nervous, or skin disturbances of any importance are observed. The study of a recent series of 62 cases enabled us to record the following observations: (1) complete remission is obtained in as much as 30—35% of cases of acute myeloblastic leukemia in children and adults, either in the initial attack of the disease or on relapse; and (2) complete remission of acute lymphocytic leukemia on relapse can be obtained, when it is refractory to other forms of treatment. There seems to be no cross resistance between this new drug and previously used drugs. For this reason, the therapeutic protocol applied in our department at the Saint-Louis Hospital associates cytosine arabinoside with methyl-GAG for acute myeloblastic leukemias. The preliminary results of this association are promising, but it would be premature as yet to draw any conclusions for the future.

The combination of these new drugs in various ways constitutes the second great source of progress in the treatment of leukemia (Table 2). At present there are two main streams of ideas in chemotherapeutical research. One is derived from the remarkable work of the American leukemia worker, SKIPPER (American Cancer Society, 1965), who has attempted to count the malignant leukemic cells in the mice he was treating and who considers that the entire problem of treatment in leukemia both in the mouse and in man is arithmetical. If, for example, the number of leukemic cells is known and is, say, 10^{12}, it may be postulated that the first drug reduced the number to 10^6, the second from 10^6 to 10^3, and so on; and when all the leukemic cells have been destroyed the disease will have been eradicated. To achieve eradication several procedures have been proposed:

(1) The first is to give the available drugs in association at the same time. Various combinations have been proposed, especially as regards acute lymphoblastic leukemia, the one that holds out most hope. The Bethesda hematologists have thus been admini-

Table 2. *Complete Remissions in Acute Lymphoblastic Leukemia of Childhood Previously Untreated*

Therapy	% Complete remissions One drug	Combination of drugs	Number of patients	References
Methotrexate	26%		48	
		44%	42	FREI, 1961
6-mercaptopurine	26%		43	
		82%	154	FREI, 1965
Prednisone				
1 mg/kg body weight	57%		72	FREIREICH, 1963
	61%		55	JEAN BERNARD, 1962
ACTH	66%		100	PIERCE, 1957
		84%	63	Acute Leukemia B, 1965
Vincristine	57% [1]		103	KARON, 1963
		95% [2]	82	JEAN BERNARD, 1965
Prednisone				
3 mg/kg body weight	74%		62	JEAN BERNARD, 1962
	62% [2]		180	

[1] Patients in first remission.
[2] Adults and children

Table 3. *Present Plan of Treatment for Initial Acute Lymphoblastic Leukemia*

Induction		Consolidation (3 weeks)	Maintenance	Reinduction
Prednisone 3 mg/kg body weight daily and Vincristine 1, then 2 mg/m² weekly i.v.	Complete remission	Methotrexate 15 mg/m² twice weekly, i.m. (one month after last injection of vincristine) and 6-mercaptopurine 2.5 mg/kg body weight daily by mouth (as soon as prednisone stopped)	Methotrexate 15 mg/m² once weekly, i.m. and 6-mercaptopurine 2.5 mg/kg body weight daily by mouth	6-monthly for the duration of the remission Prednisone 3 mg/kg body weight, daily for 15 days Vincristine on 1st, 7th and 14th days 1—2—2 mg/m² Methotrexate intrathecally 0.1—0.2—0.3 mg/kg body weight

stering together the four chief drugs: vincristine, amethopterin, mercaptopurine, and prednisone, in a therapeutic protocol known as VAMP (FREI *et al.*, 1965; SELAWRY and FREI, 1963). Variants of this protocol with less tendency to cause aplasia have recently been proposed. From the point of view of both theory and practice, the vital contribution of the VAMP method is that without any maintenance treatment it has prolonged the remission of a certain number of patients for a long time. This in itself is a new concept. When a large number of cells are destroyed at the beginning of the disease there is indeed a great risk of serious aplasia, but a fairly long remission can be obtained thereby.

(2) The second method is that of a sequence of treatments. It was first employed by ZUELZER (1963), an American pediatrician and hematologist who hit upon the idea of following up methotrexate by 6-mercaptopurine, administering each drug for a month as long as the remission lasted. This method was also employed by a

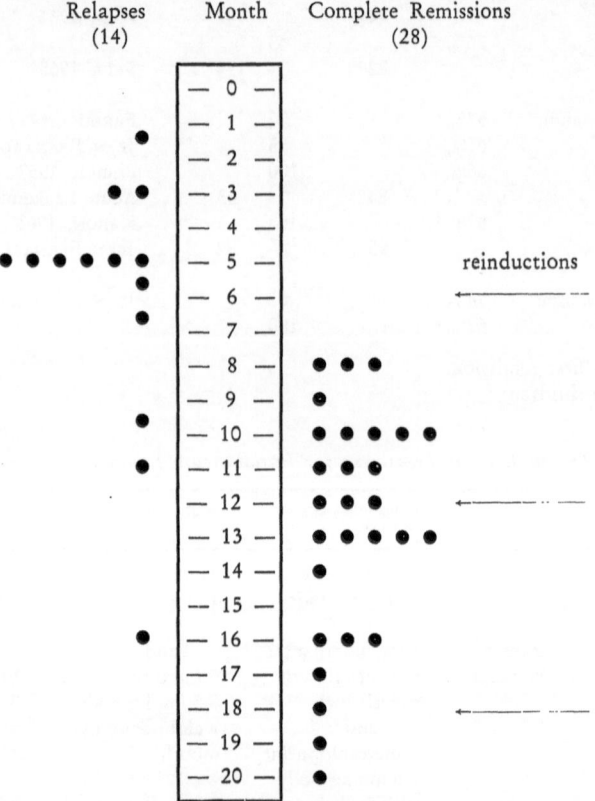

Fig. 1. Duration of Complete Remissions of Protocol 02—64
(Reinduction every six Months)

second group of research workers, led by G. MATHÉ. The five or six drugs available for the treatment of acute leukemia are given successively for a month each, after which the series is started again. The results of this group have not yet been published, but the preliminary results are encouraging.

(3) We ourselves employ a third method, known as systematic reinduction. We are a little wary of methods that tend excessively to cause aplasia, and prefer to give attack treatment again to patients when their condition is good rather than systematically select periods. The hypothesis is that some malignant cells still subsist in small numbers in the patient's body and that it is preferable to destroy them before they start multiplying. Our present schedule of treatment is therefore as follows: (1) induction treatment with prednisone and vincristine, as mentioned; complete remission is obtained in nearly all cases; (2) consolidation treatment with methotrexate in high doses and 6-mercaptopurine; and (3) maintenance with methotrexate in small doses and 6-mercaptopurine (Table 3). An interesting observation was made recently by SELAWRY (SELAWRY and FREI, 1963); he showed that methotrexate administered intermittently — the dose being divided into two injections twice a week — is much more active than when administered daily. Finally, we later reinduce, i. e., we give prednisone and vincristine systematically six months afterwards to a patient in perfect condition and good health (Fig. 1). This is the original aspect of the method.

A preliminary study of the results of this method brought out the fact that many relapses occurred in the fifth month. We concluded tentatively that we had made a mistake in reinducing at the sixth month and that it was too late. In the present series the reinduction is carried out at the third month, and so far we have had no relapse in the early period after the beginning of treatment. A considerable number of our patients are coming up to or have passed the second year of complete remission.

II. Treatment by Control rather than Destruction

Cytoregulatory Treatment

Cytoregulatory treatment is based on and guided by observation of long-term remissions in leukemia. BURCHENAL, of New York, has collected a series of 100 or more authentic cases of complete remission lasting for over four years throughout the world (BERNARD et al., 1962; BURCHENAL, 1964, 1965; DAMESHEK et al., 1965). We personally have observed 14 similar cases, all carefully checked. Of this series eight patients are still alive, one of them after a complete remission of ten years (BURCHENAL, 1964).

A study of these cases gives rise to the following observations:

(1) The usual criteria for assessing the prognosis of acute leukemia are not valid for long-term remissions. Of these 14 patients, nine have lymphoblastic and five myeloid leukemia, and eight are children and six adults. In some cases no maintenance treatment whatever was given. ZUELZER had already reported a very long remission lasting 11 years; the cyclic treatment he had proposed was administered for a year, and the next ten years passed without any treatment being given.

(2) These data are important and cast doubt upon and render disputable Skipper's arithmetical concepts. The question arises whether the destruction he proposes of all leukemic cells is (a) necessary, (b) sufficient, and (c) harmless. Is it necessary? There is no lack of examples in pathology of subjects who have lived in reasonable harmony with a certain number of cancerous cells for a very long time — it is by no means sure that it is essential to destroy all the leukemic cells in the body.

Is it sufficient? If human acute leukemia, like that of the mouse, is due to a virus, it might well be asked if it is very reasonable to destroy all the cells if the viruses remain present during the remission and are thus capable of causing a relapse. And lastly, is it harmless? This is by no means certain. Firstly, if all the malignant cells are killed it may deprive the organism of a stimulus that it needs to immunize itself. And secondly — and this is the most important point —, the treatment we administer with drugs is not solely destructive of the leukemic cells but also destroys the cells known at present as immunocompetent cells. It is possible that drugs at present both kill the leukemic cells and deprive the organism of its means of defence at a later date. This perhaps explains why complete remissions may be seen for very long periods in subjects who have not undergone such aggressive treatment as is administered at present.

Other additional data help support the views I am defending in this paper. When a very long remission of the type I have just mentioned is observed, it may be asked what has happened during the remission. There are other possible hypotheses at the present stage of our knowledge as well as the one that some remaining leukemic cells are lying dormant somewhere in the body, cells that M. BESSIS and we have proposed should be termed "quiescent" cells. Such cells raise many problems: how many are present, what is their morphology, where are they located, do they migrate, have they a low rate of multiplication, and are they affected by environmental factors? It is not possible at present to answer these questions. It should however be said that this problem is not specific for acute leukemia but applies to all cancers. For example, a woman operated on for cancer of the breast may survive for 10 to 15 years without incident, when suddenly metastases appear in the bone marrow. What were the cancer cells doing during all this time? On what basis can it be claimed that the organism has succeeded in keeping them in a quiescent state? This is indeed one of the fundamental problems of the study of cancer today.

By way of illustration of what is happening in leukemia two old cases may be mentioned. The first relates to Michael M ..., a small boy whom M. BESSIS and I treated in 1947 by exchange transfusion (BESSIS and BERNARD, 1947). Until then it had not been thought that remissions could be obtained in the treatment of acute leukemia. This procedure produced a complete remission that lasted for only a short time — two months —, but it was the first deliberately produced remission.

Another observation is related to a period a little later when the only treatment we had at our disposal was ACTH. The child treated had a very serious tumorous form of leukemia with an enormous spleen, large lymph nodes, and skin and bone tumors; the leukocyte count was 100 000, and the marrow differential count showed 100% leukoblasts. After five days on ACTH he went into remission, spleen, skin, and bone reverted to their normal state, the white cell count fell to 6000, and the myelogram was absolutely normal. ACTH is merely a stimulus and contributes nothing. It must therefore be acknowledged that this child had himself the capacity, hidden but nevertheless present, of ridding himself of his cancer, even if only momentarily.

More recently still we made another observation that also gives food for thought. A young woman of 20 years of age who fell ill of acute lymphoblastic leukemia in 1960 was treated as we were at that time treating our patients, with prednisone only, in a dosage of 3 mg/kg body weight daily for a period of 25 days. The remission was complete, and she was placed on maintenance treatment with 6-mercaptopurine; and the remission continued till 1965. Then suddenly systemic lupus erythematosus appeared, with absolutely typical clinical and biochemical signs. There are many possible hypotheses to account for this — coincidence, common ground between the two diseases, the part played by the treatment (a hypothesis that cannot be discarded), and the possibility that leukemia produces an immune response in the organism, in some cases with the happy result of bringing about a remission, in other cases, however, going to the extreme of causing lupus erythematosus.

Observations such as this are extremely rare. We have found none comparable in the literature. But they provide much thought-provoking material.

A whole series of recent research projects is directed towards finding evidence in favour of the theory postulating the existence of a reaction of the patient against his leukemia. Research is in progress in our laboratory under the direction of J. DAUSSET, F. KOURILSKY, C. DRESCH and Y. NAJEAN (KOURILSKY, 1966), in which blast cells are marked with chromium-51, the duration of the life of these cells is studied, antibodies against them are sought in the serum of patients while the disease is developing or while it is in remission, the leukemic white-cell group is determined, and virus antigens are tested against the leukemic blast cells. The preliminary results obtained may be compared with those recently obtained by KLEIN with the sera of children with Burkitt's lymphoma. This is a remarkable lymphoblastic tumor of the jaw which is found in West, Central, and East Africa, and because of Burkitt's work is considered to be very possibly due to a virus and in any case very probably transmitted by a mosquito. Using immunofluorescent methods, KLEIN observed the existence of antibodies against the blast cells in the serum of patients with Burkitt's tumour, especially during periods of remission.

Thus the first positive results are beginning to appear confirming the existence of an anti-leukemic power in the serum of patients with leukemia or lymphoblastoma. It is therefore possible to envisage the development of immunotherapeutic methods for leukemia. Three main avenues of research are open. Passive immunotherapy may be serological or cellular, exchange transfusion probably being an example of the former. The use of the serum of patients in remission, which M. BESSIS and I had already started in 1948, using the blood of leukemia patients in remission, has been revived by BURKITT and various workers in Central Africa. Successful results have recently been reported and prolonged remissions obtained by the employment of the serum of patients with Burkitt's lymphoma in remission. This passive immunotherapy may also be cellular and approximate to the "adoptive" immunotherapy proposed by G. MATHÉ, which has inspired his attempts at treatment with an allogenic marrow graft in the hope that the grafted cells would act not only on the malignant cells of the recipient but also on any virus that might exist. Other methods of immunotherapy that might be discussed are active, non-specific with BCG, and specific with cells or a virus. These methods have been employed especially in the prevention of Friend's leukemia of mice.

For a long time there has been controversy between the protagonists of methods involving cell destruction, who were in the majority, and the protagonists of methods involving cell control. The opposition between these two groups has now ceased, each side admitting that neither of the two approaches by itself will produce the results desired. It does not seem that destructive methods can cure any considerable number of cases of leukemia; nor, on the other hand, does it seem at all probable that immunotherapeutic methods by themselves can destroy the enormous numbers — as many as 10^{12} — of leukemic cells that probably exist at the outset of the disease. Viruses, if they are concerned, are very weakly antigenic, and so too are the leukemic cells themselves. It is therefore not surprising that the defense mechanisms brought into being in the organism by the leukemic cells and the viruses, if any, are weak. Nevertheless, the general view at present, the view that directs present-day research, is that every effort should be made to combine destructive methods with methods utilizing the individual's own defenses.

References

American Cancer Society and National Cancer Institute: Conference on obstacles to the control of acute leukemia, held at the Airlie House, Warrenton (Va.), March 1964. Cancer Res. **25**, 1469—1479 (1965).

BERNARD, J.: Principes généraux actuels du traitement de la maladie de Hodgkin, des lymphosarcomes, des réticulosarcomes. Rev. Prat. (Paris) **16**, 871—879 (1966).

—, M. BOIRON, Cl. JACQUILLAT, M. WEIL, and Y. NAJEAN: Un nouvel agent actif dans le traitement des leucémies aiguës: la cytosine arabinoside. Presse méd. **74**, 799—802 (1966).

— —, M. WEIL, J. P. LEVY, M. SELIGMANN, and Y. NAJEAN: Etude de la rémission complète des leucémies aiguës (analyse de 300 observations). Nouv. Rev. franç. Hémat. **2**, 195—222 (1962).

BESSIS, M., et J. BERNARD: Remarquables résultats du traitement d'un cas de leucémie aiguë par exsanguino-transfusion. Bull. Soc. méd. Paris **63**, 871 (1947).

BRUNNER, K. W., and C. W. YOUNG: A methylhydrazine in Hodgkin's disease and other malignant neoplasms — therapeutic and toxic effects studied in 51 patients. Ann. intern. Med. **63**, 69—86 (1965).

BURCHENAL, J. H.: Approaches to the aetiology and treatment of acute leukemias. Second Annual Guest Lecture, Nov. 10th, 1964. London: Queen Anne Press 1965.

— Long-term remissions of acute leukaemia — spontaneous and induced. Series Haemat., vol. **1**, 47—56 (1965).

CHEVALLIER, P. et J. BERNARD: La maladie de Hodgkin. Paris: Masson 1932.

DAMESHEK, W., T. F. NECHELES, H. E. FINKEL, and D. H. ALLEN: Therapy of acute leukaemia, 1965. Blood **26**, 220—225 (1965).

EASSON, E.: Maladie de Hodgkin. Analyse des résultats à long terme. Nouv. Rev. franç. Hémat. **6**, 55—59 (1966).

— La maladie de Hodgkin est-elle une affection curable? Nouv. Rev. franç. Hémat. **6**, 109—111 (1966).

— Possibilities for the cure of Hodgkin's disease. Cancer (Philad.) **19**, 345—350 (1966).

—, and M. H. RUSSELL: The cure of Hodgkin's disease. Brit. med. J. **1**, 1704—1707 (1963).

ENNUYER, A., P. BATAINI, et J. FRANIATE: Résultats lointains obtenus par radiothérapie dans la maladie de Hodgkin. Nouv. Rev. franç. Hémat. **6**, 76—79 (1966).

FAYOS, J., R. HENDRIX, V. MACDONALD, and I. LAMPE: Hodgkin's disease — a review of radiotherapeutic experience. Amer. J. Roentgenol. **93**, 557—567 (1965).

FREI, E., and M. KARON: The effectiveness of combinations of antileukaemic agents in inducing and maintaining remissions in children with acute leukaemia. Blood **26**, 642—656 (1965).

GARY-BOBO, J.: Résultats lointains obtenus dans la maladie de Hodgkin traitée par radiothérapie seule. Nouv. Rev. franç. Hémat. **6**, 102—104 (1966).

GILBERT, R.: Le traitement de la granulomatose maligne par la radiothérapie. J. Radiol. Électrol. **22**, 1577 (1938).

— Radiotherapy in Hodgkin's disease. Amer. J. Roentgenol. **41**, 198—241 (1939).

GLINSKA, H.: Résultats lointains du traitement de la maladie de Hodgkin. Nouv. Rev. franç. Hémat. **6**, 83—98 (1966).

GODLEE, J. N.: Résultats lointains du traitement de la maladie de Hodgkin. Nouv. Rev. franç. Hémat. **6**, 104—107 (1966).

GRACE, J. T., and A. MITTELMAN: Surgery in the management of Hodgkin's disease. Cancer (Philad.) 19, 353—355 (1966).

JELLIFFE, A. M.: Le rôle de la chimiotherapie dans les longues survies de la maladie de Hodgkin. Nouv. Rev. franç. Hémat. 6, 142—150 (1966).

JOHNSON, R. E., and K. C. BRACE: Radiation response of Hodgkin's disease recurrent after chemotherapy. Cancer (Philad.) 19, 368—370 (1966).

KAPLAN, H. S.: The radical radiotherapy of regionally localized Hodgkin's disease. Radiology 78, 553—561 (1962).

— Radiothérapie de la maladie de Hodgkin à la Stanford University School of Medicine. Résultats lointains. Nouv. Rev. franç. Hémat. 6, 73—76 (1966).

— Role of intensive radiotherapy in the management of Hodgkin's disease. Cancer (Philad.) 19, 356—357 (1966).

— Technique statistique d'analyse des résultats de la radiothérapie de la maladie de Hodgkin. Nouv. Rev. franç. Hémat. 6, 115—117 (1966).

—, et S. ROSENBERG: La radiothérapie segmentaire de la maladie de Hodgkin. Premiers résultats de deux essais thérapeutiques contrôlés. Nouv. Rev. franç. Hémat. 6, 121—133 (1966).

KARNOFSKY, D. A.: Chemotherapy of Hodgkin's disease. Cancer (Philad.) 19, 371—377 (1966).

KOURILSKY, F. M.: Etude sur la composition allo-antigénique du leucoblaste de la leucémie aiguë. Thèse. Paris: Faculté de la Médicine 1966.

LACHER, M. J., and J. R. DURANT: Combined vinblastine and chlorambucil therapy of Hodgkin's disease. Ann. Intern. Med. 62, 468—476 (1965).

LAUGIER, A. J., M. SCHLIENGER, G. JUILLARD, et R. LE FUR: Radiothérapie des lympho- et réticulosarcomes. Rev. Prat. (Paris) 16, 895—909 (1966).

LAUWERS, L., et H. DANGOT: Relation entre le degré d'activité de la maladie de Hodgkin au cours de 5 premières années et le devenir des malades survivants à 5 ans. Nouv. Rev. franç. Hémat. 6, 98—101 (1966).

LUKES, R., C. GOMPEL, et C. NEZELOF: Le diagnostic histopathologique de la maladie de Hodgkin. Nouv. Rev. franç. Hémat. 6, 11—14 (1966).

MATHE, G.: Analyse critique de la notion de "curabilité" de la maladie de Hodgkin. Nouv. Rev. franç. Hémat. 6, 118—120 (1966).

— La chimiothérapie des lymphoréticulopathies malignes chroniques. Rev. Prat. (Paris) 16, 881—892 (1966).

PAPILLON, J., J. L. CHASSARD, et A. CONTAMIN: Problème de la dose optimale dans l'irradiation de la maladie de Hodgkin. Nouv. Rev. franç. Hémat. 6, 161—163 (1966).

—, P. CROIZAT, L. REVOL, J. L. CHASSARD, J. FEROLDI, A. CONTAMIN, and L. DUTOU: Les survies de plus de 10 ans dans la maladie de Hodgkin. Nouv. Rev. franç. Hémat. 6, 79—83 (1966).

PETERS, V.: Résultats lointains du traitement de la maladie de Hodgkin. Nouv. Rev. franç. Hémat. 6, 60—73 (1966).

PIEMONTE, M.: Considérations sur la place de la radiothérapie. Nouv. Rev. franç. Hémat. 6, 107—108 (1966).

SCHWARTZ, D.: Peut-on savoir si la maladie de Hodgkin est curable? Commentaire statistique. Nouv. Rev. franç. Hémat. 6, 111—115 (1966).

SELAWRY, O. S., and E. FREI: Prolongation of remission in acute lymphocytic leukemia by alteration in dose schedule and route of administration of methotrexate (Abstract). Proc. Amer. Ass. Cancer Res. 6, 57 (224) (1965).

—, and J. HANANIAN: Vincristine treatment of cancer in children. J. Amer. med. Ass. 183, 741—746 (1963).

THOMPSON, I., T. HALL, and W. C. MOLONEY: Combination of adult acute myelogenous leukemia: experience with the simultaneous use of vincristine, amethopterin, 6-mercaptopurine and prednisone. New Engl. J. Med. 273, 1302—1307 (1965).

TUBIANA, M., A. LAUGIER, M. HAYAT, E. ATTIE et G. MATHE: Essai d'association radiothérapie-chimiothérapie dans le traitement de la maladie de Hodgkin. Nouv. Rev. franç. Hémat. 6, 134—142 (1966).

Tubiana, M., A. Laugier, M.-J. Schlienger, et G. Juillard: La radiothérapie de la maladie de Hodgkin. Rev. Prat. (Paris) 16, 911—925 (1966).
—, P. Rambert, A. Laugier, et C. M. Lalanne: Les irradiations étendues dans la maladie de Hodgkin; réactions précoces. Nouv. Rev. franç. Hémat. 6, 164—173 (1966).
Zuelzer, W. W.: Cyclic therapy and long-term survival in childhood leukemia. Blood 22, 840 (1963).

Regional Perfusion for Melanoma and Sarcoma of the Limbs

Oscar Creech, jr., and Edward Krementz

With 11 Figures

Regional perfusion was developed in 1957 to increase the tumoricidal dose of anticarcinogenic drugs without increasing its systemic toxicity. Since separation of perfused from unperfused tissues is most successful when the part can be encircled with a tourniquet, the method lends itself well to treatment of tumors of the limbs. This paper describes the operative techniques and presents the results of perfusion for melanoma and sarcoma of the limbs.

1. Techniques of Perfusion

a) Perfusion of the Upper Limb

A non-inflammable general anesthetic is used for perfusion of the upper limbs. The patient lies supine, with a small sandbag or folded sheet beneath his shoulder

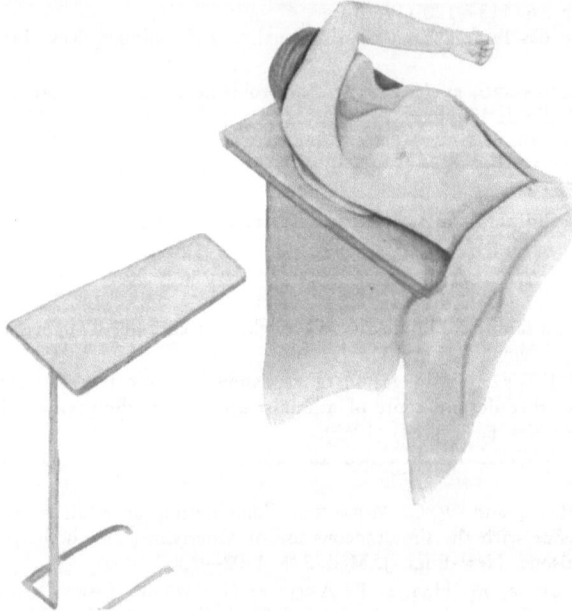

Fig. 1. The patient lies supine, with a small sandbag under the left scapula. The arm rests horizontally on a Mayo stand

on the affected side and with his forearm and hand supported in a horizontal position by a padded Mayo stand (Fig. 1 and 2). When lesions on the distal third of the forearm or on the hand are to be perfused and excised, the entire forequarter is prepared with ether and inorganic iodide solution. The hand need not be prepared for perfusion of lesions on the arm but may be wrapped in a sterile towel and covered with a stockinette roll. Sterile drapes are so placed as to ensure inclusion of the forequarter in the surgical field, free movement of the limb during the operation, and applicability of the tourniquet for isolation of the limb and axilla.

Incisions are made beginning just below the middle third of the clavicle and extending laterally and inferiorly to the anterior axillary line (Fig. 2). The precise

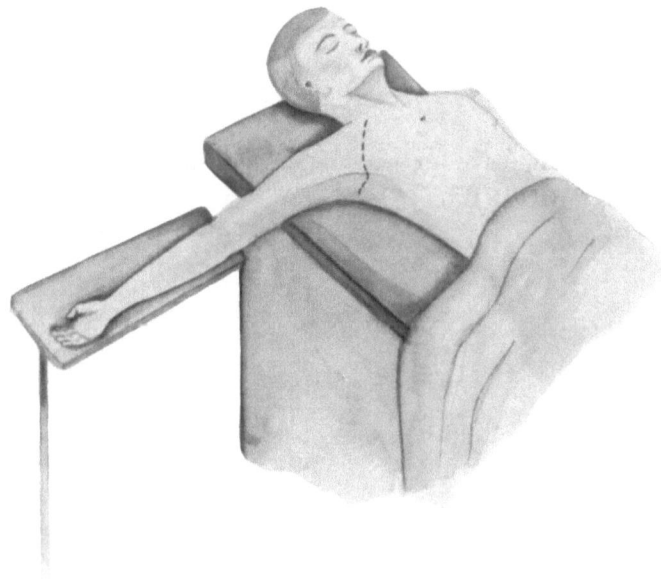

Fig. 2. The incision for perfusion begins just below the middle third of the clavicle and extends into the axilla for axillary dissection

site of incision is chosen for easy axillary dissection. The fibers of the pectoralis major muscle are exposed by carrying the incision through skin, subcutaneous tissue, and deep fascia (Fig. 3). After the skin flaps have been raised to allow retraction, the pectoralis major muscle is incised in the direction of its fibers. Next the pectoralis minor muscle is either exposed and divided at its insertion on the humerus (Fig. 4a and b), or is retracted laterally to expose the axillary artery and vein in their first or medial third (Fig. 4c). Cotton tapes are passed around these vessels, proximally and distally, and through short segments of rubber tubing to form nooses.

After heparin is given in a dose of 1.5 mg per kg body weight, the nooses are tightened, and the vessels are incised longitudinally for easy insertion of the perfusion catheters. A No. 10 and a No. 14 French plastic catheter are inserted in a distal direction into the artery and vein respectively (Fig. 4d), the tips of the catheters being allowed to extend about one inch beyond the tourniquet when

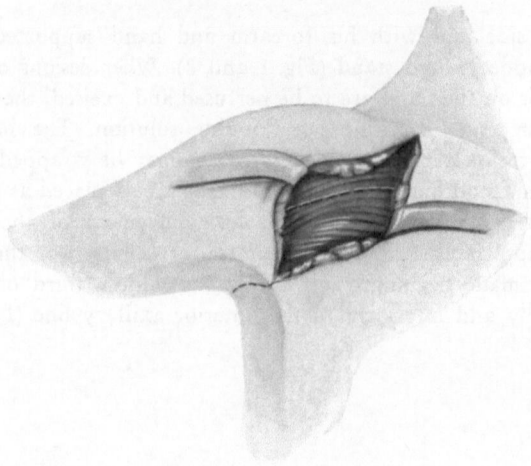

Fig. 3. The medial half of the incision is made first for cannulation of the axillary artery and vein. The skin and subcutaneous tissue are retracted laterally and medially, and the pectoralis major muscle is separated in the direction of its fibers

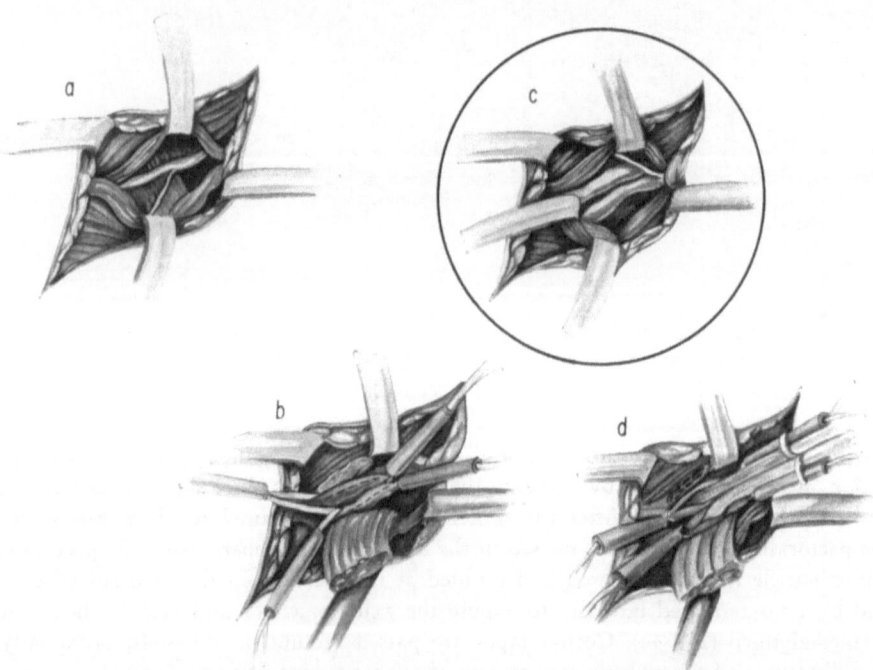

Fig. 4. (a) The fibers of the pectoralis major muscle are retracted superiorly and inferiorly to expose the pectoralis minor muscle. (b) By means of an electrocautery the pectoralis minor muscle is divided near its insertion and retracted inferiorly. Tapes are passed around the axillary artery medially and laterally and through short sections of rubber tubing to form a noose. (c) In some instances the pectoralis minor muscle need not be divided, but can be retracted laterally to provide adequate exposure of the axillary artery and vein. (d) Catheters are inserted into the axillary artery and vein in a distal direction, and the nooses are tightened proximally and distally around the catheters, which are further secured by tying them to the sections of rubber tubing

tightly applied. The catheters are securely tied to the proximal nooses to prevent their accidental movement during perfusion.

The tourniquet is fixed to the chest wall by one of two methods. In one, a No. 5/32 STEINMANN pin is inserted through the trapezius muscle at the junction of the middle and outer thirds of the clavicle, and another through the latissimus dorsi muscle about an inch below the lower margin of the axilla (Fig. 5). An Esmarch

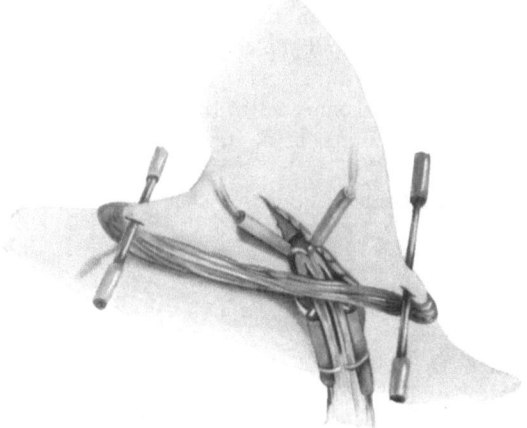

Fig. 5. A Steinmann pin is passed through the trapezius muscle above the shoulder and another through the latissimus dorsi below the axilla, and an Esmarch bandage or latex tube is wrapped tightly around the forequarter, passing over the catheters

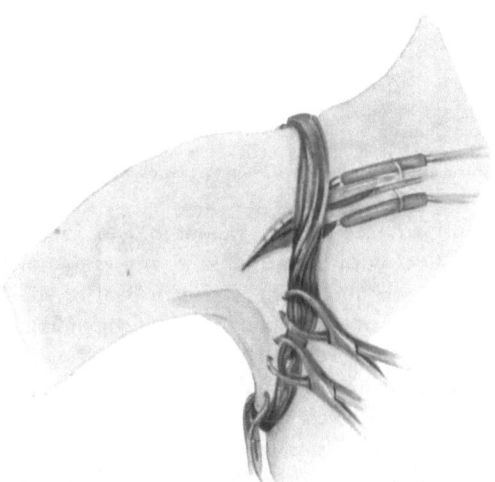

Fig. 6. By an alternative method of fixing the tourniquet to the chest wall, large towel forceps are fastened to the skin just anterior to and below the axilla, and the tourniquet is applied beneath them. The ring handles of the towel forceps can be secured to the drapes of the chest wall with sutures or with additional towel forceps

bandage is then wrapped around the two STEINMANN pins to form a noose around the forequarter. If the lower STEINMANN pin is inadvertently placed within the lower margin of the axilla, the soft tissues may yield when the tourniquet is applied and cause part of the axilla to be outside the isolated region.

In the second method of applying the tourniquet, towel forceps are inserted about an inch from the anterior, inferior, and posterior margins of the axilla (Fig. 6), and the tourniquet is applied outside these points of insertion. The tourniquet is secured in position by suturing the handles of the clips to the skin.

Before the catheters are attached to the pump oxygenator, the adequacy of the venous flow should be determined by releasing the venous catheter. If the catheter has been passed accidentally into the orifice of one of the numerous tributaries of the axillary vein or has become lodged in the cusp of one of the many valves, the venous drainage may be impeded, and the catheter will have to be repositioned to ensure that it is in the axillary vein.

When the catheters have been connected to the pump oxygenator, perfusion may be begun (Fig. 7), the first five minutes being used to warm the blood to about 98° F

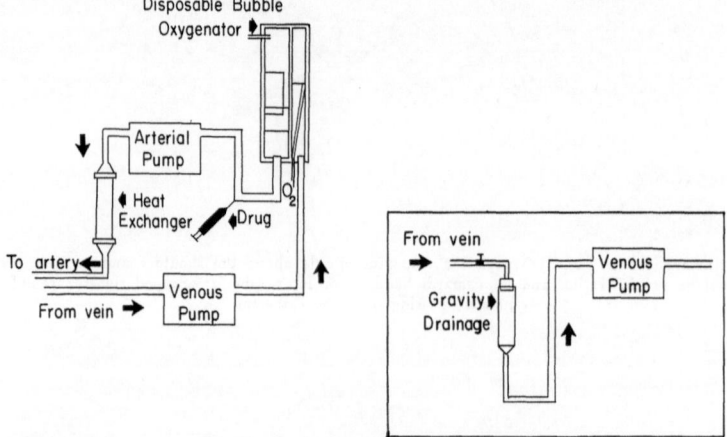

Fig. 7. Flow diagram of the extracorporal circuit. Whenever placement of the venous catheter is difficult, and particularly in perfusion of the upper limb, gravity drainage is used (inset), and a clamp is applied to the tubing proximal to the venous reservoir to control the venous outflow

and to determine the optimal rate of flow (about 100 to 150 ml per minute). The distribution of the blood flow within the limb and any escape of blood beneath the tourniquet are determined with fluorescein. Three to 5 ml of sodium fluorescein are injected into the arterial line, and the skin of the perfused region as well as that just proximal to the tourniquet is examined under ultraviolet light. Fluorescence of the skin proximal to the tourniquet is indicative of escape, and the dosage of the cytotoxic drug should be reduced accordingly. Two or more equal doses of the drug are injected at intervals of 3 to 5 minutes, and perfusion is continued for 30 to 45 minutes after injection of the last dose. At the end of the perfusion, 250 ml of dextran or whole blood are given through a side arm in the arterial line distal to the pump head while the residual drug and dextran are removed from the limb by the venous pump or by gravity drainage. The limb cannot, of course, be completely isolated, and it is therefore important not to remove more blood than the amount of dextran given.

The catheters are removed, and protamine is injected intravenously in an amount equal to that of the heparin used. Blood is allowed to flow freely from the proximal and distal ends of the vessels by momentary release of the occluding tapes. Running sutures of No. 5-0 arterial silk are used to close the arterial and venous incisions. If the axillary artery is atherosclerotic or has been damaged by cannulation, a patch graft from a tributary of the axillary vein may be needed to prevent narrowing of the artery.

Axillary lymphadenectomy is usually combined with perfusion of the upper limb. After hemostasis has been obtained, the cutaneous incision is extended across the axilla, and skin flaps are prepared. The lateral portion of the pectoralis major muscle is divided, and dissection is done as usual. The pectoralis major muscle is reapproximated with interrupted sutures of heavy silk, two drainage catheters are placed in the axilla, and the remainder of the wound is closed in layers.

b) Perfusion of the Lower Limb

A spinal anesthetic is preferable for perfusion of the lower limb, but a non-inflammable general anesthetic may also be used. With the patient supine and the buttock resting on a sandbag placed beneath the sacrum (Fig. 8), the entire hind-

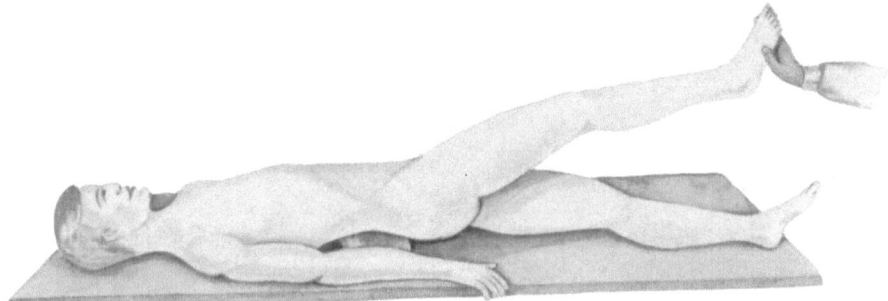

Fig. 8. For perfusion of the lower limb, the patient lies supine, with a sandbag under the sacrum so that the buttock of the affected limb is elevated

quarter is prepared with ether and aqueous solution of iodine as far above as the costal margin and as far below as 6 to 8 inches beyond the site of the primary or secondary lesion to be excised. Sterile drapes are placed beneath the buttock to include the gluteal crease well within the surgical field. If no lesions on the foot or leg are to be excised, these parts are wrapped in a sterile drape and covered with a stockinette roll.

The indication for perfusion determines the site of incision. In prophylactic perfusion in a patient with primary melanoma, regional lymph nodes will be removed simultaneously, and the external iliac artery and vein are the preferred sites of cannulation, although the common femoral vessels may be used. For recurrent or metastatic melanoma in a patient who has already had regional lymphadenectomy, the common femoral artery and vein are cannulated. In some instances, scarring in this region may necessitate cannulation through the external iliac vessels. For perfusion of clinically positive regional nodes, the superficial femoral artery and vein are cannulated in their middle third.

Primary invasive melanoma of the lower limb is treated by perfusion, wide excision of the primary lesion or its site when earlier excision has been inadequate, and regional lymphadenectomy. A vertical incision, about four inches long and centered on the inguinal ligament, is made over the common femoral vessels (Fig. 9). After division of the aponeurosis of the external oblique muscle in the direction of its fibers, the transversalis fascia is incised, and the peritoneum is retracted upward to expose the external iliac artery and vein. Nooses of silk are placed around the branches of the external iliac artery to occlude them temporarily, and tapes are

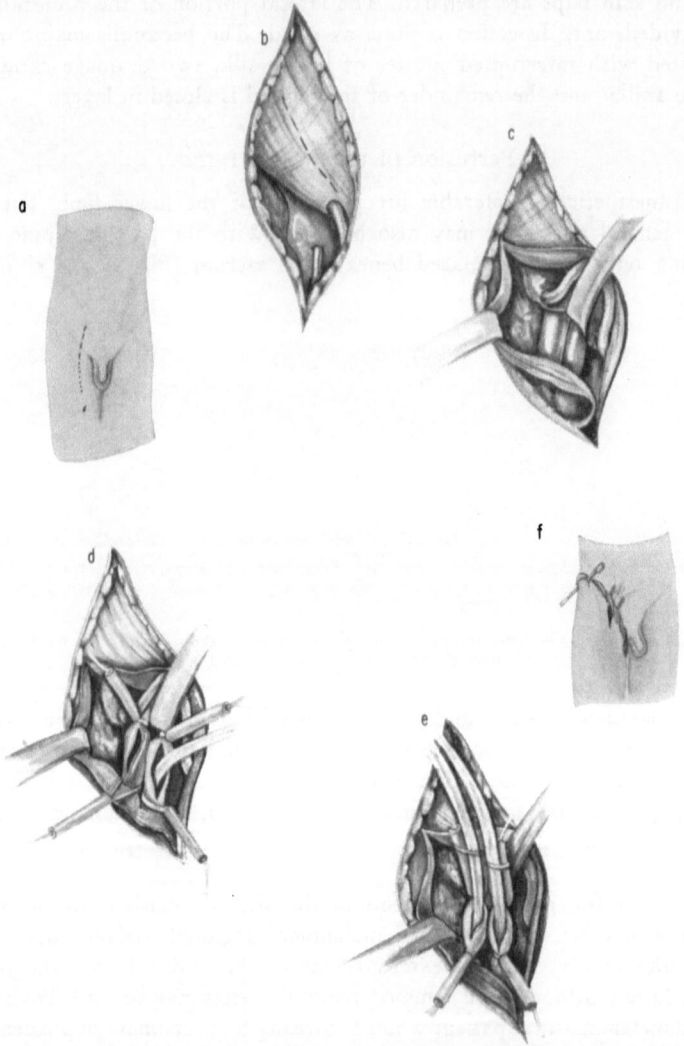

Fig. 9. (a) When perfusion is being done for primary melanoma and is to be combined with regional lymphadenectomy, an incision 4 in. (10 cm.) long, centered on the inguinal ligament, is made over the femoral vessels. (b) The aponeurosis of the external oblique muscle is divided in the direction of its fibers, and (c) the external iliac artery and vein are exposed by incision of the transversalis fascia and retraction of the peritoneum upward. Tapes are passed around the external iliac artery and vein above and below, and are inserted through segments of rubber tubes to form nooses. (d) Longitudinal incisions are made in the artery and vein, (e) catheters are inserted and secured in place, (f) a Steinmann pin is passed through the iliac crest, and an Esmarch bandage is wrapped tightly around the limb

passed around the artery and vein above and below to occlude them. Heparin is given, and the distance from the site of insertion to the midpoint of the common femoral artery and vein is marked on the catheter with a silk ligature. A No. 10 French catheter is then inserted into the artery and a No. 18 catheter into the vein. A No. 5/32 STEINMANN pin is driven through the iliac crest from inside out and, if necessary, another STEINMANN pin is passed through the obturator muscle just beneath the pubic ramus in an anterior-posterior direction. With the limb elevated and sharply abducted, an Esmarch bandage is wound around its root and secured in place by the STEINMANN pin. Proper application of the tourniquet will prevent passage of blood between the limb and the systematic circulation.

The catheters are connected to the pump oxygenator, and perfusion is begun. The temperature of the blood is allowed to reach 98 °F, and the flow through the venous and arterial pumps is adjusted to 250 to 300 ml per minute, depending upon the size of the limb. The proper position of the catheter is ensured by injection of 5 ml of sodium fluorescein into the arterial pump head and the use of ultraviolet light to determine the distribution of the dye. That the catheter is properly placed in the common femoral artery is indicated by fluorescence of the entire limb up to the tourniquet within 5 minutes after injection of the dye and by the absence of fluorescence above the tourniquet.

Multiple doses of the chemotherapeutic agent are injected at intervals of 2 to 5 minutes, and perfusion is continued for 30 to 45 minutes after injection of the last

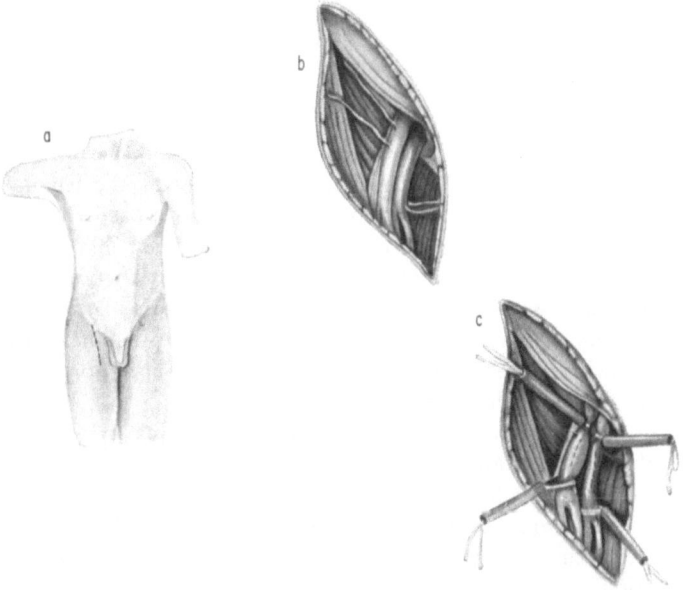

Fig. 10 a—c

Fig. 10. (a) When regional lymphadenectomy is not planned, perfusion is carried out through an oblique incision over the common femoral artery and vein, beginning at the inguinal ligament and extending inferiorly and medially for about 4—5 in. (10—12 cm.). (b) The common femoral artery and vein are exposed in the femoral trigone, and (c) these vessels are encircled with tapes. Catheters are inserted into the femoral artery and vein in a distal direction. (d) Care is taken to ensure that the catheter is in the upper portion of the superficial femoral artery rather than in the profunda. (e) When properly positioned, the catheters are secured in place by tightening the nooses and tying them to the segments of rubber tubing above dose. At the end of perfusion, 500 ml of dextran or whole blood are used to wash out the vascular system. The tourniquet is released, the catheters are removed, and the artery and vein are repaired. A dose of protamine is given, equal to that of the heparin used before perfusion.

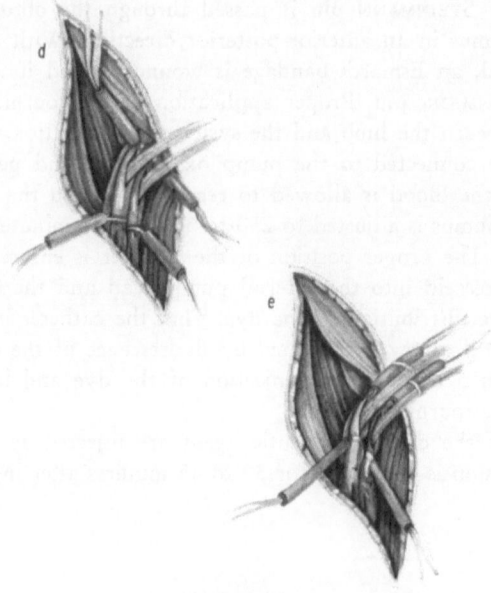

Fig. 10 d, e

If regional lymph nodes are to be removed at the time of perfusion, the incision is extended inferiorly and slightly medially to the apex of the femoral (Scarpa's) trigone (Fig. 9). Enlarged external iliac nodes are removed, but superficial inguinal and common iliac or obturator nodes are not disturbed, since their involvement indicates systemic metastasis. Since wound complications are frequent after lymphadenectomy, the inguinal ligament is sutured to the pectineus muscle to seal the incisions of the external iliac artery and vein off from the wound of the inguinal dissection. This precaution also helps prevent the formation of a hernia. The sartorius muscle is then shifted medially to cover the femoral vessels.

In patients with recurrent lesions or in-transit metastasis in whom lymphadenectomy has already been done, the common femoral artery and vein are commonly used for perfusion, although the external iliac muscle may be used (Fig. 10). Primary or secondary lesions are excised at the end of perfusion when this is necessary. A split thickness skin graft is usually needed to cover the defect in wide excision of primary lesions.

Large clinically positive nodes can sometimes be reduced in size by first perfusing them alone, and two or three weeks later removing them, with or without perfusion. An incision is made in the middle third of the thigh directly over the superficial femoral artery and vein (Fig. 11), and the sartorius muscle is retracted to expose the vessels. Two No. 10 French catheters are passed, one proximally and one distally, into the artery, and two No. 14 catheters are inserted similarly into the vein. This technique permits perfusion of the entire limb, including the affected regional nodes, without dissecting within the region of the nodes. After a tourniquet is applied over a STEINMANN pin, the operation is carried out as already described.

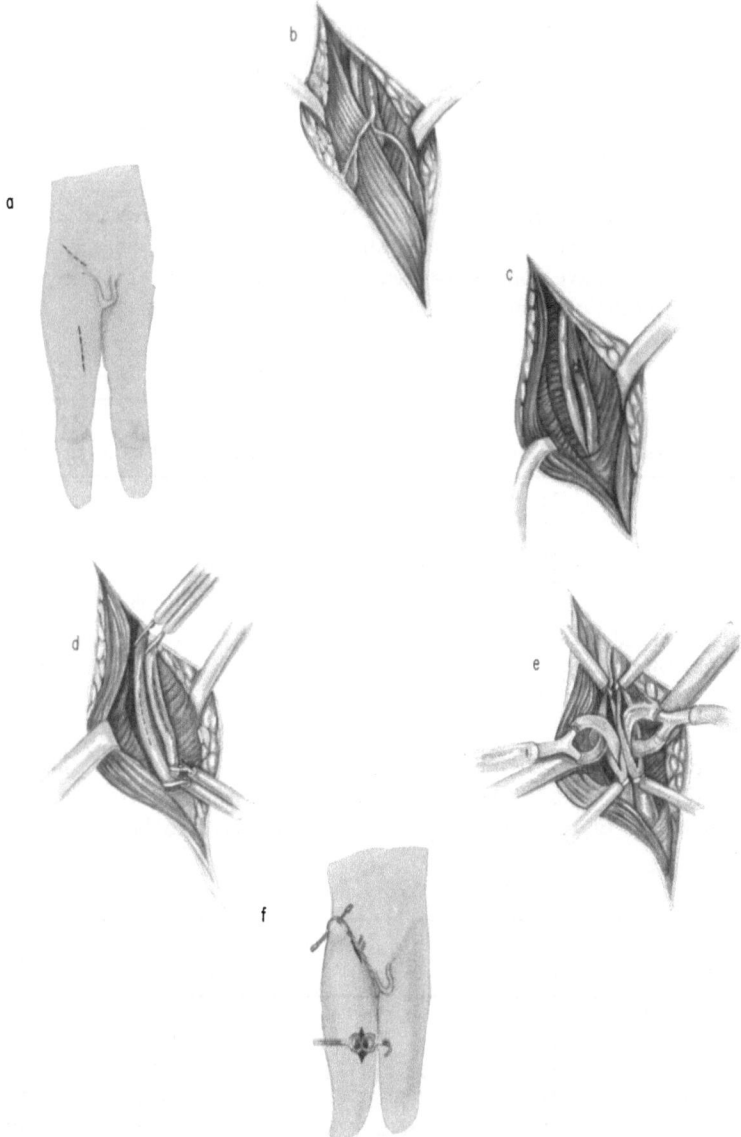

Fig. 11. (a) When large inguinal nodes are present, the femoral artery and vein are cannulated through a longitudinal incision in the midportion of the thigh. A short transverse incision is made above the inguinal ligament for exposure and occlusion of the external iliac artery and vein. (b) The sartorius muscle is exposed and (c) retracted laterally to expose the superficial femoral artery and vein. (d) Tapes are passed around these vessels, and (e) catheters are inserted into the artery and vein in proximal and distal directions. (f) A Steinmann pin is driven through the crest of the ilium, and an Esmarch bandage is wrapped tightly around the root of the limb

2. Results

a) Melanoma

Of 322 patients with melanoma treated by perfusion, 187 with melanoma of the limbs have been observed one or more years after treatment (Table 1). More than half the patients were treated for recurrent or locally metastatic melanoma, classified here as secondary melanoma. In the remainder, the perfusion was prophylactic and was combined with excision and regional lymphadenectomy.

More than half the patients treated 4 or more years ago and two-fifths of those treated 5 or more years ago have no evidence of malignant disease. Prophylactic treatment of primary melanoma is, of course, more successful than treatment of recurrent lesions and regional metastasis: 15 of 19 patients treated for primary melanoma are free of malignant disease after 5 years, whereas only 12 of 46 with secondary melanoma have apparently been cured. Results in both categories, however, are better than results of surgical treatment alone.

Table 1. *Melanoma of Limbs* [1]

Year	Primary		Secondary		Total	
	No. Patients	No. Controlled	No. Patients	No. Controlled	No. Patients	No. Controlled
1	81	72	106	45	187	117
2	63	55	86	33	149	88
3	51	41	71	26	122	67
4	33	29	57	19	90	48
5	19	15	46	12	65	27

[1] Does not include patients observed for less than one year or patients with involved iliac nodes or systemic metastases.

b) Sarcoma

Of 80 patients with sarcoma who have been treated by perfusion, 51 with sarcoma of the limbs have been observed one or more years after treatment (Table 2). In more than half of these 51, treatment was considered to be palliative because

Table 2. *Sarcoma of Limbs* [1]

Year	Adjuvant		Palliative		Total	
	No. Patients	No. Controlled	No. Patients	No. Controlled	No. Patients	No. Controlled
1	23	20	28	5	51	25
2	21	16	24	4	45	20
3	17	12	22	4	39	16
4	15	11	17	1	32	12
5	13	9	12	1	25	10

[1] Does not include patients observed for less than one year or those with systemic metastases.

of the extensiveness of the sarcoma or because of recurrence after previous excision. Almost a third of those treated 4 or more years ago and two-fifths of those treated 5 or more years ago are free of malignant disease. For almost all patients alive at the end of the fourth and fifth years, perfusion was an adjuvant to wide excision or amputation. If the patients with far-advanced sarcoma are excluded from consideration, then two-thirds of the patients were apparently cured at 5 years after treatment. These results are superior to results of excision alone.

The Mistakes Most Commonly Made in Treating Cancer

PIERRE DENOIX

Most of the mistakes made at the start of or during the treatment of cancer arise from a failure to recognize the consequences of the existence of an interaction between the cancer and its host (DENOIX, 1962). Cancer should no longer be regarded as a parasite developing inexorably in a passive host. The concept is gaining ground — and is receiving support from many experimental studies — that a malignant tumor behaves like a graft on a host that is to a greater or lesser extent capable of recognizing it as foreign to itself and thus of more or less effectively setting its own system of defence in motion against it.

A very long period — in some cases 15 or 20 years — may elapse between the initiation of the malignant process and its clinical manifestation. In comparison with this long silent period, the mean duration of untreated cancer from its clinical diagnosis is from 18 to 30 months. What occurred during the much longer silent period, it must be admitted, is what influences the course of the disease and the prognosis for the patient. The source of the mistakes described below is to be found in the failure to recognize these facts.

The traditional view was that the vital element is time and every effort should be made to prevent it from being lost. In fact, while time may in certain circumstances be an aggravating factor, it is not so always and it does not always operate in the same way. The importance of the time factor is merely relative. Reference to Table 1 will make this clear. In this table groups of malignant tumors of the

Table 1. *Survival Time in Relation to Extent of Disease in Breast Cancer*

Extent of disease in accordance with T.N.M. system	No.	less than 2 months	No.	2—5 months	No.	6—12 months	No.	over 12 months	Significance
T1 + T2	92	74%	93	67%	52	79%	33	91%	$p = 0\,05$
T3 + T4	37	49%	54	48%	57	37%	63	33%	Not significant

breast are divided into, on the one hand, group T 1 + T 2 and, on the other, group T 3 + T 4. It will be seen that, with an equal extent of spread, the latter group is little or not at all affected by the time, the seriousness increasing with the extent of the spread independently of the time. The table shows in particular that the number of T 3 + T 4 cases is greater than that of T 1 + T 2 for the longer periods of time (63 against 33) and that the greater seriousness of the group T 3 + T 4, which is the larger, affects the average seriousness of the whole series. Among the patients as a whole the seriousness of the disease increases with time, whereas when there is a constant rate of spread the time factor becomes subsidiary.

At the Institut Gustave-Roussy we have applied ourselves to the task of measuring the real significance of the time factor. We have introduced the concept of speed (LALANNE ,1962) or rate of growth, as shown in Table 2. From this table it

Table 2. *Rate of Growth in Relation to Survival after Four Years in Breast Cancer*

Rate of growth	< 6 months No.	survival	> 6 months No.	survival	Significance
Tumor stationary	127	69%	79	73%	Without significance
Developing slowly	47	45%	54	31%	Without significance
Developing rapidly	18	22%	17	18%	Without significance
Significance		$p = 0.001$		$p = 0.001$	

can be seen that what counts is the combination of time and the extent of spread, i. e., the greater or lesser amount of time taken to attain a certain degree of spread. At whatever time the patient is seen, his situation depends on the relationship between the size of his tumor and this time factor. The mistake that should not be made with a patient is to hasten events for fear of losing time and being faced with a worsening situation. If a cancer is really developing at such a speed that fresh evidence of its spread appears within a few days, it is certain that no available form of treatment could halt its progress. A few days or even a week or two give a safety margin of time that runs no risk of jeopardizing the patient's future. With such a time margin the patient can be carefully examined and all the necessary investigations carried out to determine the exact site of the tumor, the extent of its spread, and its nature and characteristics. With these data the plan of treatment can be decided upon with a full knowledge of the situation.

The concept of a rhythm of development entails consequences that, if properly grasped, may lead to the avoidance of certain mistakes. At the Institut Gustave-Roussy (DENOIX, 1965), stress has for a long time been placed on the concept of an active phase during the course of cancer. This concept accords with experimental findings, especially those of FOULDS (1965). It seems to be the rule that cancer develops in successive phases, during each of which a degree of stabilization is observed, the result of an equilibrium established between the host and the tumor. Progression from one phase to another usually means an increase in the size of the tumor, but regression is possible, though exceptional. The active phase indicates a disturbance of the equilibrium established between the host and the tumor, most often to the advantage of the tumor. It is a phase during which every effort should be made to avoid making the upset in the equilibrium worse by any excessive or untimely treatment.

So far there is no biological test in existence giving an accurate indication of whether a patient is or is not in the developing phase. From the clinical standpoint, it seemed to us that the concept of a recent and progressive increase in the size of the tumor, occurring within the space of a few weeks, was extremely valuable; but unfortunately such an increase can only be gauged in superficial tumors.

Whatever the position, if we consider the patient to be in the developing phase we reject forthwith the idea of a surgical operation, even though all the other conditions are in its favour. In these cases — and this is especially indicated in breast cancer — we prefer first to employ radiotherapy, which makes it possible to decide to what extent the lesion is developing. Sometimes the tumor becomes stabilized as a result of the radiotherapy and surgical intervention can then be considered. At other times, however, in spite of the irradiation the tumor continues to spread. In these cases operation is not a possibility; nor would they have been improved by immediate surgery. They are extremely serious cases, and immediate surgery would have had exactly the opposite effect.

In a series of 266 cases (VOGT-HOERNER et al., 1964) of malignant tumors of the breast, which would normally have been considered perfectly operable, we considered that 29 were in the developing phase. The 29 patients were treated by irradiation, the others being operated on. In the 237 patients operated on, the average survival rate after five years was 73 % (we shall cite this study later to show the difference according to whether or not there is invasion of the lymph nodes); on the other hand, in the group considered as being in the developing phase the survival rate after five years was 41 %. The clinical criteria we adopted to divide these two groups into operable and non-operable were thus significant, since the fate of the two groups was different.

Identification of these developing forms makes it possible to avoid another mistake, which is to think that increasing the skin area removed in breast cancer reduces the risk of early local recurrence in the field of operation. We practically never see any more of these rapidly spreading skin cases since we abandoned surgery for cases of cancer in the developing phase, although classically they are fit subjects for operation. These post-operative extensions and early local recurrences, when the disease spreads in a veritably fulminating fashion, took place when the patients were operated on during the developing phase, at a time when the host-tumor relationship was in disequilibrium to the advantage of the tumor.

Other mistakes can be made at the time the plan of treatment is decided on, if the decision is not the result of a discussion involving all concerned. When a patient has been carefully examined, when the extent of the tumor has been determined,[1] and when all the necessary investigations have made it possible to classify the patient as accurately as possible — this is the time for choosing the mode of treatment, which in an increasing number of cancers will be a combined treatment making use of different techniques. The mistake to be avoided is for the specialist to whom the patient has first addressed himself to embark upon treatment indiscriminately. Only too often he may utilize the resources of the techniques he is well acquainted with, without asking himself whether it might not be possible to do better with other methods, or even as well but at less expense to the patient in terms of function, psychological trauma, or even financial outlay. This is why it seems essential to aim increasingly at the establishment of teams of specialists whose task it will be to draw up a plan of treatment together before the actual treatment is begun.

The basic elements of such a team are a surgeon, a radiologist, and a physician, all with equal responsibility and supported by a pathologist. They will first consider

---

[1] With the help of the T. N. M. classification system of the International Union Against Cancer.

the findings of the clinical examination, then the therapeutic possibilites each can offer. The final plan of treatment will be chosen so as to employ the simplest forms to achieve the best possible result. This is the practice followed in certain French cancer centers, particularly the Institut Gustave-Roussy. It has proved of great benefit to the patients.

Another mistake at the time when the decision on treatment is being taken would be an over-rigid approach to the treatment — to utilize the available resources in treatment to the maximum for a cancer of a given site without asking whether a simpler approach might not be possible. The circumstances that may lead to cure or palliation in patients with cancer may certainly be very different. Thus at present it is not possible to envisage "cure" for patients with distant metastases; on the other hand, if there are no distant metastases cure can be hoped for, but the amount and the intensity of the treatment will be very different according to whether the lymph nodes are or are not involved. Absence of lymph-node involvement (N-) is an extremely favorable factor and with it cure can often be achieved by simple, limited action. If the lymph nodes are involved (N+), however, the treatment is much more intensive. If, for example, a patient has cancer of the cervix uteri with extensive regional spread (T 4) but with no lymph-node involvement (N-), this situation will enable the surgeon to attack the cancer boldly with perhaps extensive local excision or indeed in certain cases even pelvic exenteration, and the chances of cure are considerable. On the other hand, if the lymph nodes are involved (N+) it would be a serious mistake to decide on pelvic exenteration, a mutilating operation with a difficult aftermath and serious physical and psychological sequelae, without a careful weighing up of the pros and cons. Since the period of survival is short, if the local conditions are tolerable the treatment should be limited, symptomatic, and palliative. If on the other hand the tumor because of its extent either causes great pain to the patient or results in a rectovesicovaginal fistula, which is extremely unpleasant for the patient, pelvic exenteration should certainly be considered, for the patient will be more comfortable after the operation even if her survival is short.

It must therefore be fully realized that a therapeutic programme must not be decided upon in the abstract, the view merely being taken that marshalling the maximum therapeutic resources available will give the maximum chances to the patient. On the contrary, each of the methods that could be employed should be scrutinized for its validity in relation to the patient's prognosticated survival time. If this survival time is likely to be short, every effort should be made not to make his state worse functionally and psychologically. An over-systematic approach to the treatment of cancer is a lazy attitude that abolishes every stimulus towards the search for something simpler and better. At the Institut Gustave-Roussy we have discarded this over-systematic approach, and for that reason we think that we have been able to benefit a considerable number of patients; the improvements in treatment we have introduced have not always improved the prospects of cure, but they have left the patients more comfortable and subjected them to less suffering.

Another mistake that should not be committed is "static" use of what are called prognostic criteria. During the clinical examination and while treatment is being carried out, we obtain from the patient information enabling us to forecast some of what is likely to happen. It is very important not to be content with merely collecting these data, summing them up when all is over, and using them only to forecast what will happen, for some of the criteria may be used in a dynamic way when they come to light to modify the treatment.

Work done by HEROVICI (DENOIX and HEROVICI, 1962) at the Institut Gustave-Roussy, based on the staining of biopsy specimens from the cervix uteri with picropolychrome, may perhaps enable a forecast to be made of whether the lymph nodes are involved or not. It is easy to imagine how important it is to try to expand such research, for if it could be established before treatment that the nodes were not involved (N-) it would greatly simplify the treatment. With such a test for cancer of the breast its treatment too would be immensely facilitated, for simple mastectomy would be be sufficient to give a very high percentage of cures in N- cases. Hence the need to increase the number of and perfect tests like this one, so as to bring them into use at the earliest possible moment.

The prognostic criteria available are mostly obtained during treatment, and particularly during surgical operations. It would be a mistake to neglect the considerable contribution afforded by on-the-spot histological examinations during the operation to determine the extent of the disease and the condition of the lymph nodes. The information thus obtained will provide guidance on the extent to which the operation itself should be pursued.

In this connexion, another example of prognostic methods used at the Institut Gustave-Roussy deserves mention (VOGT-HOERNER et al., 1964). It is related to cancer of the outer quadrants of the breast. In these cases we carry out a thorough on-the-spot histological examination of an axillary biopsy specimen. Published statistical studies have shown that when the axillary lymph nodes are not involved, as shown by an extremely detailed histological examination (i. e., giving a percentage of N- of the order of 33 %), there is sufficient ground for believing that the internal mammary nodes are not involved. Consequently a mastectomy is often carried out in these cases without ablation of the pectoral muscles. In a series of cases belonging to the category of N- we obtained a survival rate of 92 % at five years with operation alone. These examples show how prognostic criteria can be obtained before treatment (which is ideal), or during treatment (which is still good), and how they can influence the plan of treatment.

Stress must be placed on the extremely important role of lymph-node involvement or its absence in the mode of treatment of patients and in the prognosis. We have already referred to it on several occasions, and it would be a mistake not to attribute considerable importance to it. An attempt must be made as quickly as possible to find out the state of the lymph nodes and draw practical conclusions therefrom. In work carried out at the Institut Gustave-Roussy (DENOIX and GELLE, 1955) it was shown that the likelihood of a patient with no involvement of any of the lymph-node areas around the tumor having local recurrences later is practically nil. Thus in our series of 266 breast cancers (VOGT-HOERNER et al., 1964), the only cases of recurrence that we observed in the group of 83 N- patients who had a 92 % five-year survival rate were those in which there were distant metastases but no local recurrences.

These findings appear to justify the view that in cases where the lymph-node involvement is N- surgery should not be supplemented by radiotherapy but should be the only mode of treatment. On the other hand, where the involvement is N+, radiotherapy should play an important part. It would seem to us to be a mistake to propose postoperative irradiation for patients without lymph-node involvement.

Chemotherapy is coming more and more into consideration as supplementary treatment for solid tumours. It too is the source of many mistakes in treatment. Applied over-systematically and unreasoningly, it is not without danger. The first mistake is to embark upon it at once (as unfortunately too many practitioners do) before the plan of treatment has been decided upon. This is irrational practice, only too often based on the doctor's desire to do something quickly — a desire arising from the persisting view that quick action is a necessity. Such systematic chemotherapy prior to the usual forms of treatment must be forbidden; the use of drugs must be withheld until the doctor, surgeon, and radiologist have met as a team to decide on the extent to which it is indicated.

Another mistake that is prone to occur at present is that of advocating systematic chemotherapy as a supplement to surgery or radiotherapy. In the absence of careful and controlled drug trials to establish the value of the drugs used, it would be prudent to wait until those who have the means to carry them out do so. It should be realized that the pharmaceutical products that we use may in some cases have a depressive effect on the immunological defence system; indeed, several of them are employed to prepare subjects for organ grafts. It should also be realized that in host-tumor relationships the organism's defence processes play an important part. If it is granted that N- forms of cancer provide a proof that they have been able to destroy the malignant cells appearing in the lymph nodes, the reason is that the defence mechanism has played its part. We have no information whatever on whether systematic drug treatment administered blindly might not depress the defence mechanism and facilitate the appearance of metastases that the organism would otherwise have destroyed.

The danger that systematic treatment with drugs involves will now be clear. The need for a rational approach is so great that we consider that it would be a mistake, and indeed a risk, in our present state of knowledge to supplement the usual treatment of patients rated as N- with chemotherapy.

Among the arguments adduced to justify the administration of drugs either during or immediately after surgery is the observed fact that malignant cells are present in the blood after operation. The mistake here is to consider that because a cell is mobile and will be arrested somewhere it must therefore always give rise to a metastasis there. Experience shows that in fact this is not so. What matters is not the liberation of the cells — for during the long history of all malignant tumors cells are liberated, and the first time very early indeed —, but their fate wherever they are arrested. A great number among them do not develop further, and in this respect the important point is whether the organism has or has not the capacity to destroy them, not whether the cells are liberated. It is not certain that massive and especially blind drug treatment does not have the opposite effect and facilitate the arrest and assumption of the latent state of cells that could otherwise have been destroyed by the organism's defence mechanism itself. It is therefore sensible to be extremely cautious and not to misuse drugs as a supplementary treatment when this treatment is based on a false concept of the fate of liberated cells.

A more general mistake that should not be committed is to squander therapeutic resources. This affords another argument against over-systematic treatment not based on verified clinical and experimental findings, for there is no guarantee that there will not later be malignant manifestations requiring treatment whose use and effectiveness will unfortunately be limited by the earlier over-treatment. For this reason initial radiotherapy or chemotherapy, while adequate for the purpose, should be employed sparingly. In particular, treatment should not be repeated systematically without good reason, for reserves must be kept for a future that is uncertain.

Reference has already been made to therapeutic trials and to the increasing need to subject any new treatment to a controlled statistical trial. It seems to us that the controversy about the legitimacy of these trials is based on a misunderstanding. Ethical arguments are adduced, but opponents of these trials do not for the most part push their reasoning to its logical conclusion; it would be a mistake to consider it wrong to conduct a therapeutic trial when a supposedly more effective form of treatment appears. Two attitudes are possible. If a cancer specialist judges from what he has read in the literature and from what he has been able to confirm himself that the new treatment is better than previous treatments, he clearly has no need to carry out a trial; indeed, he would be inconsistent with himself if he did carry one out. On the other hand, if he is not convinced by the literature, it is his duty to carry one out, and it would be a mistake for a cancer specialist so convinced to deny the specialist not so convinced the right to try to convince himself. This is why, in collaboration with other institutes in different parts of the world, we have begun a therapeutic trial at the Institut Gustave-Roussy. We considered that there was no evidence either in our own experience or in the literature proving or disproving that internal mammary curettage improved the prognosis in breast cancer, and that all the statistics published lacked valid control groups. In such circumstances the only appropriate course of action is a therapeutic trial, and this is in progress. We shall base our future treatment on the results obtained.

We shall conclude with certain mistakes made at a later stage in the patient's treatment, which sometimes have serious consequences. They may occur if latish clinical manifestations linked with secondary sclerosis or a radiation injury are taken for recurrences, and in such cases a mutilating operation or radiotherapy would be catastrophic. Two examples are as follows. A patient with a malignant lesion of the soft tissues of the lower limb received a strong dose of radiation and his limb was then resected, a skin graft being used. One day the graft, which had appeared to have taken perfectly, suddenly became ulcerated and disappeared, and the appearance of the stump was disquieting. Immediate amputation was advised by a physician, but when we were asked for advice we took a biopsy and found that a radiation injury had occurred, with secondary rejection of the graft from a site that was unfavourable because of previous irradiation. The second case was concerned with brawny arm some distance away from the area irradiated for cancer of the breast. Here the association was with sclerosis, and radiation injury had played the main part. Radiotherapy for such a patient would clearly be catastrophic, for it would make the lesions worse and they might extend not only to the soft tissues but also to the subjacent nervous, muscular, bony, and even pulmonary tissues.

It is therefore essential to be very cautious when fresh symptoms arise after the lapse of some time from the initial treatment. Before entertaining the hypothesis of a recurrence, pay due attention to:

1. the details of the previous treatment given, especially the radiation source, dose, and fields, and the qualifications of the persons administering the treatment; and

2. the present clinical state of the patient, especially any contrast between the symptoms and the patient's generally good condition.

In other words, the reason for the patient's state must be elucidated before recurrence is diagnosed and particularly before he is irradiated. Obviously a biopsy should be done wherever possible, though carefully, since it is a traumatic operation in a radiation injury and its interpretation is often very difficult in such circumstances.

All these mistakes are possible during the diagnosis and treatment of cancer or on the appearance of later symptoms. It is clear that all therapeutic action must be rationally based on a dynamic concept of the natural history of cancer and take into account the significant part played by host-tumor relationships, so that the various elements are given their true relative importance.

References

Denoix, P.: Importance des relations hôte-tumeur dans l'évolution des cancers humains. Rev. franç. Etud. clin. biol. 7, 242—245 (1962).
— Le traitement des tumeurs en fonction de nos connaissances concernant le rôle de l'hôte. Rev. franç. Etud. clin. biol. 10, 583—586 (1965).
—, and X. Gelle: Mode de décès des malades atteintes de tumeurs du sein en fonction de l'envahissement microscopique du système lymphatique. Bull. Ass. franç. Cancer 42, 548—555 (1955).
—, and C. Herovici: Relations entre un aspect histologique particulier "la clôture" et l'existence ou non d'un envahissement des ganglions pelviens. Etude de 100 cas de cancer du col utérin, stade I. Mém. Acad. Chir. 88, 590—593 (1962).
Foulds, L.: Some problems of differentiation and integration in neoplasia. In Harris, R .J. R. (ed.): Biological organization at cellular and supracellular levels. London and New York: Academic Press 1965.
Lalanne, C. M.: Taux d'accroissement et pronostic des tumeurs malignes du sein. Acta Un. int. Cancr. 18, 807 (1962).
Vogt-Hoerner, G., C. M. Lalanne, P. Juret, J. Lacour, F. Hourtoule, J. Roujeau, and C. Rouquette: Survie à la cinquième année de 237 cancers du sein opérés d'emblée. Mém. Acad. Chir. 90, 653—659 (1964).

Biological Factors Affecting the Prognosis and Treatment of Cancer

Umberto Veronesi

It is now universally recognized that tumor development depends mainly upon the biological characteristics of the tumor and of the host organism. The prognosis is therefore correlated with these factors. Hence the treatment may vary.

1. Age

The influence of age on the prognosis of some types of treated or untreated cancers is believed to be related to the biological condition of the host at specific ages. In this respect, malignant tumors can be roughly divided into three main groups:

tumors whose prognosis is not affected by age; tumors with a better prognosis at an advanced age; and tumors with a better prognosis at an early age. The first group comprises cancers of the gastrointestinal tract, oral cavity, larynx, and lung. In the second group, breast cancer is a tumor that shows a low rate of growth in very old women (HAAGENSEN, 1956). However, in the years immediately after the menopause the prognosis seems to be rather poor (SMITHERS and PAYNE, 1963). In females under 30 years of age the prognosis is worse than in other women: this, however, might to a certain extent be due to the inclusion of cases occurring during pregnancy and lactation. Patients over 45 years survive longer with leukemia than patients under 45, probably because acute cases are preponderant in the early years of life. In the third group, cancer of the thyroid (LINDSAY, 1960) and perhaps malignant melanomas (WHITE, 1963) should be mentioned. The causes that make thyroid cancer less malignant in young people are obscure; endocrine factors are perhaps of importance, as thyroid cancer seems to be stimulated by thyroid-stimulating hormone (TSH).

The data from many cancer registries show an inverse relationship between age and survival for most sites of cancer (Table 1). Although the cause of this relationship

Table 1. *Five-year Relative Survival Rate for Cancer (Selected Sites) by Age* [1]

Age group		under 45 %	45—54 %	55—64 %	65—74 %	75 and over %
All stages	Male	38.0	32.5	31.0	32.6	35.8
of cancers	Female	56.3	49.5	42.6	39.3	37.0
Localized	Male	71.8	68.0	63.5	63.8	64.3
cancers	Female	81.5	77.6	74.1	71.0	72.2

[1] Adapted from State of California Department of Public Health Tumor Registry: Cancer registration and survival in California, Berkeley 1963.

remains basically unknown, it is suggested that the age gradient in survival rates may be influenced by the more radical treatment given to patients at younger ages (State of California Department of Public Health, 1963).

To what extent does treatment vary with age? Although the majority of surgical and radiologic procedures do not vary with age, there are cases in which the treatment does change. A typical example is cancer of the thyroid, in which age is a determinant. As the disease is relatively benign in the child, the treatment is more conservative, and the growth can often be removed without dissection of the internal jugular vein and sternocleidomastoid muscle.

The choice of chemotherapeutic agents may likewise depend upon the age of the patient. In children certain types of malignant growths show susceptibility to some chemotherapeutic agents, while in adults they do not.

2. Sex

The available data on the end results of cancer treatment show that the prognosis is better in females than in males. This is mainly due to the fact that cancer in women occurs most frequently in the sex-specific sites, which have high survival rates. However, the comparable data for non-sex-linked tumors affecting both sexes still show a longer survival in females. Tumors of the gastrointestinal tract show little differences between the two sexes. Better survival rates have been reported in females than in males for patients with cancer of the tongue (CAMPBELL, 1963). Cancer of the stomach surgically treated seems to show a slightly better prognosis in females than in males (BUCALOSSI, VERONESI and LOMONACO, 1963). For cancer of the large intestine the data are controversial, the survival rate being higher in females in the United States of America, Denmark, and Norway, higher in males in Finland, and similar in the two sexes in England and Wales (CUTLER and LOURIE, 1963). Studies on the Connecticut material show a slightly better prognosis in females than in males, either in cancer of the large intestine or in cancer of the rectum (EISENBERG, KEOGH and FOOTE, 1963). Cancer of the thyroid has a better prognosis in females than in males and this is particularly apparent for some histological types like papillary cancer (MUSTACCHI and CUTLER, 1960). As regards malignant melanomas, WHITE (1963) showed recently that the prognosis is better in females than in males. The sex effect is less apparent after the menopause, so that a relation to cyclic ovarian function can be deduced. In the recent report on survival in California (State of California Department of Public Health, 1963), comparison of the five-year survival rate in females and males for cancer of non-sex-specific sites showed a constant better survival in females, except for bladder cancer (Table 2).

Table 2. *Five-year Survival Rates, Male and Female Cancer Cases, all Stages, 1942—1956* [1]

Site of cancer	Relative survival rate %	
	Male	Female
All sites	33.5	45.4
All sites, excluding skin other than melanoma	25.0	41.8
Selected sites		
Stomach	9.5	10.8
Large intestine	31.8	37.1
Rectum	31.8	36.1
Lung	4.3	8.0
Bladder	42.8	39.4
Melanoma of skin	41.5	58.1
Skin, other than melanoma	86.2	90.1
Lymphosarcoma	20.0	25.8
Hodgkin's disease	17.6	31.6
Leukemia	6.4	6.1

[1] Adapted from State of California Department of Public Health Tumor Registry: Cancer registration and survival in California, Berkeley 1963.

3. Characteristics of the Tumor

Extensive work has been done in past years to judge the prognosis from the biological characteristics of the tumor. The principal factor is the rate of growth of the tumor, which shows a significant correlation with the prognosis. A number of procedures have been proposed for the determination of the rate of growth, especially of breast cancer. Among them are mammography, which detects so-called malignant edema (PICARD, 1963) in rapidly expanding cases, and measurement of the skin temperature (HANDLEY, 1963). The rate of growth is also sometimes easily gauged by the clinical history. Whether the rate of growth is an intrinsic factor of the tumor or depends on the biological conditions of the host is not clear. Histological prognostic criteria have been established with many grading systems, based mainly on the degree of differentiation of the cancer cells (DENOIX, 1963).

All these prognostic criteria can affect the treatment. To give an example, the discovery by mammography of extensive edema in an otherwise operable breast cancer might lead to modification of the treatment plan and administration of a preoperative course of radiation. Modifications in the treatment of cancer of the rectum according to the grade of the malignancy have also been suggested (QUER, DAHLIN and MAYO, 1953). BRODERS (1958) underlined the importance of grading, not only as a prognostic tool but also as an aid in the choice of therapeutic procedures; for example, since grade I cancer of the lip almost never metastasizes, removal of the regional lymph nodes is not indicated.

4. Dissemination of Cancer Cells in the Blood

The extensive studies of COLE et al. (1961) led to the conclusion that 25% of patients with curable cancer and 50% of patients with incurable cancer have cancer cells in the peripheral blood. In addition, they found a sharp increase in the numbers of cancer cells in the venous blood from the tumor area during such manipulations as curettage, skin preparation, bone biopsy, rectal examination, and the operation itself.

These data, however, have not been confirmed by all investigators, and at the present time considerable disagreement still exists on the incidence of malignant cells in the peripheral blood of cancer patients, the reported rates varying from 4% to 75%. Difficulties in cytological interpretation and the varying quality of the preparations produced by the different methods of demonstrating the cells are the main causes of this disagreement.

Apart from this disagreement (which calls, however, for urgent settlement), the practical significance of the presence of cancer cells in the blood is also not clear. In particular, the viability of these cells is not firmly established. TAYLOR and VELLIOS (1958) failed in their attempt to grow cancer cells from human blood by autologous subcutaneous injection. However, G. MOORE et al. (1960) were successful in growing cancer cells isolated from the peripheral blood in vitro in three out of 64 samples. As regards the prognostic implications, ENGELL (1959) reported that 51% of patients surviving for five to nine years had had cancer cells in their blood at the time of operation. The author concluded that "in the majority of patients surviving five to nine years tumorous cells disseminated before and during operation must have perished in the bloodstream". WATNE, SANDBERG and MOORE (1960), reporting an 18-month follow-up study for a miscellaneous group of tumors, found that 54% of the 57 patients who had cancer cells in the blood survived, compared with 71% of the patients without demonstrable tumor cells. ROBERTS (in COLE et al., 1961) found no significant differences in 283 patients studied for the presence of circulating cancer cells: 18% of 197 patients with negative blood samples surviving for two to five years after treatment compared with 14% of 86 patients with positive samples. However, patients with a shower of cancer cells into the blood during operation showed a significant worsening of the prognosis as compared with patients with negative blood samples at operation.

The implications of the knowledge that cancer cells circulate in the blood as a result of cancer treatment are obvious. Since the discovery of circulating tumoral cells, and especially since the discovery that they increase at the time of surgery, many efforts have been made to provide chemotherapeutic cover against malignant cells during operation. However, the results of extensive clinical trials in this field, although not yet complete, do not seem to be encouraging, for the association of chemotherapeutic agents with radical surgery does not seem in the majority of cases to yield better long-term results than surgery alone. Two important points need clarification: first, the actual number of cancer patients with circulating cancer cells; and second, the long-term results in such patients when treated by conventional methods.

In the present state of knowledge, since no one can predict the ultimate effect of circulating cancer cells, there is no justification for altering the treatment on the ground that cancer cells have been demonstrated in a pre-operative blood sample. However, it seems reasonable to recommend that every effort should be made to prevent dissemination of cancer cells during operation.

5. Endocrine Factors

A number of benign tumors are structurally related, not only in origin but also in development, to the endocrine conditions of the host. Breast fibroadenomas and cysts and uterine myomas, for example, have been described as regressing and frequently disappearing after the menopause. This also, to a small extent, applies to malignant tumors occurring in the target organs of hormones. To give an example, cancers of the breast often change in development after either a natural or an artificial menopause; cases in which a natural menopause has produced remissions of the primary tumor lasting as long as 17 years have been described (SMITHERS, 1952), and the beneficial results of an artificial menopause are well known. The greatest endocrine variations occur in females during pregnancy, which plays an important part in modifying the development of some tumors. Cancer of the breast occurring during pregnancy or lactation shows a high degree of malignancy. WHITE and WHITE (1956) found a 50% five-year survival rate in a series of 12 patients with cancer localized in the breast, but only two of 25 patients in whom the disease had spread to the axillary lymph nodes lived for five years or more. According to the report of HOLLEB and FARROW (1962) on 193 patients with breast cancer occurring during pregnancy and lactation, the end results were poor, especially in a large group with axillary invasion (five-year survival 21%), while a small group without axillary metastases showed a five-year survival rate of 58%. Therapeutic abortion does not improve the chances of curing the disease. It is interesting that pregnancy occurring after radical treatment for breast cancer does not seem to modify the prognosis (BLOOM, 1963).

When pregnancy co-exists with a carcinoma of the uterine cervix no worsening of the prognosis seems to occur (KNICK, 1961). The same applies to leukemia (SHEEHY, 1958) and to Hodgkin's disease (BARRY, DIAMOND and GRAVER, 1962).

Interesting results have been obtained in studying the association between pregnancy and malignant melanoma. Although traditional literature contained some dramatic cases of worsening of the disease due to pregnancy, more recent and accurate investigations have led to rather opposite conclusions. GEORGE, FORTNER and PACK (1960) recently reported no differences in the 5- and 10-year survival rate in 54 pregnant and 112 non-pregnant patients with melanoma. WHITE et al., (1961), comparing 30 pregnant patients with melanoma and 31 non-pregnant patients, found a better five-year survival rate in the first group (73%) than in the second (55%). A case of regression of malignant melanoma during pregnancy has been also described by ALLEN (1955).

Studies on the endocrine condition by measurement have recently led to interesting results. BULBROOK, GREENWOOD and HAYWARD, 1960, and ATKINS (1962) found a discriminant formula based on the ratio between etiocholanone and 17-hydroxycorticosteroids to predict the response of advanced breast cancers to endocrine surgery. Moreover, the authors think that these measurements might be useful for evaluating in normal women the risk of incurring breast cancer. DARGENT et al. (1963) found a relation between FSH levels and the response of breast cancer to ablative endocrine procedures. In prostatic cancer the 17-hydroxycorticosteroid level is a valuable index to the efficacy of estrogen treatment (BONO and ZINGO, 1965).

The hormone state of the patient is of vital importance in the choice of hormone therapy. It suffices to mention the contrary effects of estrogens on breast cancer in women before and after the menopause or the different indications for endocrine surgery at the different endocrinologic stages of life. In this connexion it is interesting to note that ovariectomy in premenopausal women yields different results according to their age, and that in younger women (less than 35 years of age) its effect is very limited.

6. Host Resistance

Under the rather vague term of host resistance are included all factors that operate naturally in the host to withstand the spread of cancer. Whether this resistance is hormonal or immunological in character is not clear, but it is of importance in determining the prognosis.

There are many factors that suggest the intervention of host resistance in cancer. The most obvious are the development of many tumors with long periods of quiescence and sudden bursts of rapid growth, the occurrence of metastases 10 to 20 years after removal of a primary tumor, and the preference for certain metastatic sites.

The sudden appearance or rapid development of metastases after removal of a primary tumor have been described a long time ago (DUNPHY, 1950; CARYER and SCHMER, 1956; JACKSON, OLKON and SARRIS, 1958) and, although no statistical evidence has been obtained to rule out an explanation on a causal basis, animal experiments seem to confirm the clinical findings. Cases of rapid dissemination immediately after operations for other diseases and many years after resection of the tumors have also been constantly reported (TEMPLE, 1941; GORDON-TAYLOR, 1959).

The biological reason for these events probably lies in the fact that any operation leads to the release of growth-promoting humoral substances. These substances, whose function is to favor regeneration of the excised tissues, are not necessarily organ-specific but can also have far-reaching actions and stimulate the growth of any tumor cells that may be present in the body, as many experimental studies have shown (Paschkis, 1958; Paschkis et al., 1955; Trotter, 1961). The onset of an anemic state might also be a factor, if it is true that erythropoietin, a hormone released by the kidneys in anemic conditions, is a tumor growth-stimulating factor (Leaders et al., 1962; Leaders, Werder and Schmidt, 1964; Thorning, 1965).

The relative immunity of the spleen to secondary cancer is significant and may indicate a local immunological resistance of that organ. Miller and Milton (1965) showed that the spleen retarded and the liver enhanced the take of tumor cells when homologous transplants were grown in the spleen and liver of mice. Highly malignant tumors like those of the brain do not metastasize, yet it is not conceivable that the cells from such tumors fail to reach the bloodstream; they must surely do so and then be destroyed. Slight indications of immunity may also be shown by the reactive hyperplasia of lymph nodes.

A most significant finding is that in more than 50% of pre-invasive cancers of the cervix the disease does not proceed to invasion but either remains stationary or regresses completely. In this connexion there are rather surprising data on occult carcinomas. Cancer of the prostate appears to be present in an occult form in a large proportion of the elderly population, nor is it rare under the age of 60 years (Hirst and Bergman, 1954). The data of Mortensen, Woolner and Bennet (1955) indicate that it is not rare at autopsy to detect neoplastic foci in the thyroid gland of healthy people. From these data, and from the thyroid cancer statistics for the general population, it appears clear that the majority of these foci will never develop into actual disease. The biological factors that prevent their development are not known.

Anaplastic features are generally of grave prognostic significance and the hypothesis cannot be excluded that anaplasia is a reflexion of an inadequate host defense and not a property of the growth itself. Bloom (1963), in a study of the grading of tumors on a cytological basis, showed that cancer in women during pregnancy or lactation is of a high grade of malignancy. This shows that modification of host conditions such as is caused by pregnancy is able to increase the histological grade of malignancy, which should therefore not be considered as a fundamental and constant characteristic of the cancer. An alternative explanation is that pregnancy and lactation protect the breast from cancer, leading to selection in the sense that only highly malignant tumors can overcome this natural resistance (Berkson, 1963).

There are conditions during the development of a tumor in which there is a fall in host resistance. This is well documented for lymphoid tumors, especially Hodgkin's disease, which frequently shows a "poverty of immunological resistance". Dubin (1947) observed anergy to tuberculosis in patients with Hodgkin's disease, a low incidence of positive tests for syphilis, and inability to produce antibodies against Brucella organisms whenever these infections coexisted. In skin homograft studies, delayed homograft rejection and a number of takes equal to autografts have been observed (Kelly, Good and Varco, 1958). As the altered immunological responses are present in other lymphomas, it has been suggested that the tissue responses seen in Hodgkin's disease may be a reflexion of the degree and extension of involvement of the reticulo-endothelium and not a specific property of the disease (Hoyle, Dawson and Mather, 1954).

Morphological signs of host defense are sometimes identifiable in the tissues surrounding the tumor. BERG (1963) found a rather better prognosis in breast cancers when a plasmocyte infiltration was present around the tumor. But the real prognostic significance of "sinus histiocytosis" of the satellite lymph nodes has not yet been fully elucidated (BLACK and SPEER, 1958; MOORE, CHAPNICK and SCHOENBERG, 1960).

Decrease in resistance has been produced in experimental animals in a number of ways, such as by administration of cortisone (TOOLAN, 1953; BASERGA and SHUBIK, 1955) and chemicals including nitrogen mustard (GORE, ANDERSON and McDONALD, 1961), induction of operative (BUINANSKAS, McDONALD and COLE, 1958) and thermal (GRIFFITHS, HOPPE and COLE, 1960) stress, adrenalectomy (SLAWIKOWSKI, 1960) and liver damage (CHAN, McDONALD and COLE, 1961). Most of these experiments need confirmation. Controversial results were obtained with general anesthesia (TREVINO, 1961; SCHATTEN and KRAMER, 1958). HENGESH and McGREW (1962) have shown an increased percentage of takes in splenectomized animals inoculated intravenously with cancer cells. The role of the reticulo-endothelial system in the fate of embolic cancer cells has been summarized by STERN and WILLHEIM (1943).

Evidence of antibodies to cancer produced by human beings was demonstrated by GRAHAM and GRAHAM (1955), GRACE and KONDO (1958), GOLDMAN (1961), MELLORS (1962), MIHICH (1962), FINNEY et al. (1960), NAIRN et al. (1963) and many others. SOUTHAM, MOORE and RHOADS (1957) showed different responses of cancer patients to subcutaneous transplantation of homologous cancer tissue. While in the majority of cases the rejection of the implants occurred in a few weeks, four patients did not reject them and one had an axillary metastasis from the implanted tumor. The take of homologous cancer cells, except in these advanced cases of carcinoma, is not generally regarded as possible. However, a case of melanoblastoma transplanted from daughter to mother (aged 80) was described recently; the transplant developed very rapidly and killed the woman in 451 days (SCANLON et al. 1965).

GRACE et al. (1957) treated a leukemic patient with rabbit antiserum produced by injections of the patient's lymph-node tissue, obtaining a shrinkage of the leukemic skin lesions. NAUGESTER, BIERWALTER and KNORPP (1963) administered an ^{131}I-tagged antiserum to a patient with widespread melanoma, claiming a complete regression. SUMNER and FORAKER (1960) transfused into two patients with malignant melanoma the blood obtained from a patient who had experienced a spontaneous regression of melanoma, with encouraging results.

Encouraging results, including occasional regressions, have also recently been reported by NADLER after cross-transplants of tumors at an advanced stage followed by transfusion of small quantities of white cells.

PACK (1950) and KAMINSKI, KRINER and SEGERS (1953) mentioned the possibility that antirabies vaccine favourably influences the course of patients with melanoma, and cases of regression with this treatment have been recently reported (BELISARIO and MILTON, 1961; BURDICK, 1960; BURDICK and HAWK, 1964).

FINNEY, BAYERS and WILSON (1960) found a rise in antibody titer after radiation, indicating that the ionizing effect of radiation had resulted in disintegration of the tumor cells, with release of an antigen.

12*

7. Spontaneous Regression of Tumors

Although the magnitude of the problem is not very great and its importance only theoretical, the spontaneous regression of tumors deserves a few words. The total number of well documented cases of regression is about 120. Four types of tumors seem to show a special aptitude for spontaneous regression: neuroblastoma, hypernephroma, choriocarcinoma, and malignant melanoma (EVERSON and COLE, 1956). Eighty per cent of the regressions of neuroblastoma occur in infants less than one year old when first observed. This phenomenon, although not clear, seems to be associated with some environmental variation modifying the course of the disease (SIRTORI, ROCK and VERONESI, 1954). It must be remembered that in the first years of life there is a progressive regression of the extra-adrenal chromaffin tissue scattered in the retroperitoneal space, owing to the competitive activity of the growing adrenal medullary tissue. A hypothesis explaining the regression of neuroblastoma is that of maturation of these tumors. A few cases have been reported in which, while the patient was under clinical observation, an actively growing neuroblastoma underwent maturation to a ganglioneuroma, the most impressive case being that described by CUSHING and WOLBACH (1927) and later by FOX, DAVIDSON and THOMAS (1959), and followed for 46 years. According to WILLIS (1962), it is likely that many well differentiated ganglioneuromas were previously neuroblastomas.

The regressions of hypernephroma and choriocarcinoma described in medical literature are mainly of pulmonary metastases. The removal of the primary tumor seemed to be the major factor in the regression. Cases of melanoma are described which regressed after pregnancy or after treatment with antirabies vaccine.

References

ALLEN, A. C.: Brit. med. J. 2, 1067 (1955).

ATKINS, H. J. B.: Acta Un. int. Cancr. 18, 885 (1962).

BARRY, R. M., H. D. DIAMOND, and L. F. GRAVER: Amer. J. Obstet. Gynec. 84, 445 (1962).

BASERGA, R., and P. SHUBIK: Science 121, 100 (1955).

BELISARIO, J. C., and C. W. MILTON: Aust. J. Derm. 6, 113 (1961).

BERG, J. M.: In Symposium on the prognosis of malignant tumors of the breast. Basel: Karger 1963, p. 63.

BERKSON, J.: In Symposium on the prognosis of malignant tumors of the breast. Basel: Karger 1963, p. 69.

BLACK, M. M., and F. D. SPEER: Surg. Gynec. Obstet. 106, 163 (1958).

BLOOM, H. J. G.: In Symposium on the prognosis of malignant tumors of the breast. Basel: Karger 1963, p. 51.

BONO, A. V., and L. ZINGO: Tumori 51, 13 (1965).

BRODERS, A. C.: In PACK, G., and I. M. ARIEL: Treatment of cancer and allied diseases. Vol. I P. H. Hoeler Publ., New York, 1958.

BUCALOSSI, P., U. VERONESI, and F. LOMONACO: Acta Un. int. Cancr. 19, 1502 (1963).

BUINANSKAS, P., G. O. McDONALD, and W. H. COLE: Ann. Surg. 148, 642 (1958).

BULBROOK, R. D., F. C. GREENWOOD, and J. L. HAYWARD: Lancet 1, 1154 (1960).

BURDICK, K. H.: Arch. Derm. 82, 438 (1960).

—, and W. A. HAWK: Cancer 17, 708 (1964).

CAMPBELL, H.: Acta Un. int. Cancr. 19, 1450 (1963).

CARYER, D., and M. F. SCHMER: Cancer 9, 141 (1956).

CHAN, R., G. O. McDONALD, and W. H. COLE: Cancer 14, 111 (1961).

COLE, W. H., G. O. McDONALD, S. S. ROBERTS, and H. W. SOUTHWICK: Dissemination of cancer: prevention and therapy. New York: Appleton-Century-Crofts 1961.

CUSHING, H., and S. B. WOLBACH: Amer. J. Path. **3**, 203 (1927).
CUTLER, S. J., and W. L. LOURIE: Acta Un. int. Cancr. **19**, 1455 (1963).
DARGENT, M., M. MAYER, E. POMMATEAU, and S. POULAIN: In Symposium on the prognosis of malignant tumors of the breast. Basel: Karger 1963, p. 150.
DENOIX, P. F.: Rev. franç. Etud. clin. biol. **8**, 1039 (1963).
DUBIN, I.: Ann. intern. Med. **27**, 898 (1947).
DUNPHY, J. E.: New Engl. J. Med. **242**, 107 (1950).
EISENBERG, H., J. R. KEOGH, and F. M. FOOTE: Acta Un. int. Cancr. **19**, 1407 (1963).
ENGELL, H. C.: Ann. Surg. **149**, 457 (1959).
EVERSON, T. C., and W. H. COLE: Amer. Surg. **144**, 366 (1956).
FINNEY, J. W., E. H. BAYERS, and R. H. WILSON: Cancer Res. **20**, 351 (1960).
FOX, F., J. DAVIDSON, and L. B. THOMAS: Cancer **12**, 108 (1959).
GEORGE, P. A., J. G. FORTNER, and G. T. PACK: Cancer **13**, 854 (1960).
GOLDMAN, L.: Arch. Derm. **84**, 948 (1961).
GORDON-TAYLOR, G.: Brit. med. J. **1**, 455 (1959).
GORE, D. R., J. A. ANDERSON, and G. O. McDONALD: Proc. Amer. Ass. Cancer Res. **3**, 205 (1961).
GRACE, G. T., and T. KONDO: Ann. Surg. **148**, 633 (1958).
GRACE, J. T., F. GALLAN, W. C. TAYLOR, and R. I. CARLSON: Surg. Forum **8**, 185 (1957).
GRAHAM, J. B., and R. M. GRAHAM: Cancer **8**, 409 (1955).
GRIFFITHS, J. D., J. D. HOPPE, and W. H. COLE: Surg. Forum **11**, 55 (1960).
HAAGENSEN, C. D.: Diseases of the breast. Philadelphia: Thomas 1956.
HANDLEY, R. S.: In Symposium on the prognosis of malignant tumors of the breast. Basel: Karger 1963, p. 31.
HENGESH, J. W., E. A. McGREW, and S. NANOS: Acta cytol. scand. **6**, 143 (1962).
HIRST, A. E., and R. T. BERGMAN: Cancer **7**, 136 (1954).
HOLLEB, A. J., and J. H. FARROW: Surg. Gynec. Obstet. **115**, 65 (1962).
HOYLE, C., J. DAWSON, and G. MATHER: Lancet **2**, 1964 (1954).
JACKSON, B., H. G. OLKON, and S. P. SARRIS: Arch. Surg. **76**, 472 (1958).
KAMINSKI, A., J. KRINER, and A. M. SEGERS: Arch. argent. Derm. **3**, 509 (1953).
KELLY, W., R. GOOD, and R. VARCO: Surg. Gynec. Obstet. **107**, 565 (1958).
KNICK, R. A. H.: Amer. J. Obstet. Gynec. **82**, 45 (1961).
LEADERS, F. E., R. L. DIXON, J. W. OSBORNE, and J. P. LONG: Proc. Soc. exp. Biol. Med. **110**, 436 (1962).
—, A. A. WERDER, and C. SCHMIDT: Proc. exp. Soc. Biol. Med. **115**, 658 (1964).
LINDSAY, S.: Carcinoma of the thyroid gland. Springfield: Thomas 1960.
MELLORS, R. C.: Bull. N. Y. Acad. Med. **38**, 75 (1962).
MIHICH, E.: Cancer Res. **22**, 218 (1962).
MILLER, J. N., and G. W. MILTON: J. Path. Bact. **90**, 515 (1965).
MOORE, G., D. T. MOUNT, and A. WENDT: Surg. Forum **11**, 53 (1960).
MOORE, R. D., R. CHAPNICK, and M. D. SCHOENBERG: Cancer **13**, 545 (1960).
MORTENSEN, J. D., L. B. WOOLNER, and W. A. BENNET: J. clin. Endocr. **15**, 1270 (1955).
MUSTACCHI, P., and S. J. CUTLER: J. Amer. med. Ass. **173**, 1795 (1960).
NAIRN, R. C., J. PHILIP, T. GHOSE, I. B. PORTEOUS, and J. E. FOTHERGILL: Brit. med. J. **1**, 1702 (1963).
NAUGESTER, W., W. BIERWALTER, and C. KNORPP, quoted by M. ASWAG, and V. RICHARDS: Amer. J. Surg. **105**, 192 (1963).
PACK, G. T.: Arch. Derm. Syph. **62**, 694 (1950).
PASCHKIS, K. E.: Cancer Res. **18**, 981 (1958).
—, A. CANTAROW, J. STASNEY, and J. H. HOBBS: Cancer Res. **15**, 579 (1955).
PICARD, J. D.: In Symposium on the prognosis of malignant tumors of the breast. Basel: Karger 1963, p. 22.
QUER, E. A., D. C. DAHLIN, and C. W. MAYO: Surg. Gynec. Obstet. **96**, 24 (1953).
SCANLON, E. F., R. A. HAWKINS, W. F. WAYNE, and W. S. SMITH: Cancer **18**, 782 (1965).
SCHATTEN, W. E., and W. M. KRAMER: Cancer **11**, 460 (1958).
SHEEHY, T. W.: Amer. J. Obstet. Gynec. **75**, 788 (1958).

SIRTORI, C., T. ROCK, and U. VERONESI: Atti Soc. lombarda Sci. med.-biol. 9, 161 (1954).
SLAWIKOWSKI, G. T.: Cancer Res. 20, 316 (1960).
SMITHERS, D. W.: J. Fac. Radiol. (Lond.) 4, 89 (1952).
—, and P. M. PAYNE: In Symposium on the prognosis of malignant tumors of the breast. Basel: Karger 1963, p. 115.
SOUTHAM, C. M., H. MOORE, and C. P. RHOADS: Science 125, 158 (1957).
State of California Department of Public Health Tumor Registry: Cancer registration and survival in California, Berkeley 1963.
STERN, K., and R. WILLHEIM: Biochemistry of malignant tumors. New York: Chemical Publishing Co. 1943.
SUMNER, W. C., and A. G. FORAKER: Cancer 13, 79 (1960).
TAYLOR, F., and F. VELLIOS: Surgery 44, 453 (1958).
TEMPLE, L. J.: Brit. med. J. 2, 511 (1941).
THORNING, E. B.: Acta path. microbiol. scand. 65, 481 (1965).
TOOLAN, H. W.: Cancer Res. 13, 389 (1953).
TREVINO, E.: In W. H. COLE, G. O. McDONALD, S. S. ROBERTS, and H. W. SOUTHWICK: Dissemination of cancer: prevention and therapy. New York: Appleton-Century-Crofts 1961.
TROTTER, N. L.: Cancer Res. 21, 778 (1961).
WATNE, A. C., A. A. SANDBERG, and G. E. MOORE: Cancer Res. 20, 160 (1960).
WHITE, L. P.: Ann. N. Y. Acad. Sci. 100, 115 (1963).
—, G. LINDEN, L. BRESLOW, and L. HARZFELD: J. Amer. med. Ass. 177, 51 (1961).
WHITE, T. T., and W. C. WHITE: Ann. Surg. 144, 384 (1956).
WILLIS, R. A.: The pathology of tumours of children. London: Oliver and Boyd 1962, p. 11.

The Organization of Cancer Treatment

PIERRE DENOIX

With 2 Figures

Before the various possibilities for the treatment of cancer available in highly specialized cancer centers or general hospitals are considered, an attempt should be made to define the qualities requisite in cancer specialists deciding on the plan of treatment and the conditions needed for satisfactory treatment of cancer patients. To begin with, a cancer specialist should be able to take part in the devising of a plan of treatment that combines the various forms of therapy available to a varying extent but in a way suited to each patient. For a constantly increasing number of cancers and because of the growing multiplicity of technical possibilities, a single individual can no longer command the extremely wide range of knowledge required, either clinical and biological on the one hand or technical on the other; to do so he would have to be at one and the same time a physician, a surgeon, a radiologist, a pathologist, etc. Since this is impossible for one person, the knowledge must be provided by a team containing representatives of the various specialties mentioned. For each member of the team to play his part as an associate, he must have four special qualities:

1. He must obviously be fully competent in his own specialty, as a surgeon, say, or a radiologist.

2. He must have a wide knowledge of the biology — the "natural history" — of cancer and of everything needed for an understanding of the development of human cancer, especially host-tumor relationships.

3. He must have an adequate knowledge of techniques other than his own. Thus the surgeon must have extensive knowledge of radiology, chemotherapy, and pathology. During the discussion with his colleagues from other specialties on how the patient is to be treated, he must be able to produce arguments and — if it appears to be a better solution — to accept the arguments adduced in favour of treatment by specialist techniques other than his own.

4. He must be able to work along with the team and accept the sharing of responsibility on a footing of equality with different specialists.

The decision on treatment, which should be taken jointly, will commit the members of the team to a shared responsibility for the possible consequences of the plan agreed on.

Nevertheless, the surgeon, for example, will be fully responsible for the carrying out and for the consequences of any operation performed as part of the plan jointly decided on. There is, however, another level of responsibility: one that is shared with the physician and the radiologist if, for example, radiotherapy and surgery were linked and the treatment turned out to be mistaken, even though both the irradiation and the operation had been carried out correctly. Responsibility thus exists at two levels: total and individual for each specialist action specific to the person carrying it out, and shared for the individual plan of treatment as a whole.

If cancer is to be treated in satisfactory conditions, for each case there should be a meeting of at least a physician, a surgeon, and a radiologist, with the help of a pathologist and often of other specialists such as plastic surgeons and stomatologists. Such a team should operate on the footing of full equality and joint responsibility. The members are not there in their personal capacity but as representatives of their specialty, and all possible forms of treatment are discussed. The team should not consist of a leader and two (or more) assistants, for this would risk giving the leader's specialty a predominance that might jeopardize the fairness of the hearing given to the other specialties. Each specialist should feel that he is sharing fully in the discussion. If the discussion takes place in this way, the chances are that the plan of treatment agreed on by the team will give the patient the simplest, as well as the most effective, therapy.

An example will illustrate this. If a patient with cancer of the lip goes first to a surgeon, the latter may consider himself in a position to decide on the form of treatment by himself. If so the chances are that he will consider a resection, which may entail plastic surgery. He will cure his patient, but at the price of a series of operations that will confine him to bed for a fairly long time. On the other hand, if the same patient had been made the subject of a discussion between a surgeon, a radiologist, and a physician, the decision would very probably have been that the patient should be treated with interstitial radiation, which would be as likely to cure as resection but would cause infinitely less immobilization of the patient and infinitely less local change. On the other hand, if there were palpable and mobile lymph nodes, the team would decide in favour of cervical lymph node resection.

It is obviously necessary that the team's discussion should be based on a joint clinical examination of the patient carried out before any treatment is started. Such a joint examination enables a balance to be achieved between the pessimistic and optimistic tendencies of the team members. There can be no doubt that when a physician, a surgeon, and a radiologist have agreed on the clinical classification of a patient's cancer, they will be as near to the truth as they can be. The use of the T. N. M. classification of the International Union Against Cancer in such a case is indicated, both to enshrine their agreed view and to serve as a foundation for the decision on treatment.

Suppose, for example, that in the series of possible treatments for cancer of the breast the existence or absence of incomplete adherence to the pectoralis major is the crux of the question whether there should be pre-operative radiotherapy or immediate operation. If such a decision were left in the hands of the surgeon alone, it is conceivable that he would, more or less unconsciously, minimize the limitation of mobility; if it were left in the hands of the radiologist alone his tendency would be the opposite. With both these findings confronting each other and a third team member, the physician, taking part (the physician's role as a regulator is essential), the chances of arriving closer to the truth would be enhanced.

The primary role of such a team is therefore to select the plan of treatment. A usual complementary role is that of taking joint responsibility for the prolonged follow-up of the patient. With this system the patient has the best chances of receiving the simplest and most appropriate plan of treatment.

While a team of this kind should be fundamental to any organization for the treatment of cancer, it can find a place in very different structures, in a specialized institution as well as in a general hospital. We shall now deal with the team in such various backgrounds.

In a specialized cancer center a team is easy to organize since, especially in France, such a center is by definition an institution where the various techniques concerned with cancer treatment are all found under the same roof — the medical, surgical, radiological, and pathological specialties being basic but having possibly their own internal subdivisions, as for example that of surgery into general, ENT, thoracic, etc. In radiology all the radiation sources — external radiotherapy, interstitial radiotherapy, etc. — may be available.

A fully-equipped cancer center should be able to furnish from its own resources all the specialist techniques required to treat cancer of any site whatever. In such a center, it may be expected that the medical staff consisting of the specialists of the various branches will be divided up into a certain number of teams of three (consisting of a physician, a surgeon, and a radiologist). At the Institut Gustave-Roussy these teams are called "site committees", each team being in charge of the cancers of a specific organ or region. The center usually has specialist departments of medicine, surgery, radiology, etc., and each department appoints a permanent representative as one of the three-man teams forming the "site committees". Each team has as its responsibility to receive and examine the patient and come to a decision on the treatment he is to be given; and in his turn each member of the team takes responsibility for the part of the plan that concerns the specialist department he represents. The team is also responsible for the lengthy follow-up of the patient. Thus a fully equipped cancer center has two levels of activity: a lower executive level at which the technical means and the hospital beds are available to all; and a higher level at which the teams take decisions and can make use of the whole range of specialist techniques of the centre (see Fig. 1).

The number of teams or committees will depend on the number of patients and the number of specialists the center has at its disposal. A big center with an adequate staff could limit the number of organs for which a team was to be responsible, thus

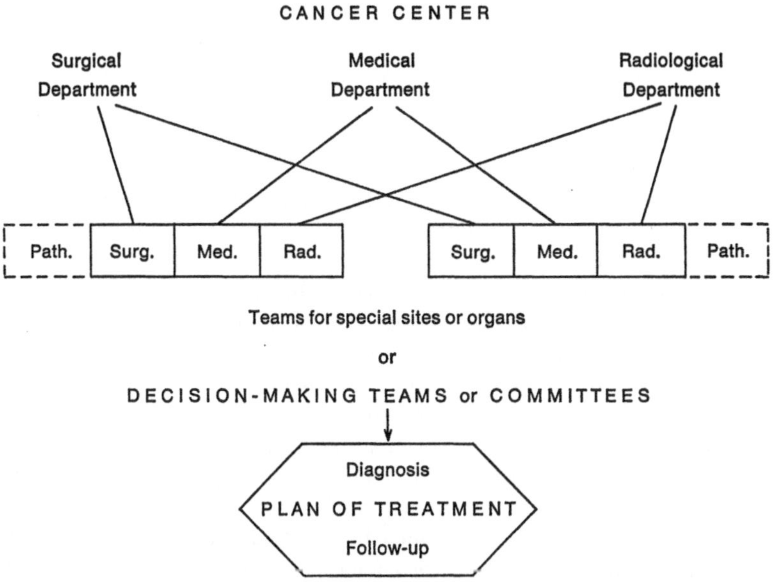

CANCER CENTER

| Surgical | Medical | Radiological |
| Department | Department | Department |

| Path. | Surg. | Med. | Rad. | | Surg. | Med. | Rad. | Path. |

Teams for special sites or organs

or

DECISION-MAKING TEAMS or COMMITTEES

Diagnosis
PLAN OF TREATMENT
Follow-up

Fig. 1

increasing the specialization. There may be a whole range of variations, from the single team in a small center responsible for all the sites to the thirteen teams among which the patients at the Institut Gustave-Roussy are distributed.

A structure of this kind, which gives natural expression to the idea of teamwork, is the opposite of any set-up placing in juxtaposition autonomous departments with a monopoly over any kind of patient. So far is it from such a set-up that the patient during his treatment, whether he goes to hospital or not, will pass through the various specialist departments of the center. In such a center, for example, there will be no ENT department whose head will decide both whether surgery will be undertaken and whether irradiation or chemotherapy will be carried out. The department of head and neck surgery will appoint a representative to the team responsible for tumors of the larynx; and in that team will also be found representatives for radiology and chemotherapy. Together they will decide on the plan of treatment, and the relevant part involving ENT techniques will be carried out in the head and neck surgery department.

The special statute of the French cancer centers was drafted so as to set up the structures most suitable for this kind of teamwork. They have been pushed to their most logical conclusion at the Institut Gustave-Roussy, where one of the main points of organization has been the drafting of a "protocol of treatment" for each team or committee. This document is prepared by the team or committee and submitted by the medical director of the center to a specialist committee consisting of all the heads of the specialist departments. When the document has been given its final form, accepted by everyone, it is approved by the director and becomes the team's working document. It consists of three parts.

The first part contains a description of the clinical extent of the disease in terms of the T. N. M. system of the UICC as applied to the sites for which the team is responsible.

The second part specifies the technical methods to be used during treatment. The methods are described in a very general way (maximum dose, extent of excision, etc.), obviously not in the detail with which the methods are to be applied, since the detailed execution of the instructions fall within the province and responsibility of the specialized department concerned.

The third part contains the indications for treatment which, in respect of each T. N. M. category of the clinical classification, will present the ideal plan of treatment sought to be applied.

When a patient appears for the first time at the Institut Gustave-Roussy, he is directed at once to a representative of the team or committee, whose duty it is to take charge of him. The representative has the preliminary examinations carried out according to a prearranged schedule, and when they are completed he presents the patient to the committee, the members of which examine him jointly and then after due deliberation decide on the plan of treatment, referring to and attempting to follow the provisions of the protocol of treatment. It may be that the committee's examination brings to light a contraindication making the patient's case an exception; it will then have to be fully justified by the findings. Because of this defined and recorded policy it will be easy, when some years later the results of a series of cases are being assessed, to understand the justification for the decisions about treatment at a given moment.

One of the duties of a specialized center is to elaborate new methods of treatment so that the medical community can take advantage of them. To be able to assess the value of what is done, it is necessary to accept the discipline involved, which makes it possible to treat a sufficient number of patients quicker and in a uniform way. The center that has succeeded in making a new method of treatment known becomes interested in seeking fresh advances. There will therefore always be a time lag between what the center has just recommended and what it is doing at the moment.

By dint of using the system, we perceived that the fact that the committee was given a written document was of great advantage in maintaining uniformity of policy. With such a reference document the indications are kept within the confines of the plan laid down; whereas if each member of the committee had been given his freedom to do whatever he "thought" best at any time, he would — as experience has shown — be tempted by something he had recently read to propose some new method. Each of the members in turn might have acted in the same way, and in such circumstances there would never have been any consistent policy that would have been susceptible of assessment. A structure like this, based on three-man teams, is an excellent foundation for controlled clinical trials, which are the only method of judging of the value of a method of treatment.

Our experience has showed us that there is no difficulty in progressing from a team's protocol of treatment to a plan for a therapeutic trial. The working habits of the team correspond to those required for the execution of a satisfactory trial.

We have seen how this teamwork can be organized in a specialized cancer center. It remains to be seen how it would fare in a general hospital, the same principle being observed of a joint plan of treatment drawn up by a team before treatment is begun. In the general hospital the same specialized services are found as in the cancer center; thus, for example, there are an ENT department, a gynecological department, a medical department, and a radiology department. The range of technical possibilities at the disposal of the general hospital is thus of the same order as that of the cancer center, and indeed it is sometimes more complete. On the other hand, there is no level at which a joint decision can be taken on the plan of treatment.

In the general hospital it is unfortunately the rule that the first treatment given to a patient when he is seen by a consultant is that of the consultant's particular specialty. All that the specialty is capable of doing is done without concern about the possibility of doing better, because more simply, with a different technique. What often happens then is that, when the possibilities of the first specialist's department have been exhausted and it is decided that there is still something more to be done, the patient is then directed to another department for additional treatment. The regrettable thing is that this associated treatment was not decided beforehand by a representative from each department, the position being that the order of treatment has been imposed on the second department by the decision of the first.

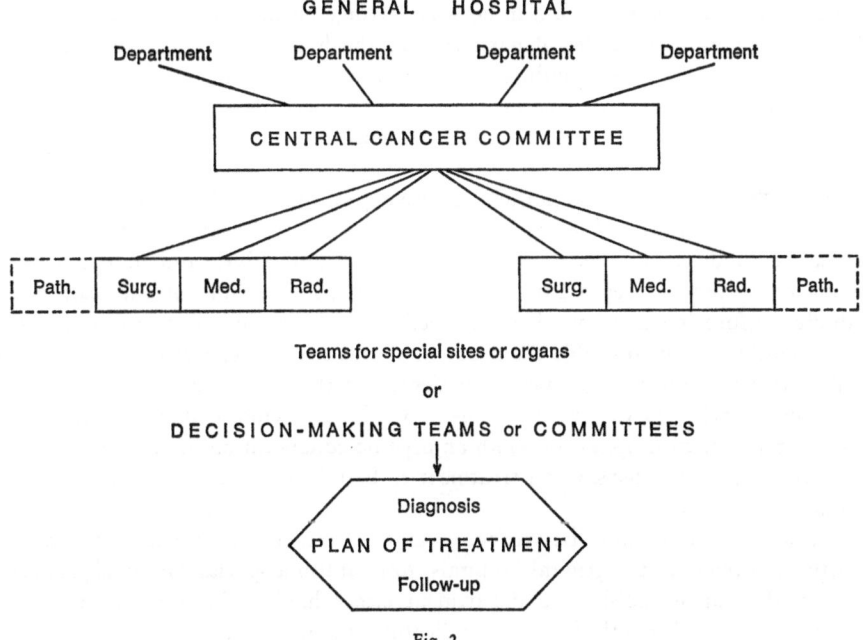

Fig. 2

This is the essential defect of general hospitals. The situation can nevertheless be considerably improved without introducing a new service. It would be enough to bring in the system of a decision-making team (Fig. 2). It is perfectly possible to arrange for each specialized (or unspecialized) department in a general hospital to delegate a representative to a central cancer team. The team would see all patients suspected of cancer appearing in any department of the hospital. Such a central team or committees could be broken up into a certain number of decision-making teams, each made responsible for the cancers of certain organs or sites, each set up in terms of the technical aspects of cancers of those organs or sites. Thus, for example, the surgeon on the team dealing with cancer of the urinary tract would be delegated by the hospital urological department.

The decision-making teams would take over the care of the patients falling to their lot, see that the preliminary investigations to establish the diagnosis and the clinical classification of the tumor were carried out, and draw up the plan of treatment for the individual patient. They would then see to it that the various departments of the hospital concerned dealt with that part of the plan of treatment allotted to them.

The central team or committees would play a co-ordinating role, and have the necessary secretarial assistance to enable each of the teams to exercise regular supervision over the patients in the various departments, so that they received the specialized treatment decided for them and the treatment was given at the appropriate times. When the departments administering treatment had checked the immediate results, the central team would take over the follow-up of the patient on behalf of the various people concerned, who would be kept abreast of the situation.

A structure such as this would in no way infringe on the usual technical independence of the various specialist departments of the hospital or derogate from their legitimate rights and responsibilities in respect of treatment. The essential thing, however, is that the plan of treatment would have been drawn up jointly through each department delegating its powers to its representative on the decision-making team.

At least in theory, there is nothing to prevent an organization of this kind from being set up. The problem is essentially a psychological one. Each departmental head must agree to delegate some of his powers and prerogatives and accept a team decision of a kind of "supranational" team. The working rules of the team could be drafted before it started work by a meeting of the various departmental chiefs, and it would no doubt resemble the protocol of treatment of cancer centers.

Thus two possibilities are open to patients: on the one hand the cancer center, very compact, with its various departments working in close collaboration; and on the other the general hospital, in which an organic collaboration between the departments would enable a decision on treatment to be taken in common and before any treatment is undertaken.

It would in our opinion be wrong, given the present psychological state of the departmental chiefs in the general hospitals, to establish a special cancer department. This would mean establishing a department either having the various specialized techniques at its disposal and so duplicating techniques and facilities already available in the hospital, or else with a single technique, which would have the major drawback that a single department in the hospital would be called the cancer department and yet not have the means of doing everything expected of it. It would probably arouse the hostility of its neighbouring departments, which would not accept its monopoly, and if it were the place where the co-ordinating team met there would be the risk of maneuvering for the advantage of the specialty concerned. The decisions of the co-ordinating committee and the decision-making teams would be more acceptable to all if they were taken on neutral and common ground.

A final problem is that of the training of physicians and specialists who may be appointed as representatives of the departments not specialized in cancer in the decision-making committees. It is necessary that they should have some knowledge of cancer and its treatment so as to be able to make an active contribution to the decision. For this they must receive training, and this should be done within departments presided over by professors of cancerology. In France at present there are professorships in most of the large towns with medical faculties, and they are linked with cancer centers. The centers should have the means of training cancer specialists, not only to fill posts within the centers but, more important still, to fill posts in departments not specialized in cancer in general hospitals. This suggests the establishment of a diploma in cancer studies that would qualify anyone holding it for appointment as representative of whatever department he is attached to in a general hospital to the central co-ordinating committee dealing with cases of cancer.

A system like this is at present adumbrated in France by the "advanced consultations" that the specialized cancer centers hold in towns other than those in which they are situated. Most centers, at least once a month, send a physician or a team who examine, generally at the chief hospital, the patients sent by the doctors of the area, follow up patients who have been treated at the center, and look into the treatment of patients they have seen earlier. There are sixty towns in which this system is operative.

In some hospital centers the departmental chiefs in the hospital are present at the consultation and bring from their departments the patients for whom they want advice on treatment. The physician from the cancer center then plays the exact part of a consultant, since he is there to give his advice on what should be done.

In most cases the patients are treated locally with the available resources but according to the plan of treatment advised by the center physician. In this set-up there is a foretaste of the decision-making team of the general hospital, and it functions in a great many cases to the satisfaction of all.

It is exceptional for the special center to take over a patient for part of the treatment, and even more for the whole of the treatment. This happens only when the necessary specialist resources are not present locally and the local specialists agree. It would not happen in a general hospital, since by definition the resources of such a hospital would be at least as complete as those of a cancer center. The drawback that — for staffing reasons — most advanced consultations can be carried out by only one person, who cannot be omniscient, would not occur in a general hospital, for there the decision-making team would consist of several persons, each representing the specialties existing in the hospital. Where the advanced consultant cannot suggest a plan of treatment after examination of the patient and discussion with the doctor presenting him, he usually takes the case record away to the cancer center, where he seeks the advice of colleagues more specialized in such cases.

It seems therefore perfectly possible to envisage a cancer campaign in any region based upon two elements. One is the specialized cancer centers, which are not intended to take in all cancer patients but constitute pilot centers where new forms of treatment are elaborated and cancer specialists are trained. The other is a special form of collaboration at the general hospitals, into which specialists educated at the specialized centers are gradually introduced.

We conclude by again stressing that in cancer the essential thing is to establish in advance a co-ordinated plan of treatment employing the resources available to the best possible advantage by adoption of the simplest and most effective solution. Opportunities of receiving treatment on such a basis can be offered to cancer patients both in specialized cancer centers — which are necessary regionally — and in general hospitals.

A Look into the Future

NIKOLAI N. BLOKHIN *

The present monograph, written by eminent specialists representing various countries of the world, sets out clearly the modern treatment of malignant tumors and demonstrates the considerable amount of success achieved in recent decades in the field of cancer detection and treatment.

A large portion of the achievement can be attributed to the organization of cancer control. While organizational procedures and methods of cancer detection as well as of cancer education naturally vary in different countries, the main ideas and ideals are undoubtedly the same. The teaching about precancerous lesions and their detection and treatment has become one of the links in a chain of cancer control activities.

Advances in epidemiological research introduced many new ideas about the prevalence of the various forms of cancer in different countries of the world and opened up wide possibilities for the study of factors contributing to the development of certain kinds of tumors in man.

Cancer epidemiological data coupled with laboratory and field study of various carcinogenic agents in the human environment provide a basis for the development of methods of cancer prevention.

The modern state of surgery and anesthesiology permits operative removal of tumors of any localization. Such procedures as removal of the lung, esophagus, or stomach and resection of liver lobes are no longer unique and daring but, on the contrary, rather commonplace. Even such operations as removal of the lower half of the body have become possible nowadays in cases where there is no other practical way of getting rid of malignant tumors. The development of transplantation surgery opens up new vistas for surgical oncology.

The results of different kinds of radiotherapy employed separately or in combination with surgery are encouraging. The effectiveness of radiotherapy has increased still further with the introduction of sources of high energy and the selective application of radioactive isotopes.

_____

* President of the Soviet Academy of Medical Sciences, President of the International Union against Cancer, Director of the Herzen Institute for Cancer, Moscow.

Hormone therapy in certain kinds of tumors and a great number of antitumor chemotherapeutic preparations add to the successful new treatments now being developed.

All these methods of cancer control have been based on theoretical and experimental research, which acquire ever greater scope and significance.

The health and vital statistics of many countries reveal a marked reduction in the number of patients with advanced forms of cancer of the skin, cervix and mammary gland. This is undoubtedly the result of work on the early detection of cancer. In economically developed countries the death rate from cancer of the skin is negligible; and the immediate and longterm results of treatment of a number of malignant tumors improve steadily (owing to the efforts of surgeons, radiologists, and therapeutists).

None the less, cancer is still one of the most frequent causes of death. A very great task thus awaits us in the future — to change the situation in the field of cancer and reduce the mortality.

Despite all the activities of health agencies many cases of cancer are detected late in life, when modern medicine is powerless to give any practical help. The reason lies in the nature of the disease, which has few symptoms in its initial stages. Whatever the successes of surgery, too, many operations turn out to be insufficiently radical, while in other cases the advance of the disease excludes any possibility of surgical intervention. Nor can a cure that exacts a toll of severe infirmity and mental discomfort be regarded as an ideal way out; hence the attempts to find other methods of treatment. Radiotherapeutic methods are not free from side effects resulting in damage to healthy tissues and a general adverse effect upon the organism. The response of different malignant tumors to radiotherapy varies greatly; that is why the effectiveness of treatment is usually far from constant. Many factors are responsible for this situation, among them the site of the tumor and its accessibility to radiation. Though the drug therapy of cancer gains daily in popularity, it cannot be regarded as the long-awaited solution to the treatment of cancer. More often than not drugs are used only for palliative purposes. The complete disappearance of tumors in a number of patients as a result of drugs is mostly temporary in nature. Moreover, all active antitumor chemotherapeutic compounds exert a considerable toxic effect. In order to increase the absorption by the tumor of the preparation introduced intravenously directly at the site, we are obliged to resort to complex and ingenious techniques such as regional perfusion, so as to safeguard the organism from the side effects of the compound. These complex methods are not free from serious faults, and the subsequent occurrence of complications places emphasis on the unsatisfactory character of existing chemotherapeutic measures — unsatisfactory because of their lack of specificity and their high toxicity.

In spite of all the limitations and drawbacks of the methods of treatment applied at present, considerable success can be achieved when sound therapeutic combinations are employed. The cure is not always complete, and sometimes it is far from complete, but in many cases the treatment results in prolongation of the patient's life and the creation of better living and functional conditions for what time is left to him. Cancer continues, however, to be the second major cause of death in economically developed countries, and so far all efforts to change this situation have failed.

As for the prospects in cancer, what ways are there of increasing the effectiveness of cancer control methods and when can results be expected?

To answer these questions, we should first of all look at the history of medicine and at previous experience in controlling some other diseases of equal and at times perhaps even greater significance to humanity than cancer.

In most cases the solution of the problem is linked with studies of the nature and cause of the disease. Rare exceptions do not contradict but rather confirm this general rule. Such an exception was Jenner, who introduced preventive immunization against smallpox long before elucidation of the nature and pathogenesis of the disease.

Progress of medicine in disease control usually follows the successes of major sciences such as physics, chemistry, and biology. The invention of optical instruments made possible the study of the microscopic world and laid the foundation stone of microbiology. Since the time of Pasteur, Koch, Ehrlich, Ivanovsky, Mechnikov and others, microbiology has achieved control over many infections. The development of chemistry provided new opportunities to synthesize various drugs; that of the biochemistry of nucleic acids has led to modern knowledge of the cell, the cell hereditary mechanism, and the viruses. Malignant tumors fall within the domain of cell pathology and have causal relationships, at least in certain groups of tumors, with viruses. This makes their study complex enough to require advanced research techniques, which have become available only because of the progress of physics and chemistry during the course of the last few decades.

Despite the fact that from time immemorial cancer has taken its toll of human lives, data as a rule have been very inexact. Various inflammatory processes causing swelling of tissues were often recorded as cancer, and *vice versa;* and diseases of undoubtedly carcinogenic origin such as leukemia were only recently recorded under that head. It must be remembered, however, that scientific oncology did not come into existence until the second half of the XIXth century, when the microscopic study of tumors began. (Yet even then surgeons rendered help by removing tumors from accessible sites.) It was only in the eighteen-seventies that M. Novinsky of Russia succeeded in inducing tumors in animals, thus giving a start to experimental oncology.

X-rays were discovered in 1895, and were destined to play a unique role in the diagnosis and treatment of cancer. Shortly afterwards, the Curies discovered radium. Radioactive isotopes, however, appeared only in the nineteen-thirties. The discovery of the first virus tumors by Ellerman and Bang (the avian leukoses) dates from 1908; and of the virus of Rous's sarcoma from 1911. In the XIXth century something was known about the so-called carcinogenic compounds, yet it was only in 1917 that Jawagiwa and Ichikawa showed the carcinogenic effects of coal-tar; and chemical research into the carcinogenicity of hydrocarbons was not undertaken by Kennaway until the thirties. Hormones began to appear in the treatment of certain forms of cancer in the forties, which also saw the first examples of the so-called chemotherapy of tumors.

As a science, therefore, oncology has been in existence for less than a hundred years, and practically everything worthwhile in research has been discovered in the last few decades. From the point of view of the historical development of science, this is a very short space of time.

This brief review of the history of cancer studies is relevant to the question of their development in the near future. Within a very short time each of the main lines of research in the field of oncology has developed considerably. At the beginning of the century there were only speculations on the possible role of viruses in tumors, but now the viral origin of many animal tumors has been established. The discovery of the chicken sarcoma virus (ROUS) was quickly followed by that of virus tumors in the rabbits studied by SHOPE, the Bittner virus of mammary gland cancer, various viruses causing leukoses in mice and rats (GROSS, MAZURENKO, and others), and the polyoma virus (STEWART, EDDY), which causes various forms of tumor in different kinds of laboratory animals. The ability of tumorigenic viruses to overcome the barrier of species differentiation is shown with great clarity by the long-known Rous virus, which now has turned out to be pathogenic for rats, rabbits, lizards, snakes, monkeys, and probably man as well, for it causes transformation of human cells in tissue culture (SWET, MOLDAVSKY, ZILBER, and others). Tumors have been induced in laboratory animals by adenoviruses isolated from the body of a healthy individual. At this stage, however, the viral origin of human cancer cannot be regarded as firmly established, but the situation should be clarified within the next few years. It is to be hoped, indeed, that viruses will turn out to be of etiological importance in most, if not all, human tumors, for then humanity will have before it the prospect of specific tumor prophylaxis by means of antivirus immunization.

Immunology has also been gaining ground in cancer research. The demonstration of the existence of specific tumor antigens (L. ZILBER) was a prerequisite to the development of cancer immunology. The possibility of immunization against tumorigenic viruses inhabiting the body from birth, so preventing the appearance of tumors, as recently shown by G. DEITSCHMAN in hamsters and rats induced with SV_{40} virus, shows that in man, if the role of viruses in the genesis of cancer is confirmed and viruses are isolated, prophylactic antivirus immunization against malignant tumors may become feasible.

Within a short space of time another concept closely connected with the problem of cancer prevention has gained wide popularity; that of carcinogenic agents (L. SHABAD, HUEPER, and others). However, the further prospects for this concept are not very promising. In spite of intensive work in many countries in an attempt to control carcinogenic agents in food and contamination of air, water, soil, etc., it is difficult to ascertain the effect achieved on the reduction of the incidence of cancer. This, however, does not preclude the necessity for a continuing campaign against hazardous agents as well as for publicity designed to minimize the adverse effects of, for example, smoking. If the theory that cancer is diverse in its etiology is accepted, too many inside and outside factors may be of carcinogenic significance, their multiplicity hampering cancer prevention.

Detection and removal of precancerous lesions are also of great importance in cancer prophylaxis, though not all precancerous conditions lend themselves easily to treatment. In this context it is enough to mention achlorhydric gastritis.

In speaking about the future it is difficult not to give one's own subjective views. I think that virological and immunological research holds out the greatest promise and may be able to strike a decisive blow by opening up an era of specific cancer prophylaxis. Immunological methods of study deserve careful attention because of the peculiarities of tumorigenic processes in different patients, a phenomenon that is undoubtedly associated with different resistance in different organisms. If by means of antivirus immunization we succeed in preventing at least some serious lesions, particularly leukoses, this will be a solution to one of the most important questions in cancer.

Study of the tumor cell, its peculiarities, and its genetic problems has great significance for the further development of cancer treatment procedures, especially for chemotherapy and immunotherapy.

The surgical treatment of cancer is somewhere near its limit. More often than not unsatisfactory results are due not to the lack of possibilities in modern surgery but to the inadequate results attained in the course of treatment. The reason for this lies in the disease itself, its obscure pattern, peculiarities, and capacity for producing metastases and becoming generalized. Even the greatest successes of transplantation surgery will not change this situation; they will be of significance to a few patients only.

Radiotherapy still has considerable prospects. The introduction of high-energy protons and then negative mesons may be regarded as offering the possibility of a more exact and powerful effect on tumor cells, with minimal damage to neighbouring healthy tissues. These new methods may improve the results of radiotherapy of deep-seated tumors, as of the lungs, or esophagus. Radioactive isotopes also have a part to play in the treatment of certain tumors.

Nevertheless, radiation methods are by no means effective in all forms of tumor, and they have considerable adverse side effects. It is impossible to regard either radiotherapy or surgery as the complete solution to the problem of cancer treatment for both methods have in common an inhibitory influence upon certain organs and tissues, though of a local character.

One more method of cancer treatment is of special interest in our days — the administration of chemotherapeutic compounds and hormones. It is fully justified to regard antitumor chemotherapy as feasible, on the ground that chemotherapy means the selective inhibitory effect of a drug on tumor cells. The term itself was introduced into medical practice by EHRLICH to define a means of exerting such as selective influence on pathogens. Therefore the question of its suitability for application to tumors may be disputable.

In addition, the selectivity of action of existing antitumor drugs is insufficient. The side effects of alkylating agents on hematopoiesis and of antimetabolites on the epithelium of the gastrointestinal tract as well as on hematopoiesis explain why complicated techniques such as perfusion are employed.

Though the chemotherapy of cancer is in its infancy, it has already produced good results. The first series of preparations belonging to the group of alkylating compounds has been developed, and some of them — HN_2, thiophosphamide, sarcolysin, endoxan, etc. — are in common use. The so-called antimetabolites, which rather are imitators of normal metabolites (purines, pyrimidines, and folic acid) are of considerable interest. Such compounds as 6-mercaptopurine, 5-fluorouracil, and methotrexate have been widely adopted and help many patients. Antibiotics are at present of less importance, though actinomycin C and D, mitomycin C, and chrysomallin are among the compounds that have undoubtedly proved their value. The use of hormones is limited to a comparatively small group of tumors. Nevertheless, hormone treatment shows that an inhibitory influence can be obtained upon tumors indirectly through the regulating systems of the organism, as well as directly upon the tumor cells.

In sum, tumor treatment with drugs evidently has a promising future. Very soon we may expect to see new antitumor preparations, among them compounds belonging to new groups of chemical substances. The development of more effective drugs with greater selectivity of action and fewer side effects will in general render unnecessary complex methods of regional drug administration, though they may perhaps remain in use for some special forms and localizations of tumors. Various combinations of chemotherapeutic preparations of different mechanisms of action will be widely studied. It has been observed that alkylating agents are characterized by some lymphotropism, which explains their more pronounced effect on metastases in lymph nodes than on the primary tumors themselves. On the other hand, such preparations as 5-fluorouracil, when used for tumors of the digestive tract, are most effective against the primary tumors, and have less effect on the normal epithelium of the digestive tract and least on metastases in lymph nodes. The combined administration of substances of different "profiles" clearly ought to be developed.

Combined treatment using drugs, surgical measures, and radiotherapy will be extended. Immunotherapeutic preparations will be administered as a supplement to surgical intervention, with a view to preventing the development of recurrences and metastases after radical operation.

The future for the systematic administration of chemotherapeutic compounds is rather dubious, though nowadays this idea has many protagonists. The reason for doubt is the evidence for the inhibitory influence of the existing compounds upon the immunological capacity of the organism — a quality, however, that makes them useful in transplantation surgery for the prevention of the immunological rejection of homologous tissue and organ grafts. The effect of these compounds upon the immunity mechanisms may create conditions favorable for the development of recurrences and metastases, thus leading to results directly opposite to those sought.

In the field of cancer diagnosis, X-ray diagnostic techniques will doubtless be improved, as well as isotope, endoscopic, and cytologic methods. These, however, are all methods for the local diagnosis of tumors; general methods have not yielded the results expected. I think it unwise to pin too many hopes on the discovery in the near future of a biochemical method for the early detection of cancer. But among diagnostic tests there are quite a number that give a correct answer in 80—90% of cases. We are at present engaged in subjecting large groups of people, including cancer patients, to ten selected tests. Processing the available material by means of an electronic computer should yield objective data on the value of each test. Perhaps diagnostic possibilities can be extended by such an application of selected tests and by mathematical analysis of the findings.

A full study of the problems of cancer requires the international co-operation of research workers. Recent years have showed a tendency for co-operation throughout the world to increase considerably. The International Union Against Cancer has for a long time been a centre for personal contact between scientists of different countries engaged on the cancer problem. International cancer congresses, being unquestionably very useful, enjoy much popularity and draw thousands of participants from all over the world. Much organizational work is carried out by the World Health Organization, and the recently established International Agency for Research on Cancer promises further research developments, primarily in the epidemiology of cancer, on an international level. If international bodies were to succeed in organizing research on the basis of common standards, this would be of decisive importance for the provision of comparable data. Common principles for epidemiological research need to be developed and put into practice; and a single clinical and morphological classification of tumors is required. In this connexion, the contributions of DENOIX and HAMPERL in this field of cancer control are worthy of high praise.

The governments of many countries give valuable assistance to investigations in oncology, not only by supporting national research but also by participating in international agencies and yearly remitting considerable sums to finance their work.

The present situation in the scientific world is thus favorable for the progress of cancer research. The development of physics and chemistry and of modern engineering makes it possible to study cell pathology and the particularly obscure aspects of the cancer problem. The scope of specialized research and the close attention paid to the problems of pathology, if considered along with the international co-operation of men of science, give ground for hope that the solution of the problems of cancer will be found in the years to come. A look back at the development of scientific oncology shows how quickly and in what a short space of time progress has been made and encourages an optimistic attitude towards the future of oncology. Forecasting the future is not an easy task; nevertheless I think that, young though cancer research is, we may hope that it will provide a solution to the problem of cancer within this century.

Subject Index

The numbers printed in *italics* refer to detailed descriptions in the text

Monographs already published

SCHINDLER, R., Lausanne: Die tierische Zelle in Zellkultur (Volume 1).

Neuroblastomas — Biochemical Studies. Edited by C. BOHUON, Villejuif (Volume 2, Symposium).

HUEPER, W. C., Bethesda: Occupational and Environmental Cancers of the Respiratory System (Volume 3).

GOLDMAN, L., Cincinnati: Laser Cancer Research (Volume 4).

METCALF, D., Melbourne: The Thymus. Its Role in Immune Responses, Leukaemia Development and Carcinogenesis (Volume 5).

Malignant Transformation by Viruses. Edited by W. H. KIRSTEN, Chicago (Volume 6, Symposium).

MOERTEL, CH. G., Rochester: Multiple Primary Malignant Neoplasms. Their Incidence and Significance (Volume 7).

New Trends in the Treatment of Cancer. Edited by L. MANUILA, S. MOLES and P. RENTCHNICK, Genève (Volume 8).

LINDENMANN, J., Zürich / A. KLEIN, Gainesville, Florida: Immunological Aspects of Viral Oncolysis (Volume 9).

In production

NELSON, R. S., Houston: Radioactive Phosphorus in the Diagnosis of Gastrointestinal Cancer (Volume 10).

FREEMANN, R. G., and J. M. KNOX, Houston: Treatment of Skin Cancer (Volume 11).

In preparation

CHIAPPA, S., Milano: Endolymphatic Radiotherapy in Malignant Lymphomas.

DENOIX, P., Villejuif: Le traitement des cancers du sein.

FISHER, E. R., Pittsburgh: Ultrastructure of Human Normal and Neoplastic Prostate.

FUCHS, W. A., Bern: Lymphography and Tumordiagnosis.

GRUNDMANN, E., Wuppertal-Elberfeld: Morphologie und Cytochemie der Carcinogenese.

HAYWARD, J. L., London: Cancer of the Breast: Hormonal Changes.

IRLIN, I. S., Moskva: Mechanisms of Viral Carcinogenesis.

KERN, G., Köln: Carcinoma in situ.

KOLDOVSKY, P., Praha: Transplantation Tumor Specific Antigen (TTSA).

LYNCH, H. T., Omaha: Cancer Genetics: Study of Cancer Families.

MARTZ, G., Zürich: Hormonbehandlung der Tumoren.

MATHÉ, G., Villejuif: L'Immunothérapie des cancer.

NEWMAN, M. K., Detroit: Neuropathies and Myopathies Associated with Occult Malignancies.

ODARTCHENKO, N., Lausanne: Prolifération cellulaire érythropiétique.

PACK, G. T., New York: Clinical Aspects of Cancer Immunity and Cancer Susceptibility.

PACK, G. T., New York / A. H. ISLAMI, New York: Tumors of the Liver.

RITZMAN, S. E., Galveston / W. C. LEVIN, Galveston: The Syndrome of Macroglobulinemia.

STEWARD, J. K., Manchester: Tumors in Children.

WEIL, R., Lausanne: Biological and Structural Properties of Polyoma Virus and its DNA.

ZILBER, L. A., Moskva: Virogenetic Theory of Cancer Origin.